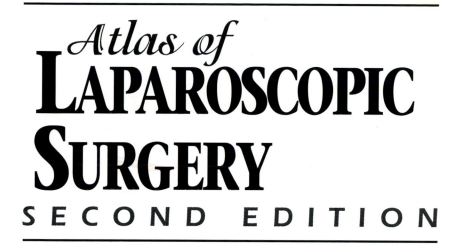

Atlas of
LAPAROSCOPIC
SURGERY

SECOND EDITION

Atlas of LAPAROSCOPIC SURGERY

SECOND EDITION

Theodore N. Pappas
Professor of Surgery
Duke University Medical Center
Duke University Medical School
Durham, North Carolina

Edward G. Chekan
Laparoscopic Fellow
Department of Surgery
Duke University Medical Center
Duke University Medical School
Durham, North Carolina

Steve Eubanks
Assistant Professor of Surgery
Director of Surgical Endoscopy
Duke University Medical Center
Duke University Medical School
Durham, North Carolina

With 43 contributors

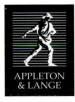

APPLETON
& LANGE

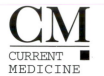

Current Medicine, Inc.
400 Market Street
Suite 700
Philadelphia, PA 19106

Managing Editor . . . . *Mary Kinsella*
Developmental Editor . . . . *Leslie Sell, PhD*
Editorial Assistant . . . . *Lisa M. Janda*
Cover Design and Layout . . . . *Christine Keller-Quirk*
Illustrators . . . . *Nicole Mock, Debra Wertz, Marie Dean, Wiesia Langenfeld,*
Christopher Burke, Rob Gordon, Claudia Grosz, Nancy Kaplan,
Tanya Leonello, Sarah McQueen, James Perkins, and Susan Tanner
Art Director . . . . *Jerilyn Kauffman*
Illustration Director . . . . *Debra Wertz*
Production Manager . . . . *Lori Holland*
Production Assistant . . . . *Constance Copeland*
Index . . . . *Alexandra Nickerson*

Atlas of laparoscopic surgery / [edited by] Theodore N.
   Pappas, Edward G. Chekan, Steve Eubanks. - 2nd ed.
        p.   cm.
      Includes bibliographical references and index.
      ISBN 0-8385-0408-6 (alk. paper)
   1. Endoscopic surgery Atlases. I. Pappas, Theodore N., 1995-
        II. Chekan, Edward G., 1965- . III. Eubanks, Steve, 1959-
        IV. Title: Atlas of laparoscopic surgery.
      [DNLM: 1. Surgical Procedures, Laparoscopic-methods Atlases.   WO
   517 D877 1999]
   RD33.53.A86   1999
   617'.05-dc21
   DNLM/DLC
   for Library of Congress   94-24984
                                                                    CIP

ISBN   0-8385-0408-6

Printed in the United States by Imago

10 9 8 7 6 5 4 3 2 1

DISTRIBUTED WORLDWIDE BY APPLETON & LANGE

Foreword

Laparoscopic surgery continues to progress at a remarkable pace. Less than fifteen years after the first laparoscopic cholecystectomy was performed, a number of new techniques and applications have been, and continue to be, developed. New material found in this edition includes: mini-laparoscopy, laparoscopic ventral herniorrhaphy, the laparoscopic approach to periampullary tumors, laparoscopic adrenalectomy, thoracoscopic lung volume reduction, laparoscopic anterior exposure for spinal fusion, and laparoscopy in the pregnant patient.

The laparoscopic approach has several unique advantages for many surgical procedures. Laparoscopic procedures are often cost effective despite the cost of the specialized laparoscopic equipment, due to shorter hospital stays. They are also less invasive and less traumatic to tissues and organs, are associated with less postoperative discomfort, and contribute to a more rapid rate of patient recovery.

The Duke/US Surgical Endosurgical Center at the Duke University Medical Center continues to provide an environment for the authors of this text to add to their breadth of experience. It is a site of significant research that has led to the development of innovative instrumentation as well as novel procedures. The center also has an outstanding plan for conducting clinical outcome studies that are of extreme importance when evaluating the effectiveness of a specific laparoscopic procedure. This combination of facilities and services, coupled with a dedication to scientific research, has led to significant advances in the laparoscopic surgical procedures detailed in this text.

The *Atlas of Laparoscopic Surgery* is composed of 27 chapters with clear illustrations of a number of laparoscopic operations. Each chapter includes a thorough discussion of the procedure combined with a complete, appropriate description of the corresponding anatomic, pathophysiologic, and differential diagnostic features. In addition, the surgical techniques are graphically depicted by a combination of intraoperative illustrations and selected photographs. The legends accompanying each of these illustrations provide unusually clear descriptions of each step. A selected bibliography that follows each chapter contains the most pertinent citations in the literature.

Occasionally a text appears that makes an exceptional impression. The second edition of the *Atlas of Laparoscopic Surgery* continues the tradition established in the first edition. It carefully details a number of procedures that can be effectively achieved by laparoscopy, is an invaluable reference written by talented and dedicated authorities, and is a must for laparoscopic surgeons. The authors deserve considerable praise for this outstanding atlas.

David C. Sabiston, Jr., MD

Preface

The second edition of the *Atlas of Laparoscopic Surgery* continues to represent the cumulative thoughts of a group of surgeons, predominantly from Duke University Medical Center. Since the publication of the first edition, the field of laparoscopic surgery has dramatically expanded. Many of the earliest laparoscopic approaches, such as cholecystectomy and antireflux procedures, have been refined. In addition, many approaches have gained increasing acceptance. To simplify the broadening scope of laparoscopic surgery, the table of contents has been subdivided by the various surgical subspecialties.

We have chosen the word "laparoscopic" in the title of this book as a generic term to include both laparoscopy and thoracoscopy. The text will be most beneficial for the minimally invasive general surgeon who occasionally does thoracoscopic work. Furthermore, as advanced laparoscopic techniques become increasingly integrated into surgical residency programs, the need for didactic exposure to laparoscopy has become more apparent. Therefore, we have also targeted the text of this atlas for general surgery residents and laparoscopic fellows. As a result, many of the basic operations, such as the laparoscopic cholecystectomy and laparoscopic gastrostomy and jejunostomy, are specifically detailed to reduce the learning curve for these procedures as much as possible. Clearly, mastery of the basic laparoscopic procedures such as cholecystectomy, hernia repair, and appendectomy (that are presently integrated into most residency programs) is necessary prior to attempting more advanced techniques, such as laparoscopic solid organ removal, antireflux procedures, and colon resection.

In addition to updating existing chapters, several new chapters have been added. The new material that is contained in this edition includes: mini-laparoscopy, laparoscopic ventral herniorrhaphy, the laparoscopic approach to periampullary tumors, laparoscopic adrenalectomy, thoracoscopic lung volume reduction, laparoscopic anterior exposure for spinal fusion, and laparoscopy in the pregnant patient.

The editors would like to thank Dr. David C. Sabiston, Jr. for his updated Foreword and for his immense support in the development of endosurgery at Duke University Medical Center. We also thank Dr. Robert W. Anderson for his current leadership and guidance. The editors also would like to thank US Surgical Corp. for their ongoing philanthropic support of the Department of Surgery at Duke Hospital and our efforts to advance our knowledge of endosurgery. Finally, we thank those who have carefully read and specifically critiqued the first edition in an effort to clarify and revise the scope of the second edition.

It is our sincere hope that this atlas will simplify and organize surgical thought for both the student laparoscopist as well as for those with advanced laparoscopic experience. It is intended that the reader of this atlas will be more fully prepared to provide the patient with a safe and effective endosurgical operation.

Theodore N. Pappas, MD
Edward G. Chekan, MD
Steve Eubanks, MD

Contributors

Shahab A. Akhter, MD
Senior Assistant Resident
Duke University Medical Center
Durham, North Carolina

B. Zane Atkins, MD
Resident
Department of Surgery
Duke University Medical Center
Durham, North Carolina

Fredrick Brody, MD
Assistant Professor
Department of Surgery
Ohio State University
Columbus, Ohio
Staff Surgeon
Cleveland Clinic Foundation
Cleveland, Ohio

William R. Burfeind, Jr., MD
Senior Assistant Resident
Department of General and Thoracic Surgery
Duke University Medical Center
Durham, North Carolina

Robert R. Byrne, MD
Senior Resident
Department of Surgery
Division of Urology
Duke University Medical Center
Durham, North Carolina

Paul J. Chai, MD
Senior Resident
Department of Surgery
Duke University Medical Center
Durham, North Carolina

Edward G. Chekan, MD
Laparoscopic Fellow
Department of Surgery
Duke University Medical Center
Durham, North Carolina

Lisa A. Clark, MD
Resident
Department of Surgery
Duke University Medical Center
Durham, North Carolina

Philipp Dahm, MD
Senior Resident
Department of Surgery
Division of Urology
Duke University Medical Center
Durham, North Carolina

Thomas A. D'Amico, MD
Assistant Professor
Department of General and Thoracic Surgery
Duke University Medical Center
Durham, North Carolina

Larkin J. Daniels, MD
Chief Resident
Department of General and Thoracic Surgery
Duke University Medical Center
Durham, North Carolina

R. Duane Davis, Jr., MD
Associate Professor
Department of Surgery
Division of Thoracic Surgery
Duke University Medical Center
Durham, North Carolina

Pierre DeMatos, MD
Senior Resident
Department of Surgery
Duke University Medical Center
Durham, North Carolina

Steve Eubanks, MD
Assistant Professor
Department of Surgery
Director of Surgical Endoscopy
Duke University Medical Center
Durham, North Carolina

John P. Grant, MD
Professor
Department of Surgery
Duke University Medical Center
Durham, North Carolina

David H. Harpole, Jr., MD
Associate Professor
Department of Thoracic Surgery
Chief
General Thoracic Surgery
Duke University Medical Center
Durham, North Carolina

Thomas Z. Hayward, III, MD
Senior Assistant Resident
Department of Surgery
Duke University Medical Center
Durham, North Carolina

Charles Hoopes, MD
Chief Resident
Department of Surgery
Duke University Medical Center
Durham, North Carolina

G. Chad Hughes, MD
Research Fellow
Department of Surgery
Duke University Medical Center
Durham, North Carolina

Alan P. Kypson, MD
Senior Assistant Resident
Department of Surgery
Duke University Medical Center
Durham, North Carolina

Kevin P. Landolfo, MD
Assistant Professor
Department of Surgery
Duke University Medical Center
Durham, North Carolina

Christine L. Lau, MD
Resident
Department of General and Thoracic Surgery
Duke University Medical Center
Durham, North Carolina

Henry L. Laws, MD
Clinical Professor
Department of Surgery
University of Alabama
Director
Department of Surgical Education
Carraway Methodist Medical Center
Birmingham, Alabama

Jeffrey H. Lawson, MD, PhD
Assistant Professor
Department of Surgery
Duke University Medical Center
Durham, North Carolina

Cleveland W. Lewis, MD
Senior Assistant Resident
Department of Surgery
Duke University Medical Center
Durham, North Carolina

Andrew J. Lodge, MD
Resident
Department of Surgery
Duke University Medical Center
Durham, North Carolina

Kirk A. Ludwig, MD
Assistant Professor
Department of Surgery
Duke University Medical Center
Durham, North Carolina

Samuel M. Mahaffey, MD
Associate Professor
Department of Surgery
Chief
Division of Pediatric Surgery
Duke University Medical Center
Durham, North Carolina

Paul J. Mosca, MD, PhD
Resident
Department of General and Thoracic Surgery
Duke University School of Medicine
Durham, North Carolina

Robert B. Noone, MD
Senior Assistant Resident
Department of Surgery
Duke University Medical Center
Durham, North Carolina

Mark W. Onaitis, MD
Resident
Department of Surgery
Duke University Medical Center
Durham, North Carolina

Theodore N. Pappas, MD
Professor
Department of Surgery
Duke University Medical Center
Durham, North Carolina

David T. Price, MD
Assistant Professor
Department of Surgery
Division of Urology
Duke University Medical Center
Durham, North Carolina

Aurora D. Pryor, MD
Research Fellow
Department of Surgery
Duke University Medical Center
Durham, North Carolina

R. Lawrence Reed II, MD
Professor
Department of Surgery
Loyola University Medical Center
Maywood, Illinois

James D. St. Louis, MD
Chief Resident
Department of Surgery
Duke University Medical Center
Durham, North Carolina

Mark W. Sebastian, MD
Assistant Professor
Department of Surgery
Duke University Medical Center
Durham, North Carolina

Ashish S. Shah, MD
Resident
Department of General and Thoracic Surgery
Duke University Medical Center
Durham, North Carolina

John T. Soper, MD
Professor
Department of Obstetrics and Gynecology
Duke University Medical Center
Durham, North Carolina

G. Robert Stephenson, Jr., MD
Resident
Department of Surgery
Duke University School of Medicine
Durham, North Carolina

J.E. Tuttle-Newhall
Assistant Professor
Department of Surgery
Duke University Medical Center
Durham, North Carolina

Steven N. Vaslef, MD, PhD
Assistant Professor
Department of Surgery
Duke University Medical Center
Durham, North Carolina

Bryan C. Weidner, MD
Chief Resident
Department of Surgery
Duke University Medical Center
Durham, North Carolina

Contents

1. Laparoscopic Instrumentation and Basic Techniques

Christine L. Lau and Steve Eubanks

2. Laparoscopic Evaluation of Abdominal Trauma

James D. St. Louis, Mark W. Sebastian, R. Lawrence Reed II, and Steven N. Vaslef

3. Laparoscopic Inguinal Herniorrhaphy

Shahab A. Akhter and Steve Eubanks

4. Laparoscopic Ventral Herniorrhaphy

Paul J. Chai and Edward G. Chekan

5. Laparoscopic Antireflux Procedures

B. Zane Atkins and Theodore N. Pappas

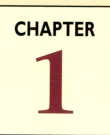
$\mathcal{L}$aparoscopic Instrumentation and Basic Techniques

Christine L. Lau
Steve Eubanks

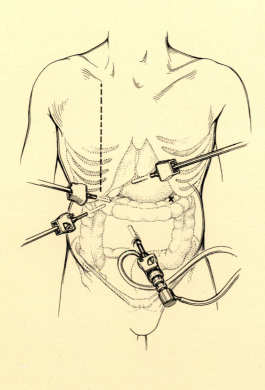

The initial success of laparoscopic cholecystectomy has stimulated surgeons and engineers to design instrument systems and surgical procedures with ever-increasing clarity and complexity. Once consigned only to the gallbladder, the laparoscope is now applied to nearly every organ system in the abdomen, chest, and mediastinum. New instrumentation is being designed and introduced at an exponential rate. To perform safe and effective procedures, surgeons must familiarize themselves with the application as well as the potential drawbacks of these new tools. This chapter provides general guidelines for the use of laparoscopic and thoracoscopic instrumentation and describes the more recent developments at the forefront of videoscopic surgery.

The Operating Room

Perhaps no single factor is more important in videoscopic surgery than the proper training of operating room personnel in the set-up, use, and troubleshooting of the video system. It has been our practice to employ a fully trained individual whose sole responsibility is equipment purchase and maintenance and who has no daily operating room assignment. This limits often-encountered frustrations with new or faulty equipment and also saves a significant amount of operating room time.

Exact details of the design of the laparoscopic operating room obviously depend on the procedure being performed. Nonetheless, some basic concepts are generally applicable and warrant consideration. The success of any videoscopic procedure depends on the spatial relationship among the surgeon, first assistant, and video monitors. In general, the primary surgeon's monitor should be placed so that the surgeon is facing both the video monitor and the organ of interest. Monitors must be unobstructed by electrical cords, tubing, anesthesia equipment, and so forth, and it is well worth the time and effort to move the patient or equipment so that the surgeon may enjoy a comfortable and unencumbered view of the screen. A secondary monitor should be placed in a similar manner for the first assistant. Other monitors placed for nurses or observers should be well away from the operating table. Whenever possible, the assistant and surgeon stand facing the same direction so that both can work in the same line of orientation.

Most hospitals choose to modify existing operating rooms for videoscopic procedures. Designs are available, however, for construction of dedicated videoscopic surgical suites with ceiling-mounted cameras and other specialized equipment. Ceiling-mounted arms have been developed with attached cabinets for the housing of monitors, light sources, video cassette recorders, and insufflators (Figure 1-1). These dedicated videoscopic suites reduce wear and tear on equipment, decrease turn-around time in the operating room and decrease procedure time secondary to constant location of equipment.

Imaging Systems

Almost 200 years ago, endoscopy began with a candle and tin tube [1–3]. It was the development of the Hopkin's Rod-Lens systems in 1966, however, that began the evolution toward current video systems. The first simultaneous visualization of the abdominal cavity by all members of the operating team was accomplished through the attachment of a computer chip television camera to a laparoscope in 1986. This set the stage for the development of modern laparoscopy.

Laparoscopes

Today, laparoscopic procedures are performed by using a descendant of the original Hopkin's Rod-Lens system. Most surgeons use a dedicated viewing laparoscope using a 0°, 30°, or 45° angle lens. Ten millimeter remains the most commonly used laparoscope size, although 5-mm scopes and smaller miniendoscopes are being used more frequently (Figure 1-2).

The authors prefer to use a 30° laparoscope when performing most advanced procedures; this allows for manipulation of the

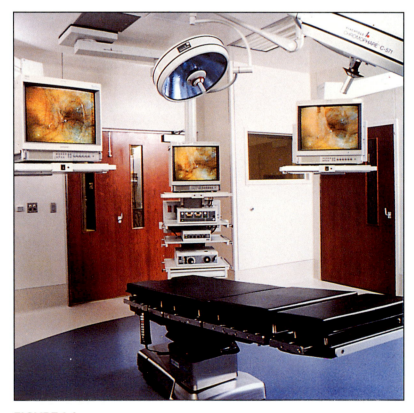

FIGURE 1-1.
Duke University Medical Center videoscopic surgical suite

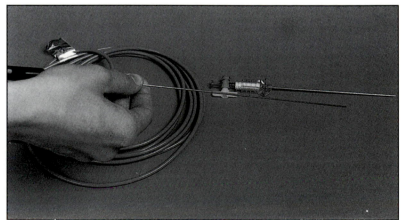

FIGURE 1-2.
Photograph of a microendoscope (Pixie scope; Origin Medsystems, Menlo Park, CA).

angle of view and broadening of the visual field accessible through a single port. This ability makes potentially dangerous maneuvers, such as retroesophageal dissection during Nissen fundoplication, much safer when performed under direct visualization. Laparoscopic suturing can be more readily performed by using an angled lens system because the laparoscope can be manipulated in a manner that limits obstruction during needle placement. The proper use of an angled lens laparoscope does, however, require slightly more dexterity and experience than does use of a 0° scope.

Light Source

A high-intensity light source is essential for adequate illumination of the abdominal or thoracic cavity. Modern systems allow fiberoptic transmission of light from source to laparoscope to operative field with a negligible loss of intensity. The clarity of the video image depends on the quality of light transmission. Meticulous maintenance of the fiberoptic light cable, including replacement when fibers are damaged, is essential for safe operation.

Despite separation of the light source from the fiberoptic cable by a heat shield, the intensity of the light may be transmitted as heat at the end of the laparoscope. Care must be taken to prevent thermal injury that may occur when the exposed end of a fiberoptic cable or laparoscope comes in contact with objects or personnel within the operative field.

Video Camera

The camera is the optical/electronic interface that attaches to the laparoscope. The camera and laparoscope are linked to a microprocessor that receives and transmits the image. One-chip cameras (560 horizontal lines per inch of resolution) provide adequate visualization for most laparoscopic operations. Three-chip cameras (900 horizontal lines per inch) are considered optimal, however, for advanced laparoscopic procedures and provide markedly improved resolution.

Video Monitors

High-resolution video monitors enable the accurate reproduction of images produced by the fiberoptic light source and video camera. The monitor should match the camera in quality, because the resolution is a product of the least accurate element. Advances are being made in flat-panel displays, a potential area of future development.

Most monitoring systems are connected to a video cassette recorder or a photographic printer. Hard copies of laparoscopic images provide surgical documentation as well as a valuable record of the gross pathology encounters. A great deal of controversy remains regarding the filming of procedures and the creation of permanent documentation, however. Many surgeons are reluctant to record these procedures because of the potential legal implications should an intraoperative complication occur. There is no legal mandate that procedures must be recorded or that, if the procedure is recorded, the tape must be included as part of the medical record.

Three-Dimensional and High-Definition Television

Three-dimensional (3-D) laparoscopic systems have been developed in an attempt to provide depth perception as an adjunct to traditional two-dimensional images. The loss of depth perception seems to be most apparent during attempts to perform precise maneuvers such as suturing. The initial 3-D systems were an advance in concept, but a regression in image quality. Most systems provided a central "hot spot" (area of high light intensity) surrounded by a darker periphery. The resolution of the image is currently more comparable to that of a one-chip than to that of a three-chip system. In addition, all members of the operating team must wear specially designed goggles that polarize the image in conjunction with the video image. Although recent advances markedly improved image quality and ease of use, the limitations of 3-D television (goggle requirement, poor color reproduction, and decreased resolution) have resulted in poor reception of these devices in the marketplace and, in turn, waning interest.

High-definition television (HDTV) provides an image with outstanding resolution and a sense of depth perception. Unfortunately, the camera size required for HDTV is unacceptably large and the currently produced systems are cost prohibitive. The future acceptance of HDTV at a consumer level is likely to make these systems more affordable, however.

Equipment

Insufflation

Visualization of the peritoneal cavity requires distension or retraction of the abdominal wall, creating an operative field for instrumentation and manipulation. Although creation of a pneumoperitoneum by insufflation of gas has traditionally been used to establish the operative field, an adequate cavity may be achieved by mechanical retraction of the abdominal wall ("gasless laparoscopy"). Two small randomized studies of laparoscopic cholecystectomies suggest that the abdominal wall lift technique used in gasless laparoscopy provides less of a neuroendocrine response and is safer and quicker than the conventional insufflation techniques [4,5]. However, gasless laparoscopy is not widely used; the standard remains insufflation of gas. An automatic insufflation device that provides continuous flow of gas as well as intra-abdominal pressure regulation was developed by Dr. Kurt Semm almost three decades ago and is the most popular system in use.

Various gases have been used for insufflation, including air, oxygen, nitrogen, nitrous oxide, helium, argon, and carbon dioxide. Carbon dioxide is the most popular gas for insufflation because of its suppression of combustion, high solubility, availability, and low cost. Carbon dioxide has the disadvantage of absorption from the peritoneum with the theoretical potential for metabolic acidosis. Patients with impaired pulmonary function may experience unacceptable levels of carbon dioxide retention during laparoscopic procedures. In addition, concern about cancer seeding in laparoscopy incisions has recently been attributed to the use of carbon dioxide gas insufflation [6].

Insufflators are designed to deliver carbon dioxide through a regulator at variable flow rates and constant cavity pressures.

The optimal intra-abdominal pressure maintained in the adult human during laparoscopic surgery is 12 to 15 mm Hg. Excessive pressure within the peritoneal cavity may lead to hemodynamic instability secondary to venous compression and should prompt immediate release of the pneumoperitoneum and consideration of conversion to an open procedure. Early models of insufflators delivered up to 3 L/min, while the second-generation insufflators were capable of 8 to 10 L/min delivery. More recently designed "high-flow" systems can operate at a rate of 15 to 20 L/min, which allows for the maintenance of adequate pneumoperitoneum even in the face of continuous gas leaks from trocar sites. The insufflator must be equipped with a working pop-off valve and alarm to avoid excessive abdominal distension.

The entire operating room team should be familiar with the controls and gauges of the insufflator. The pressure and flow rate should be observed during the initial insufflation of the peritoneal cavity and periodically checked thereafter. A high flow rate and low initial pressure (less than 5 mm Hg) should be evident if the Hasson cannula is properly positioned. Initial readings of elevated pressure and low flow rates indicate an improperly positioned trocar, a closed valve, kinked insufflation tubing, or inadequate anesthesia causing a Valsalva reaction. Abnormal initial pressures should prompt the immediate cessation of gas flow in order to prevent infusion of gas into the extraperitoneal or intravascular space. Optimal abdominal pressures in unusual settings, such as pregnancy, have not been established.

Insufflation Needles

Most insufflation needles are based on the design of Veress, in which a spring-loaded, blunt-tipped obturator is advanced past a sharp needle tip as it enters the abdominal cavity. The spring-loaded system has the advantage of covering the exposed sharp edge of the needle immediately after penetration. Insufflation needles are available in reusable and disposable styles. A significant advantage of the disposable needle is that the tip is always sharp; as a result the amount of force required for insertion is standardized.

Initially, the technique for placing the Veress needle involved elevating the abdominal wall with towel clips and inserting the needle into the abdominal cavity with considerable force.

The authors prefer an open or Hasson technique in most patients (Figures 1-3 to 1-8). Although studies have demonstrated that complication rates from both the open and closed techniques are similar, the types of complications may be markedly different. While injury to the bowel may occur with the Hasson technique, great vessel perforation is unlikely. Most life-threatening and fatal complications of laparoscopic procedures have occurred by aberrant placement of the Veress needle or initial trocar, resulting in an air embolus or major vascular injury that is not immediately controlled.

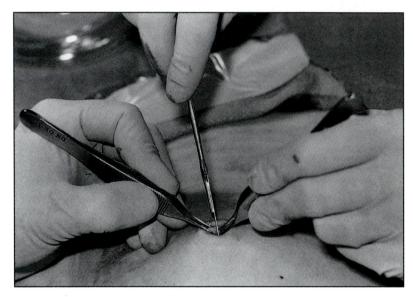

FIGURE 1-3.

Hasson trocar technique. A 10-mm vertical skin incision is made within the umbilicus. The deepest point within the umbilicus serves as the center of the incision.

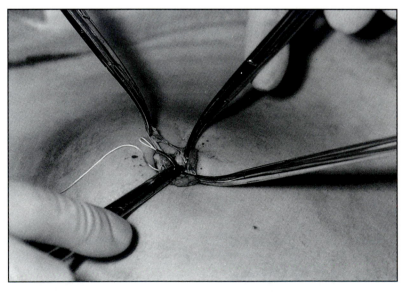

FIGURE 1-4.

The tissues are grasped between clamps, elevated, and divided until the peritoneum is entered. A stay suture is placed through the fascia on each side of the incision.

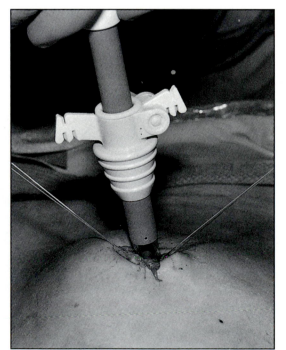

FIGURE 1-5.

The stay sutures are are elevated as the Hasson cannula is inserted into the abdomen.

Trocars

Trocar/cannula systems allow for insertion of instruments and the laparoscope. They are available in disposable and reusable styles. Much emphasis has been placed on trocar safety, and most single-use trocars now have safety shields or retractable tips. These safety devices have reduced the number of trocar-related complications but do not totally eliminate the occurrence of catastrophic events (Figure 1-9).

Secondary trocars (trocars other than those housing the laparoscope) should almost always be placed without complications because these trocars are placed under direct laparoscopic visualization. The peritoneal surface should be examined for the presence of the epigastric vessels underneath the proposed site of trocar placement. Additionally, the abdominal wall may be transilluminated to identify and avoid superficial veins. Trocar tips must be sharp, and their placement should be performed smoothly. The requirement of excessive force to place a trocar indicates that an improper technique is being used. Excessive resistance should cause the surgeon to examine the skin incision for adequacy and to check the trocar to be certain that it is properly loaded in a way that allows the sharp tip to be exposed. Placement of secondary trocars should be done by using a "J-maneuver." This technique involves placing the trocar under direct visualization at a 90° angle to the abdominal wall. The trocar is advanced until the trocar tip penetrates the peritoneum. The hand controlling the trocar is then lowered so that the tip of the trocar is elevated and the cannula is advanced in a direction parallel to the peritoneal surface of the abdominal wall. Adherence to this technique can be expected to minimize visceral or retroperitoneal injury.

Optimal spacing and positioning of the cannulae are important for the successful completion of laparoscopic procedures. Cannulae should be spaced 7 to 10 cm apart (or one hand's breadth apart). Trocars should be triangulated away from yet directed toward the target organ. This allows the surgeon to work using two hands along the same axis as the laparoscope. One should avoid trocar placement that will require the sur-

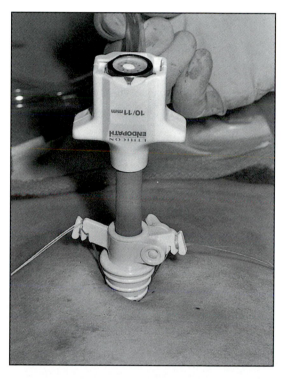

FIGURE 1-6.

The stay sutures are used to secure the cannula to the fascia. The insufflator tubing is attached to the cannula.

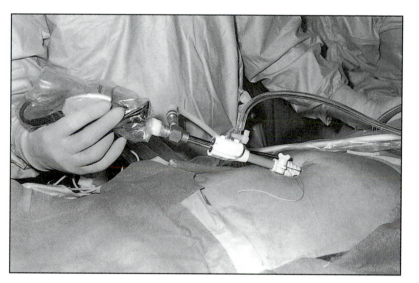

FIGURE 1-7.

The laparoscope is inserted and a 360° evaluation of the peritoneal cavity is performed.

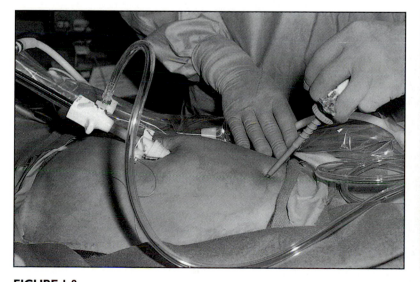

FIGURE 1-8.

A secondary trocar/cannula is inserted under laparoscopic visualization.

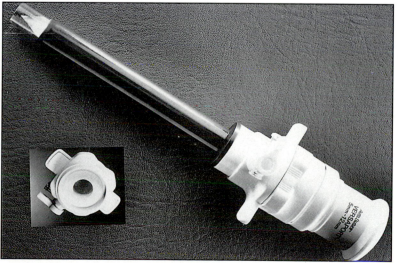

FIGURE 1-9.

Photograph of the Versaport trocar (US Surgical Corp., Norwalk, CT).

geon or assistant to work directly against the visual axis of the laparoscope.

Irrigation/Aspiration

A wide variety of irrigation systems are available, ranging from manually pumped systems to pressurized irrigation systems that provide a high-flow irrigation and aspiration. High-flow systems are essential for advanced laparoscopic procedures where one needs to rapidly clear blood that is obscuring the field. Flow rates depend on several factors, such as the pressure placed on the bag of fluid, the resistance within the tubing, and the diameter of the irrigation/aspiration wand (Figure 1-10). High-flow insufflation devices (15 to 20 L/min) should be in place when an advanced irrigation/aspiration system is being used because the suction will deflate the pneumoperitoneum rapidly.

Several systems include fluid warmers to maintain homeostatic patient temperatures. Other recent advances in irrigation/aspiration device design include the ability to place instrumentation such as cautery, graspers, and scissors through the suction irrigation port.

It is important that bleeding be rapidly controlled during laparoscopic procedures. A small amount of blood within the peritoneal cavity can absorb a great deal of light, thus making visualization suboptimal. This blood can also obscure tissue planes. The authors use 8000 units of heparin in each bag of irrigation in an attempt to prevent pooled blood from clotting. This dose of heparin within the peritoneal cavity does not cause systemic anticoagulation. Additionally, changing the position of the operating table allows one to collect pooled fluids and to assess the color of the irrigant for the presence of ongoing hemorrhage.

Instruments

A variety of instruments used to grasp tissue are available, many of which have been designed to mimic standard surgical instrumentation. Graspers can be divided into those that are atraumatic or those that contain teeth on the tissue handling surface (Figure 1-11). The authors prefer to use atraumatic graspers in almost all circumstances, with the exception of removal of a specimen from the abdominal cavity.

Endoscopic scissors are also produced with a variety of tips. The most commonly used scissors have curved tips analogous to Metzenbaum scissors (Figure 1-12). Other types of scissors have been designed for specific purposes, such as hook scissors or micro-scissors for use on the cystic duct (Figure 1-13). Most endoscopic scissors may be attached to the electrosurgical unit for simultaneous cutting and cautery.

Several types of instrumentation are unique to endoscopic surgery. The endoscopic hook cautery is frequently used to

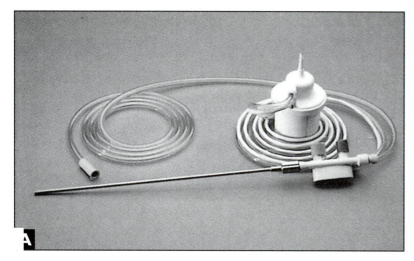

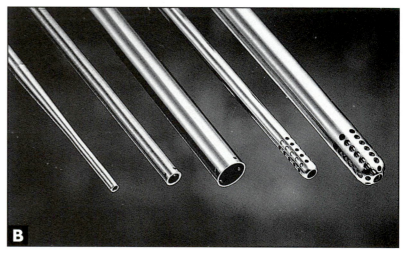

FIGURE 1-10.
A, Photograph of StrykFlow (Stryker Endoscopy, Santa Clara, CA).
B, Close-up view of various suction-irrigation cannulas.

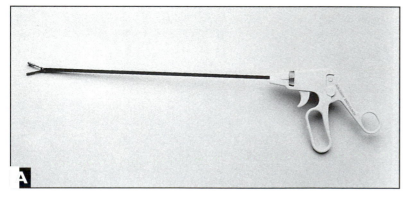

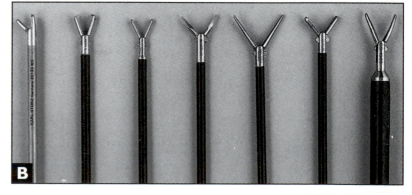

FIGURE 1-11.
A, Photograph of Endo Clinch (US Surgical Corp., Norwalk, CT).
B, Close-up view of graspers, atraumatic and those that contain teeth.

divide the peritoneal attachments between the gallbladder and the liver (Figure 1-14). As in open procedures, exposure is crucial for the safe performance of an operation. Endoscopic retractors such as the Endo Paddle and Endo Retract (US Surgical, Norwalk, CT) have been designed with a variety of shapes and sizes (Figure 1-15). The endoscopic knot pusher is essential for the placement of extracorporeal tied sutures (Figure 1-16). Single-use laparoscopic sutures are available with an attached knot pusher (Figure 1-17). The Endo Stitch (US Surgical, Norwalk, CT) represents a significant innovation in laparoscop-

ic instrumentation. This device greatly facilitates laparoscopic suturing (Figure 1-18). Conventional sutures may be used for endoscopic purposes when placed by using an endoscopic needle driver (Figure 1-19).

Endoscopic stapling devices are expensive instruments that facilitate the performance of laparoscopic procedures in a time-efficient manner. The endoscopic hernia stapler is considered essential by most laparoscopic surgeons for the placement of mesh during an endoscopic hernia repair (Figure 1-20). The endoscopic clip applier is one of the most frequently used

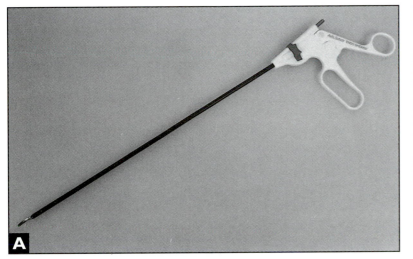

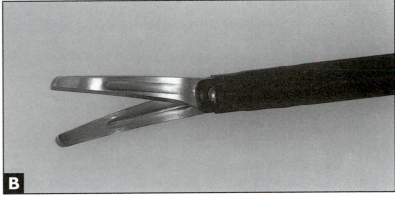

FIGURE 1-12.

A, Photograph of Endo Shears endoscopic scissors (US Surgical Corp., Norwalk, CT). **B**, Close-up view of same scissors.

FIGURE 1-13.

Photograph of three types of endoscopic scissors showing the variety of tips.

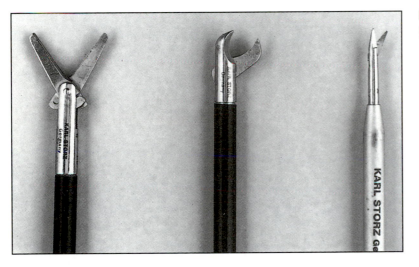

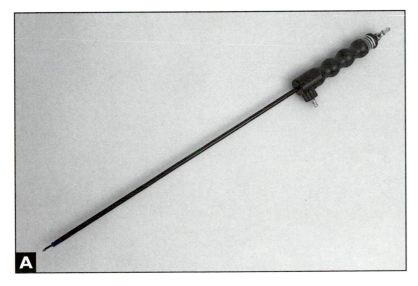

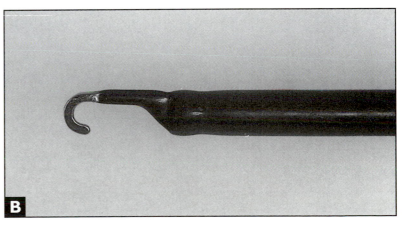

FIGURE 1-14.

A, Photograph of an endoscopic hook cautery. **B**, Close-up view of the hook cautery.

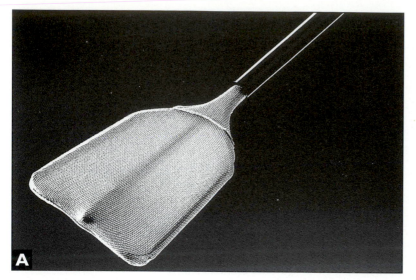
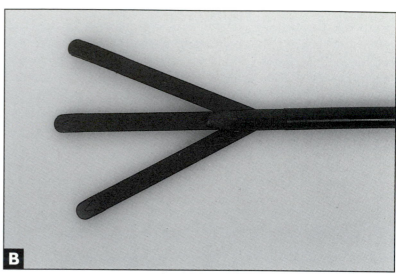

FIGURE 1-15.

A, Photograph of Endo Paddle (US Surgical Corp., Norwalk, CT). **B**, Photograph of Endo Retract endoscopic retractor (US Surgical Corp., Norwalk, CT).

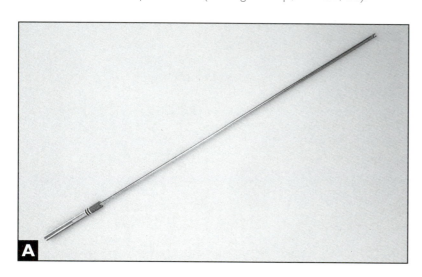
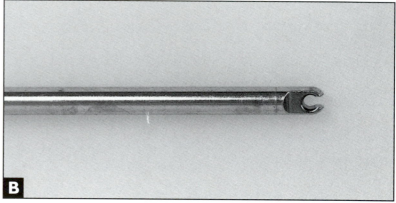
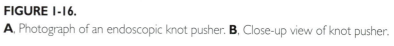

FIGURE 1-16.

A, Photograph of an endoscopic knot pusher. **B**, Close-up view of knot pusher.

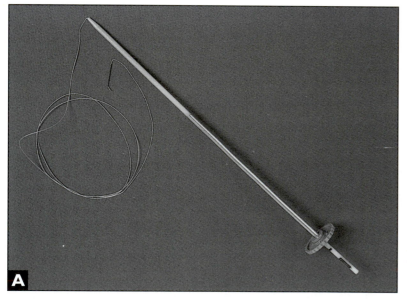
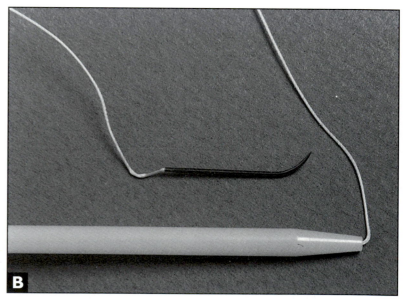

FIGURE 1-17.

A, Photograph of a single-use laparoscopic suture with an attached knot pusher (US Surgical Corp., Norwalk, CT). **B**, Close-up view of suture and pusher.

FIGURE 1-18.

Photograph of the Endo Stitch (US Surgical Corp., Norwalk, CT) device for laparoscopic suturing.

laparoscopic instruments. This device plays a significant role in the rapid acceptance of laparoscopic cholecystectomy because of the ease with which the surgeon can control the cystic duct and vessels with surgical clips. Endoscopic stapling devices, such as the Endo GIA and Endo TA (US Surgical Corp., Norwalk, CT), are applied to tissues and used in a manner analogous to that of their conventional counterparts (Figure 1-21). Endoscopic atraumatic bowel clamps are used by surgeons wishing to perform anastomosis via laparoscopic techniques (Figure 1-22).

In addition, concern about cancer seeding in laparoscopy incisions has recently been attributed to the use of carbon dioxide gas insufflation [6].

Mini-Laparoscopy

Mini-laparoscopy is an emerging facet of minimally invasive surgery. In contrast to conventional laparoscopic instruments, which are 5 to 10 mm in size, these smaller instruments are 1.7

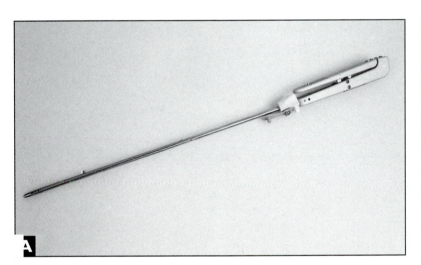

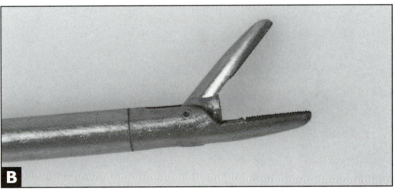

FIGURE 1-19.

A, Photograph of an endoscopic needle driver (Snowden-Pencer, Tucker, GA). **B**, Close-up view of the needle driver.

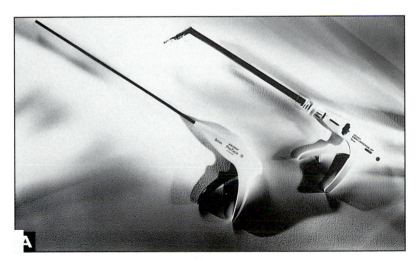

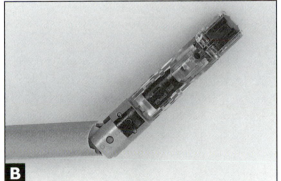

FIGURE 1-20.

A, Photograph of Endo Universal 65 hernia stapler and ProTack (US Surgical Corp., Norwalk, CT). **B**, Close-up view of the stapler.

to 3.0 mm. Technical advances have led to the development of endoscopes or mini-laparoscopes with smaller diameters. Smaller laparoscopic instruments have been developed in an effort to accomplish the same surgical task while minimizing abdominal-wall trauma. The optimal size of the mini-laparoscopic instrumentation has not been precisely determined; it may turn out that multiple sizes will be used according to the exact requirement. The smallest instruments could be used for certain tasks, whereas a procedure requiring a sturdier device could use a slightly larger instrument.

Mini-laparoscopy is most commonly used for diagnostic purposes, and it can be done under local anesthesia [7]. Local anesthesia with intravenous sedation is also used. Mini-laparoscopic instruments may, for example, be useful in patients with right-lower-quadrant pain being evaluated for acute appendicitis. For most diagnostic procedures, at least two ports are required: one for the scope and the other for another instrument to use for retraction or manipulation.

The most common procedure performed with smaller instruments is the mini-laparoscopic cholecystectomy. There are many reasons why this procedure has adapted to mini-laparoscopic techniques, including the anatomy in the right upper quadrant and the familiarity of many surgeons with the standard laparoscopic cholecystectomy. The successful completion of this minimally invasive approach is proper selection of patients and instruments. Numerous advanced procedures are also amenable to mini-laparoscopic techniques and have been performed by this less invasive approach. The surgeon using these smaller instruments often at least initially uses a combination of the smaller and regular-sized laparoscopic instruments for procedures. Procedures that incorporate mini-laparoscopic instruments include splenectomy, adrenalectomy, fundoplication, bowel resection, hernia repair, gynecologic procedures, tumor biopsy, and excision of masses. The experience and skill of the laparoscopic surgeon dictate the appropriateness of these instruments in the procedures performed.

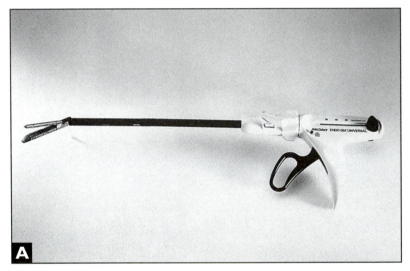
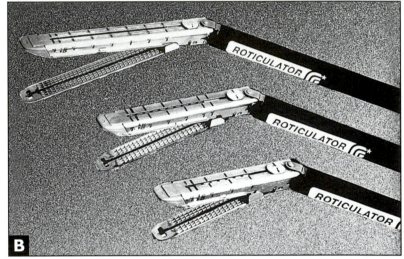

FIGURE 1-21.
A, Photograph of the Autosuture Endo GIA Universal endoscopic stapler (US Surgical Corp., Norwalk, CT). **B**, Close-up view of the stapler.

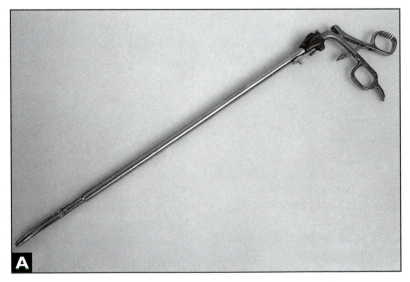
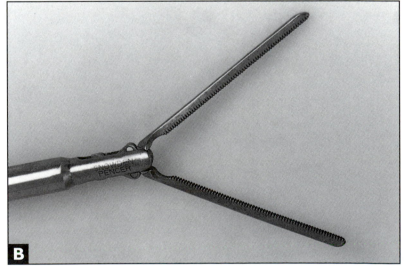

FIGURE 1-22.
A, Photograph of an endoscopic bowel clamp (Snowden Pencer, Tucker, GA). **B**, Close-up view of the clamp.

Complications, such as bleeding or injury to adjacent structures, occur with the mini-laparoscopic procedures as they do with conventional laparoscopic approaches. When significant bleeding is encountered, the ability to control it with these smaller instruments is suboptimal. Clip appliers are not yet available in smaller sizes, and control of bleeding requires reliance on preformed loops or suturing techniques. In addition, the extremely small suction devices do not clear blood as readily as the standard 5-mm suction irrigation devices.

Despite rapid progress in the technology of these mini-endoscopes, they remain unable to provide the same bright, high-resolution panoramic view of the abdomen as the conventional 5- to 10-mm scopes. During critical maneuvers, the difference in quality with these mini-laparoscopes may compromise visualization. Thus, the conventional scopes are still used for many of the more advanced laparoscopic procedures. However, mini-endoscopes are being incorporated in these procedures during times when an additional larger instrument, such as a clip applier or stapler, is required; they can be used through the larger laparoscopic port.

Mini-laparoscopic techniques provide entry into the next level of minimally invasive surgery. Research in the areas of safety, impact, cost-effectiveness, and feasibility of mini-laparoscopy is needed; few studies in this area have been published. With proper training, continued improvements in instrument design, and prudent application, mini-laparoscopy is certain to provide patients with significant benefits.

Training and Credentialling

Laparoscopic surgery requires a knowledge base and specific skills in addition to general surgical training. Laparoscopic procedures should be performed only by those capable of performing the same procedures in an open manner. However, technical expertise in conventional operations does not translate into technical competency in laparoscopic procedures. An increasing effort is underway to integrate laparoscopic surgery as an essential component of residency training and many surgeons completing general surgery residencies are opting for advanced training in laparoscopic techniques as fellows in this area. However, a tremendous need remains for the training of practicing surgeons in these techniques, and the need exists for the introduction of evolving techniques and technology.

No nationally accepted standards for the credentialling of surgeons in laparoscopic surgery exist. The Society of American Gastrointestinal and Endoscopic Surgeons (SAGES) has published recommendations for the training and credentialling of surgeons in laparoscopic surgery. However, the medical/legal burden of credentialling surgeons rests at the level of the individual hospital.

The essential components of training in order to meet credentialling standards for most institutions include the attendance by the surgeon at a laparoscopic training course that includes didactics and hands-on laboratory training. The surgeon must participate as an observer or as an assistant in a specified number of cases. The surgeon must perform a specified number of cases in the presence of a preceptor, an individual previously credentialled for this same procedure who serves as a teacher or mentor. The surgeon must then perform a specified number of cases in the presence of and be approved by a proctor. A proctor is an unbiased individual who observes the surgeon performing laparoscopic procedures without intervening or instructing during the operation. The proctor then makes a recommendation to the hospital regarding the surgeon's competency to perform this type of operation. The final stage of credentialling is the review and approval by the hospital credentialling committee. The number of cases required at each stage varies greatly between institutions. SAGES will provide guidelines for training and credentialling of surgeons in laparoscopic surgery upon request; their address is as follows: Suite 3000, 2716 Ocean Park Boulevard, Santa Monica, California, 90405.

References

1. Berci G: History of endoscopy. In *Endoscopy.* Edited by Berci G. New York: Appleton-Century-Crofts; 1976:xix–xxiii.

2. Knyrim K, Seidlitz H, Vakil N, Classes M: Perspectives in "electronic endoscopy" past, present, and future of fibers and CCDs in medical endoscopes. *Endoscopy* 1990, 22(suppl 1):2–8.

3. Hunter JG, Sackier JM, eds.: *Minimally Invasive Surgery.* New York: McGraw-Hill, Inc.; 1993.

4. Kitano S, Iso Y, Tomikawa M, *et al.*: A prospective trial comparing pneumoperitoneum and U-shaped retractor elevation for laparoscopic cholecystectomy. *Surg Endosc* 1993, 7:311–314.

5. Koivusalo AM, Kellokumpu I, Scheinin M, *et al.*: Randomized comparison of the neuroendocrine response to laparoscopic cholecystectomy using either conventional or abdominal wall lift techniques. *Br J Surg* 1996, 83:1532–1536.

6. Matthew G, Watson DI, Rofe AM, *et al.*: Wound metastases following laparoscopy. *Br J Surg* 1996, 83:1087–1089.

7. Bruhat MA, Goldchmit R: Minilaparoscopy in gynecology. *Eur J Obst Gynecol Reprod Biol* 1998, 76:207–210.

Laparoscopic Evaluation of Abdominal Trauma

James D. St. Louis
Mark W. Sebastian
R. Lawrence Reed II
Steven N. Vaslef

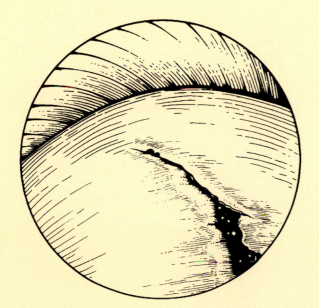

Background

Trauma is the leading cause of death in the United States among individuals between the ages of 1 and 44 years. It accounts for approximately 150,000 deaths annually [1]. Fifty-seven million people were accidentally injured in 1985. There is an annual injury incidence of once for every four people [2]. Today's politically motivated environment dictates that cost-effective, dependable diagnostic methods be used for the evaluation of the trauma patient. Finding these tools is a prime challenge for the trauma surgeon.

The introduction of diagnostic peritoneal lavage (DPL) in 1965 by Root and colleagues [3] revolutionized the approach to abdominal trauma. It has proved to be a safe and accurate technique, with an accuracy of greater than 95%. The procedure is easily mastered, can be performed on a patient within minutes of arrival to the emergency department, and gives immediate results. Although DPL has become a gold standard, its high sensitivity coupled with a low specificity is recognized as a drawback. It is apparent that a substantial number of nontherapeutic laparotomies have been performed for insignificant injuries, such as nonbleeding splenic or liver lacerations. The incidence of nontherapeutic laparotomies after a positive DPL is reported to be 5% to 14% for blunt trauma and as high as 50% for penetrating injuries [4].

Over the past two decades, reports of the use of computed tomography (CT) in the diagnosis of abdominal trauma have flooded the literature [5–7]. With the development of more sophisticated scanners, many trauma surgeons are more comfortable with nonoperative management of stable patients with solid organ injuries. Scanning with CT provides a good evaluation of retroperitoneal injuries, which are invaluable by DPL. This test also provides an excellent way to more precisely identify a source of bleeding. Yet, there are concerns about the use of CT in trauma. When applied within the first few hours of blunt injury, abdominal CT may miss as many as 50% of visceral injuries, particularly pancreatic injuries. Scanning is time consuming, although the newer-generation scanners have become much faster. Many argue that taking a potentially unstable patient away from a controlled environment is dangerous. Finally, the routine use of CT scanning produces a tremendous financial burden, with an average cost of $1000 per study.

With the evolution of laparoscopic technique and equipment, the examination of abdominal injuries with laparoscopy not only provides an accurate and inexpensive diagnostic tool [8]; it is also effective in avoiding nontherapeutic laparotomies [9,10]. Laparoscopic inspection of the abdominal cavity after trauma was initially advocated by Gazzaniga and coworkers [11] and Carnevale and coworkers [12]. Carnevale and coworkers reviewed 20 patients who were evaluated with laparoscopy before exploratory laparotomy. Laparotomy was avoided in 12 of the 20 patients who had sustained abdominal trauma. Several other reviews have recently appeared in the literature (Table 2-1).

With the advent of more sophisticated equipment and increasing experience by general surgeons, laparoscopy is increasingly used to evaluate both penetrating and blunt abdominal trauma (Tables 2-2 and 2-3). Although commonly performed in

Table 2-1. Laparoscopy in abdominal trauma

Study	Year	Patients, n	Type of trauma
Gazzaniga and coworkers [11]	1976	37	Mixed*
Carnevale and coworkers [12]	1977	20	Mixed*
Berci and coworkers [13]	1991	150	Blunt
Salvino and coworkers [17]	1993	75	Mixed*
Fabian and coworkers [18]	1993	182	Mixed*
Sosa and coworkers [15]	1995	121	Penetrating
Smith and coworkers [16]	1995	133	Mixed*
Zantut and coworkers [14]	1997	510	Mixed*

*Combination of blunt and penetrating injury.

Table 2-2. Frequency of organ injury in penetrating abdominal trauma*

Organ or system	Occurrence, %
Liver	37
Small bowel	26
Stomach	19
Colon	17
Major vascular	13
Retroperitoneal	10
Mesentery	10
Spleen	7
Diaphragm	5
Kidney	4
Pancreas	4
Duodenum	2
Biliary system	1
Other	1

*From Greenfield and coworkers [19]; with permission.

Table 2-3. Frequency of organ injury in blunt abdominal trauma*	
Organ or system	**Occurrence, %**
Spleen	25
Intestine	15
Liver	15
Retroperitoneal	13
Kidney	12
Urinary bladder	6
Mesentery	5
Pancreas	3
Diaphragm	2
Urethra	2
Vascular	2

*From Greenfield and coworkers [19]; with permission.

the operating room, laparoscopic evaluation may be accomplished in the emergency department.

Several potential complications are associated with the use of laparoscopy for trauma. Several series have reported tension pneumothoraces associated with diaphragmatic injuries and pneumoperitoneum, although no adverse outcomes have been reported [12]. Gas embolization is also a theoretically possible complication, although this has not been reported in the recent literature. The three major limitations of laparoscopy in evaluation of abdominal trauma are 1) failure to visualize the spleen, 2) inability to reliably evacuate blood clots; and 3) inability to fully examine the small bowel [13].

Surgical Technique

Figures 2-1 through 2-20 depict the surgical technique for laparoscopic evaluation in abdominal trauma.

Set-up

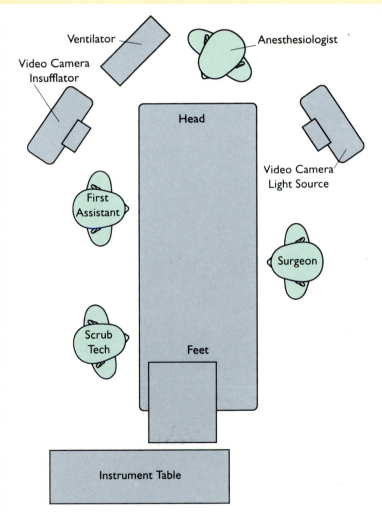

FIGURE 2-1.

Initial operating room set-up for laparoscopic exploration for abdominal trauma. Preoperative antibiotics are generally administered in the emergency department. Nasogastric and Foley catheters should also be placed in the emergency department. The initial positioning of the surgeon is similar to that for laparoscopic cholecystectomy. The surgeon must be sure that the patient is placed on an operating table that is easily and reliably moveable by the anesthesiologist. The first assistant must be prepared to take control of the camera as the exploration progresses. Both the operating room staff and the operating surgeon must keep in mind that flexibility in positioning the patient and equipment is critical during such exploration.

Set-up

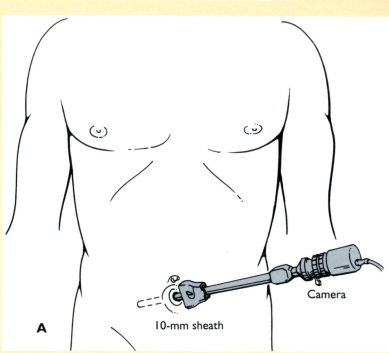

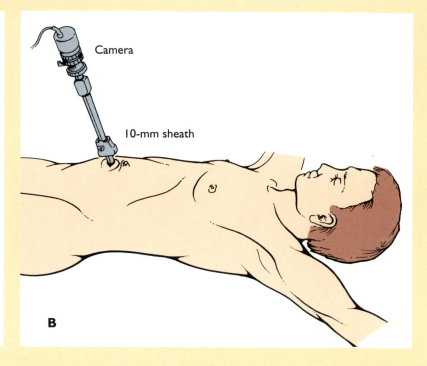

FIGURE 2-2.

A and **B**, The patient is initially positioned with the head down by 30° with the arm extended at the side. Access to the peritoneal cavity is gained infraumbilically using a 10-mm sheath via a closed (Veress needle) or open (Hasson trocar) technique. After insufflation with either carbon dioxide or nitrous oxide to a pressure of 15 to 20 mm Hg, the laparoscope is inserted via the 10-mm sheath. At this point, the peritoneal cavity is thoroughly inspected, with special attention to areas of known or possible peritoneal violation.

Procedure

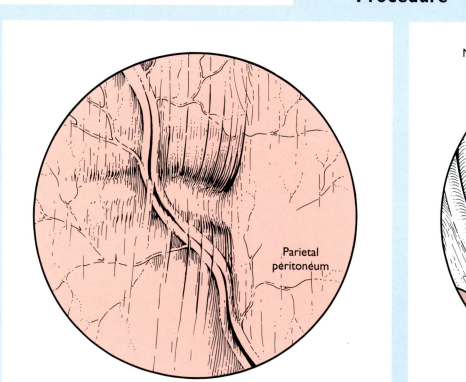

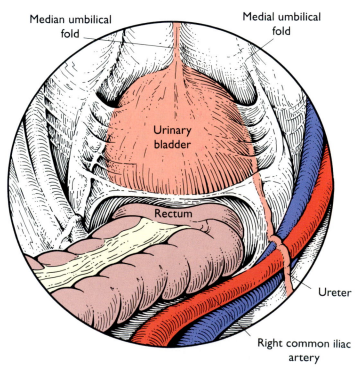

FIGURE 2-3.

Initial exploration consists of a complete evaluation of the parietal peritoneal surface of the anterior abdominal wall. This should be accomplished with the operating table flat. Particular attention is paid to known sites of external injury (penetrating entrance wounds).

FIGURE 2-4.

Once the parietal peritoneal surface has been inspected, the surgeon begins a systematic and complete exploration of the abdominal cavity. This technical description will begin with viewing the pelvis. The surgeon should first give special attention to the presence of free fluid in the pelvis. The patient should be placed with the head down by 30°, allowing the small bowel to fall cephalad.

Procedure

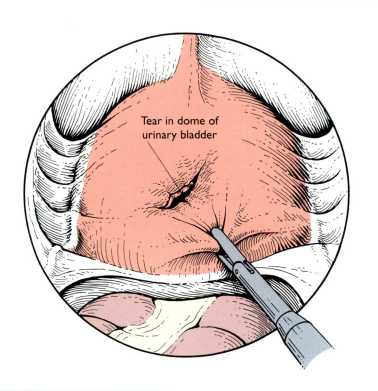

FIGURE 2-5.

The bladder is inspected for penetration by looking for ecchymosis of the bladder wall or the free flow of urine. At this point, a 5-mm trocar may be placed in the right upper quadrant. A fine grasper is placed through the sheath. This allows the surgeon to place traction on the bladder for a better evaluation of the pelvis.

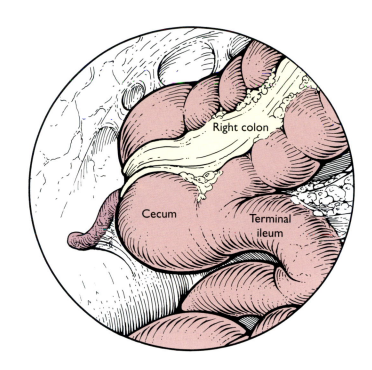

FIGURE 2-6.

The exploration is continued by examining the right lower quadrant. The patient is kept in 30° of the Trendelenburg position, but the table is rotated in the long axis 30° to the left. This allows better exposure to the right lower quadrant. The surgeon now pays special attention to the cecum and right (ascending) colon. Penetrating injuries to the anterior surface of the colon are evaluated. Bleeding, extravasation of bowel contents, and ecchymosis all indicate injury to the colon.

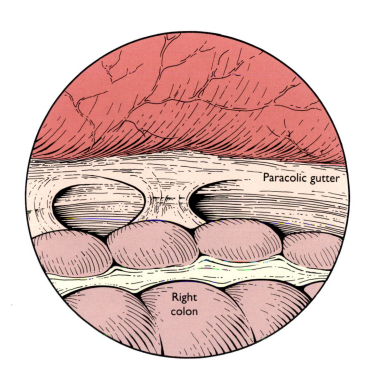

FIGURE 2-7.

The right paracolic gutter is evaluated for evidence of retroperitoneal injury. Ecchymosis is an important clue to injury in this region. If retroperitoneal injury is anticipated (which is suggested from knowledge of the entry wound), freeing up of the retroperitoneal portion of the ascending colon is recommended.

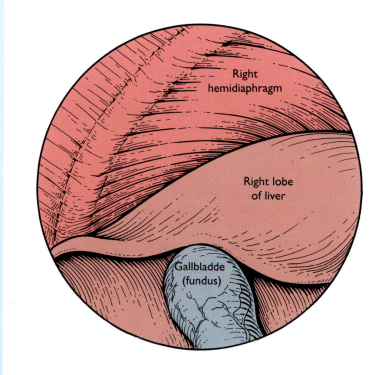

FIGURE 2-8.

The liver and contents of the right upper quadrant are now evaluated. The operating table should be flattened. The liver can best be evaluated with the aid of the grasper. The anterior and lateral surfaces of the right lobe may be easily explored with minimal effort.

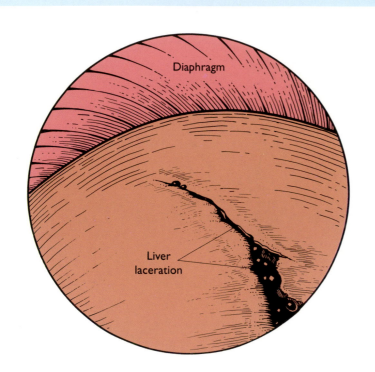

FIGURE 2-9.

Penetrating injuries (lacerations) and parenchymal fractures to the surface of the liver can be evaluated for active bleeding. Cauterization of bleeding sites may be attempted; if initial attempts fail, the procedure should be converted to open laparotomy.

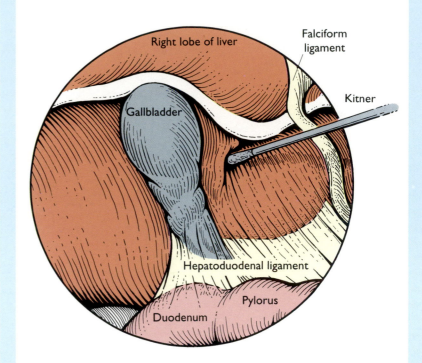

FIGURE 2-10.

The inferior surface of the right lobe of the liver and gallbladder are next evaluated. This is accomplished by simply elevating the right lobe with an endoscopic Kitner probe. One must be aware that isolated injury to the inferior surface of the liver is uncommon. Thus, the surgeon should reevaluate the liver for additional injuries if a laceration is found on the inferior surface.

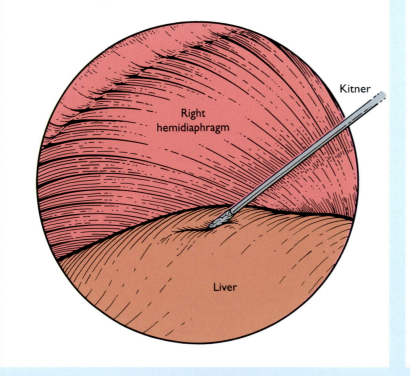

FIGURE 2-11.

Once the right lobe has been completely evaluated, the exploration can then be continued by examining the right hemidiaphragm. The operating table is now placed with the feet down 30°, leaving it rotated to the left. A Kitner probe may be used to shift the liver medially. The anterior and central portions of the diaphragm can be explored without difficulty. The surgeon must be aware that a thorough evaluation of the posterior portion of the diaphragm using laparoscopy is difficult.

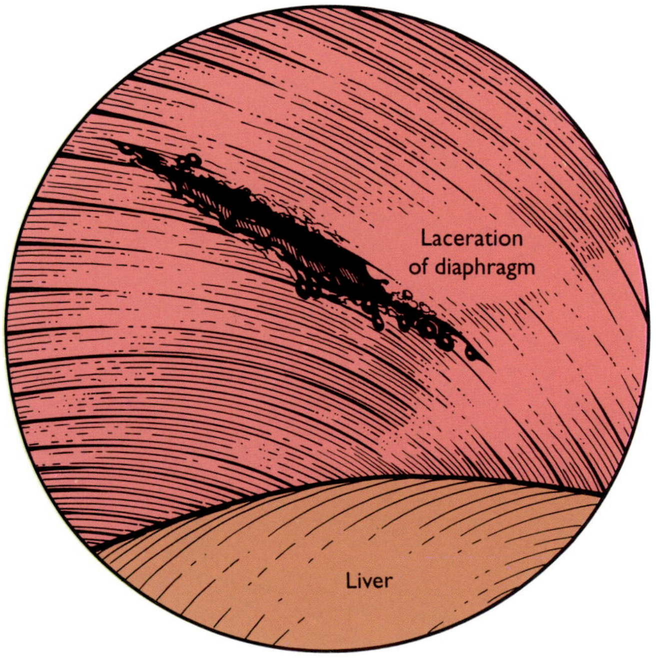

FIGURE 2-12.

Lacerations to the diaphragm can be seen without difficulty, especially in the anterior and central portions.

Procedure

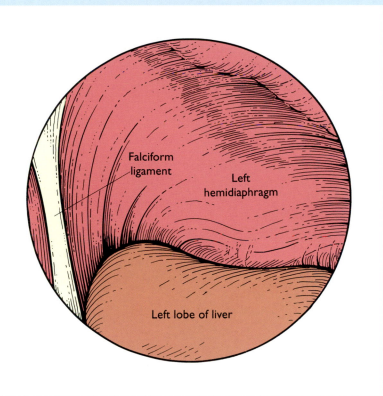

FIGURE 2-13.

The left upper quadrant is now examined. The operating table is rotated 30° in the long axis to the right, leaving the patient's feet down. The left lobe of the liver and left hemidiaphragm are evaluated.

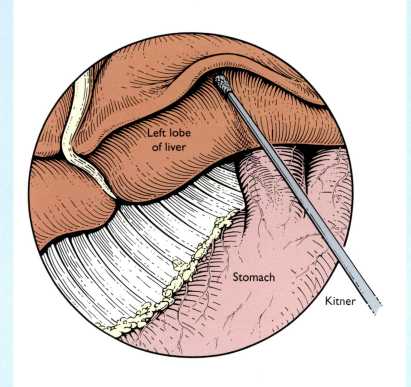

FIGURE 2-14.

A Kitner probe may be used to elevate the liver to view its inferior surface. The anterior surface of the stomach is also explored at this time.

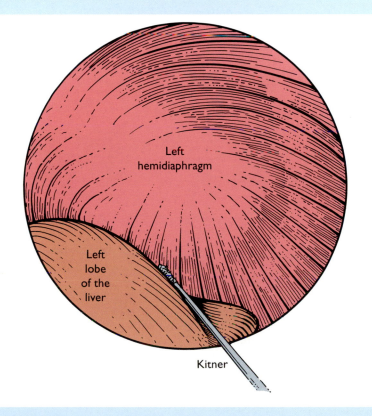

FIGURE 2-15.

The left hemidiaphragm is viewed as before. The grasper is used to shift the left lobe of the liver to the right.

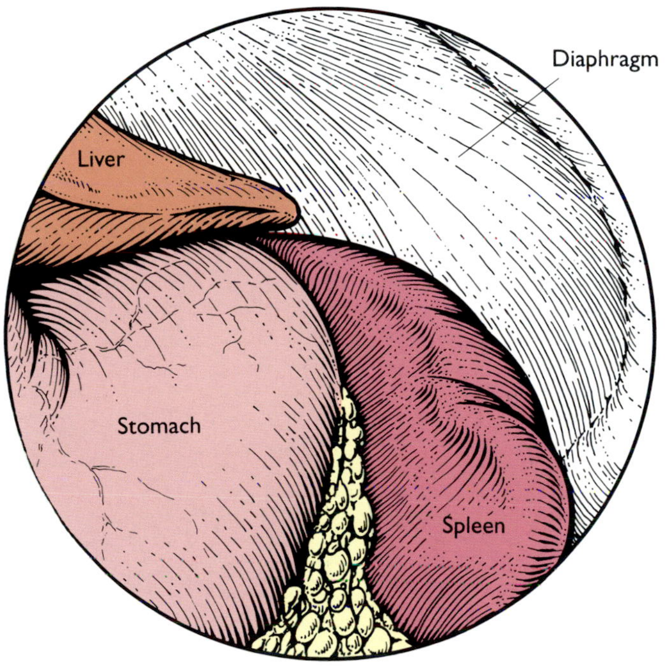

FIGURE 2-16.

The spleen is next evaluated for injuries. It is impossible to visualize the entire spleen because of its posterior position. The anterior aspect of the inferior portion of the spleen is inspected.

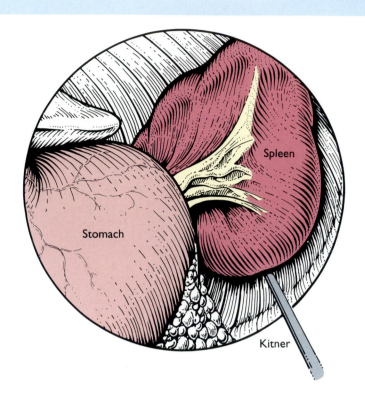

FIGURE 2-17.

A Kitner probe may be used to gently elevate the spleen to visualize the posterior surface. Extreme care must be used to avoid iatrogenic injury.

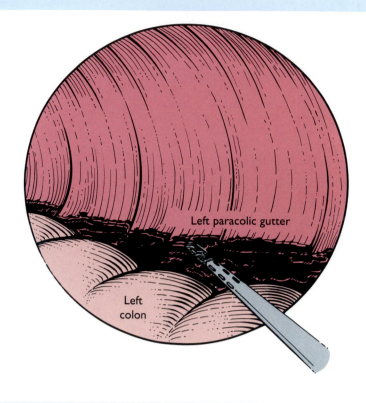

FIGURE 2-18.

Although complete visualization of the spleen is not possible with the laparoscope, injury can be surmised by the presence of blood in the left paracolic gutter. The blood is evacuated and the region is evaluated for reaccumulation. Reaccumulation of blood indicates active bleeding and is an indication for conversion to open laparotomy.

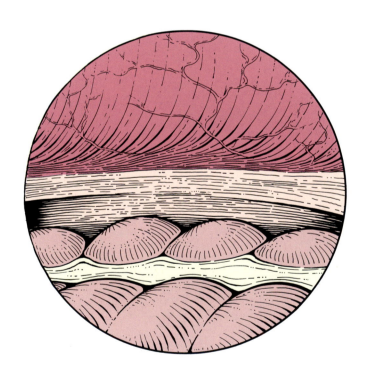

FIGURE 2-19.

The left (descending) colon and left paracolic gutter are now examined. The colon is evaluated for penetrating injuries. The paracolic gutter is examined for ecchymosis, indicating retroperitoneal injury.

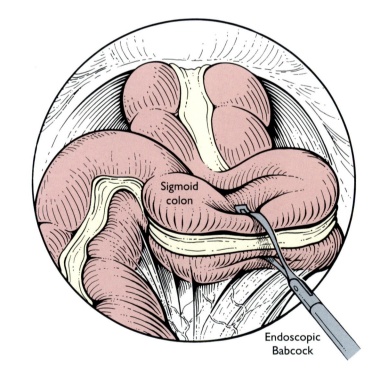

FIGURE 2-20.

The sigmoid colon is now explored for injuries. This may be best accomplished with the aid of endoscopic Babcocks. Because this is a redundant structure, it is possible to examine both anterior and posterior surfaces.

References

1. Rice DP, Mackenzie EJ, *et al.*, eds.: *Cost of Injury in the United States: A Report to Congress.* Atlanta: Centers for Disease Control; 1989.

2. Baker CC, Oppenheiner L, Stephens B, *et al.*: Epidemiology of trauma death. *Am J Surg* 1980, 140:144–150.

3. Root HO, Hauser CW, McKinley CR, *et al.*: Diagnostic peritoneal lavage. *Surgery* 1965, 57:633–637.

4. Oreskovich MR, Carrico CJ: Stab wounds of the anterior abdomen. *Ann Surg* 1983, 4:411–419.

5. Matsubara TK, Fong HMT, Burns CM: Computed tomography of the abdomen in the management of blunt abdominal trauma. *J Trauma* 1986, 26:585–592.

6. Sorkey AJ, Farnell MB, *et al.*: The complementary roles of diagnostic peritoneal lavage and computed tomography in the evaluation of blunt abdominal trauma. *Surgery* 1989, 106:794–800.

7. Meyer DM, Thal ER, *et al.*: Evaluation of computed tomography and diagnostic peritoneal lavage in blunt abdominal trauma. *J Trauma* 1989, 29:1168–1172.

8. Marks JM, Youngelman DF, *et al.*: Cost analysis of diagnostic laparoscopy vs laparotomy in the evaluation of penetrating abdominal trauma. *Surg Endosc* 1997, 11:272–276.

9. Kelling G: Uber Oesophagoskopie, Gastroskopie und Koelioskopie. *Munch Med Wochenschr* 1901, 49:21. In *Surg Clin North Am* 1992, 72:997–1002.

10. Jacobaeus HC: Kurze Ubersicht Uber meine Erfahrunger mit der Laparothorakoskopie. *Munch Med Wochenschr* 1911, 57:2017. In *Surg Clin North Am* 1992, 72:997–1002.

11. Gazzaniga AB, Stanton WW, Barlett RH: Laparoscopy in the diagnosis of blunt and penetrating injuries to the abdomen. *Am J Surg* 1976, 131:315–318.

12. Carnevale N, Baron N, Delany HM: Peritoneoscopy as an aid in the diagnosis of abdominal trauma: a preliminary report. *J Trauma* 1977, 17:634–641.

13. Berci G, Sackier JM, Paz-Partlow M: Emergency laparoscopy. *Am J Surg* 1991, 161:332–335.

14. Zantut LF, Ivantury RR, *et al.*: Diagnostic and therapeutic laparoscopy for penetrating abdominal trauma: a multicenter experience. *J Trauma* 1996, 42:825–829.

15. Sosa JL, Arrillaga A, *et al.*: Laparoscopy in 121 consecutive patients with abdominal gunshot wounds. *J Trauma* 1995, 39:501–504.

16. Smith RS, Fry WR, *et al.*: Therapeutic laparoscopy in trauma. *Am J Surg* 1995, 170:632–636.

17. Salvino CK, Esposito TJ, *et al.*: The role of diagnostic laparoscopy in the management of trauma patients: a preliminary assessment. *J Trauma* 1993, 34:506–515.

18. Fabian TC, Croce MA, Stewart RM, *et al.*: A prospective analysis of diagnostic laparoscopy in trauma. *Ann Surg* 1993, 127:557–565.

19. Greenfield LJ, Mulholland MW, Oldham KT, Zelenock GB, eds.: *Surgery: Scientific Principles and Practice.* Philadelphia: J.B. Lippincott; 1993.

Laparoscopic Inguinal Herniorrhaphy

Shahab A. Akhter
Steve Eubanks

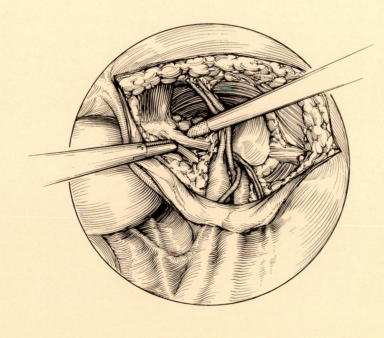

Inguinal herniorrhaphy has a rich history dating back to the origins of surgery (Table 3-1). Approximately 750,000 inguinal hernias are repaired annually in the United States, making it one of the two most common procedures performed by general surgeons. The estimated annual cost of hernia repair in this country is approximately $28 billion, which represents 3% of the nation's health care costs [1]. Conventional open hernia repair has been associated with recurrence rates of 5% to 10%.

Morbidity, including incisional pain and convalescence, can be significant. The best approach for repair of inguinal hernias has always been controversial, and laparoscopic inguinal herniorrhaphy is the latest technique to be introduced (Table 3-2). At least six conceptually different methods have been described to date. This chapter describes two laparoscopic mesh repairs: transabdominal preperitoneal placement (TAPP) and totally preperitoneal placement (TOPP).

Table 3-1. The abbreviated history of hernia surgery

Year	Investigator and study	Location	Contribution
			Anatomic era
1556	Pierre Franco [37]	France	First recorded description of an operation for strangulated hernia
1756	Percival Pott [3]	England	Published treatise on hernia including the first description of the congenital nature of indirect hernias
1778	August Gottlieb Richter [38]	Germany	First description of hernia with partial enterocele ("Richter's hernia")
1793	Arbos Gimbernat [39]	Spain	Described lacunar ligament ("Gimbernat's ligament")
1804	Sir Astley Paston Cooper [40,41]	England	Described superior pubic ligament, transversalis fascia, and shutter mechanism of internal oblique and transversus abdominis
1806	Franz Caspar Hesselbach [42,43]	Germany	Described iliopubic tract and "Hesselbach's triangle"
1809	Antonio Scarpa [44,45]	Italy	Published classic treatises on cremasteric fascia ("Scarpa's fascia") and sliding hernia
			Early surgical repairs
1871	Henry O. Marcy [46,47]	Boston	Stressed importance of ligation of the hernia sac with internal ring repair as well as introduced antiseptic ligatures
1884	Edoardo Bassini [48]	Italy	Described reconstruction of the inguinal floor by approximation of the transversalis fascia and inguinal ligament ("Bassini repair")
1889	William S. Halsted [49]	Baltimore	Described reconstruction of inguinal floor with transposition of the spermatic cord ("Halsted I Procedure")
1898	Georg Lothaissen [50]	Austria	Described Cooper's ligament repair
1942	Chester B. McVay [51,52]	South Dakota	Reintroduced and popularized Cooper's ligament repair ("McVay repair")
			Preperitoneal repair
1920	Sir George Lenthal Cheatle [53]	England	Introduced preperitoneal repair
1936	Arnold Kirkpatrick Henry [54]	Chicago	Rediscovered preperitoneal repair
1960s	Lloyd Nyhus [26,28]	Seattle, Chicago	Popularized iliopubic tract preperitoneal repair
1975	Rene E. Stoppa [29,55]	Dublin, Cairo	Reported "giant prosthetic repair"
			Contemporary repairs
1969	Edwin W. Shearburn and Richard N. Myers [56]	Canada	Described continuous, multilayer repair of inguinal floor ("Shouldice repair")
1970	Irving L. Lichtenstein [57]	Los Angeles	Popularized ambulatory hernia surgery
1989	Irving L. Lichtenstein [58]	Los Angeles	Introduced "tension-free" primary mesh repair

Table 3-2. History of laparoscopic inguinal herniorrhaphy

Year	Study	Contribution
1990	Ger and coworkers [4]	Reported laparoscopic closure of indirect hernia sac in dogs
1990	Schultz and coworkers [6]	Described "plug and patch" laparoscopic inguinal herniorrhaphy
1991	Spaw and coworkers [59]	Described detailed anatomy with respect to laparoscopic approach
1991	Toy and Smoot [12]	Described intra-abdominal onlay patch technique
1992	Gazayerli [14]	Described laparoscopic "anatomic repair" and patch technique
1992	Dion and Morin [15]	Described transabdominal preperitoneal patch (TAPP) technique
1992	McKernan [30,60,61]	Described totally preperitoneal patch (TOPP) technique
1993	MacFayden and coworkers [5]	First large review of complications and results
1995	Fitzgibbons and coworkers [21]	Multicenter trial comparing TAPP, TOPP, and onlay mesh techniques

Anatomy

Figures 3-1 and 3-2 depict the anatomy of the groin.

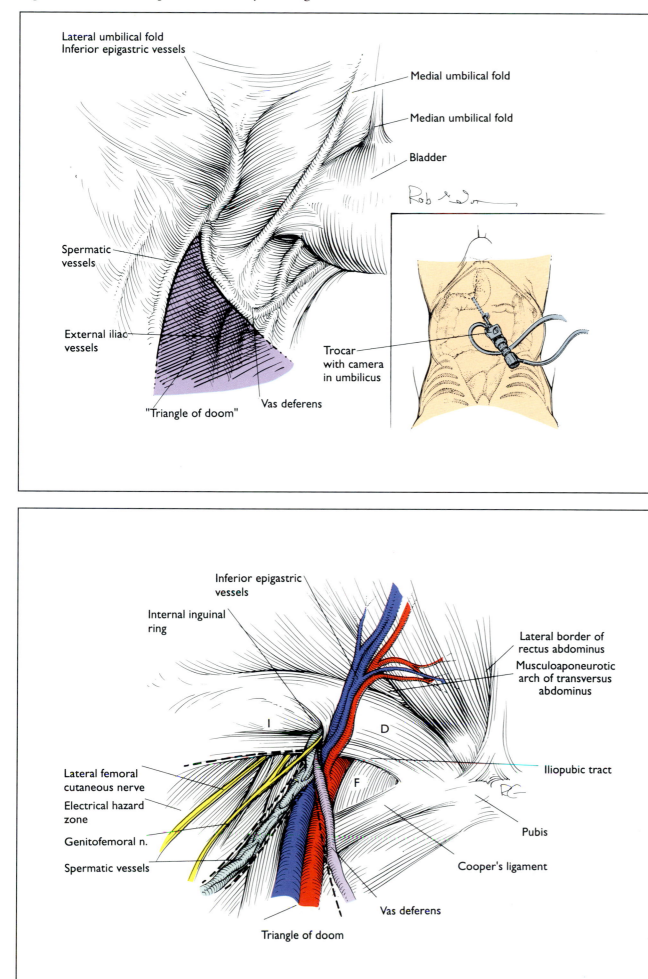

FIGURE 3-1.

Laparoscopic view of the left male groin with intact peritoneum. The laparoscope offers the surgeon a new perspective on the anatomy of the groin. On initial inspection of the left male groin with the peritoneum intact, the following landmarks are identified: 1) the bladder and median umbilical fold (urachus remnant) defining the midline; 2) the medial umbilical fold; 3) the lateral umbilical fold identifying the location of the inferior epigastric vessels; 4) the spermatic vessels; and 5) the vas deferens. The "triangle of doom" is bounded by the spermatic vessels and vas deferens and identifies the area under which lie the external iliac vessels and femoral nerve [3].

FIGURE 3-2.

Laparoscopic view of the left male groin with peritoneum removed. With the peritoneum removed, the topographical anatomy is more clearly apparent. The following structures are important: 1) Cooper's ligament, pubis, lateral border of rectus abdominis, and musculoaponeurotic arch of the transversus abdominis, the structures to which mesh is affixed during hernia repair; 2) the iliopubic tract, a thickening of the transversus abdominis aponeurosis that lies immediately posterior to the inguinal ligament; 3) the inferior epigastric vessels, the last branches of the external iliac artery and vein before its passing beneath the inguinal ligament; 4) the spermatic vessels and vas deferens; and 5) the "electrical hazard zone," which contains the lateral femoral cutaneous nerve and the genital and femoral branches of the genitofemoral nerve. The locations of the various hernia types can now be readily identified and include the indirect (I), direct (D), and femoral (F) variants.

Pathophysiology, Presentation, and Differential Diagnosis

Direct hernias appear to result from a primary defect in the inguinal floor; this is the deepest layer of abdominal fascia and is composed of the transversus abdominus aponeurosis and transversalis fascia. Most direct inguinal hernias are thought to develop through the aging process and to be aggravated by intermittent increases in intra-abdominal pressure, as occurs with coughing, constipation, prostatic hypertrophy, and obesity. Biochemical studies indicate that in adults, reduced collagen synthesis is a causal factor in the development of inguinal herniation [2].

Indirect inguinal hernias occur as a result of herniation through the internal ring through which the gonadal vessels and vas deferens course (or round ligament in females). After testicular descent during fetal development, the testes are normally covered by a rim of peritoneum (tunica albuginea) in continuity with the abdomen proper via the processus vaginalis. Normally, the processus vaginalis involutes separating the peritoneum from the scrotum. An indirect hernia will result if the processus vaginalis remains patent and, with increased intra-abdominal pressure, slips through the internal inguinal ring and enters the scrotum. Therefore, most indirect inguinal hernias are felt to be congenital in origin.

Femoral hernias arise from defects in the floor beneath the inguinal ligament alongside the femoral vessels and should therefore be classified separately from direct and indirect hernias. Their pathogenesis is probably similar to the direct variant and involves weakness of the reflected fibers of the iliopubic tract where the femoral vessels penetrate the fascia.

Inguinal hernias usually present as an intermittent or persistent bulge with or without localized pain. These complaints are often precipitated or exacerbated by standing or physical activity. The complete history should include a discussion of contributing factors such as chronic obstructive pulmonary disease, constipation or other forms of low-grade bowel obstruction, bladder outlet obstruction, and cirrhosis with ascites. Alleviation of these conditions will be important to ensure the durability of the repair.

Physical examination will usually reveal the diagnosis. The patient should be examined initially while standing and then supine. The groin is visually inspected for a mass. The testes and spermatic cord are inspected and palpated in order to reveal the presence of herniated viscera or tenderness. The inguinal floor is palpated during Valsalva in order to identify a direct component. Elicitation of pain on straining suggests the diagnosis but is not confirmatory. Many conditions cause pain or a mass in the groin and should be investigated if the symptoms or findings are atypical (Table 3-3). In selected cases, exploration may be performed in the absence of physical findings when the history is strongly suggestive.

Indications for Laparoscopic Repair

Several large studies have been conducted to compare the benefits of laparoscopic inguinal herniorrhaphy with those of conventional open inguinal herniorrhaphy. As a result, particular indications for each procedure have also been derived. Primarily on the basis of outcome and cost, the laparoscopic approach is best indicated for men with bilateral or recurrent inguinal hernias. For bilateral hernias, both sides can be repaired in a single operation, with no significant difference in postoperative pain or recovery time. The open approach may require two separate operations and is associated with prolonged recovery time. With recurrent hernias, the laparoscopic approach enters through a new plane away from most of the scarring of the previous repair. Laparoscopic hernia repair for unilateral primary hernia may be an acceptable or preferred repair in properly selected patients and in the hands of a surgeon experienced with these techniques.

Laparoscopic repair is relatively contraindicated for pediatric patients and high-risk patients who cannot tolerate general anesthesia. Previous prostate, bladder, or abdominal surgery is a relative contraindication; in these cases, the surgeon's experience plays a large role. With large scrotal hernias, managing the large sac may be difficult and the potential for hematoma formation in the remaining space is increased.

Surgical Technique

At least six conceptually different approaches to the laparoscopic repair of inguinal hernia have been reported. The initial method involved simple clip plication of the indirect hernia sac and internal ring. Results in an experimental model were first reported by Ger and colleagues [4] in 1990 and early clinical experience was described as part of a multi-institutional review in 1993 [5]. This technique did not include a floor repair and its application in adults has been limited.

The second approach, the "plug and patch" technique, was first described by Schultz and colleagues [6] in 1990 and subsequently by numerous other clinicians [7–10]. Although each author's method varies slightly, all include placement of one or more mesh plugs (usually polypropylene) directly into the hernia followed by coverage of the orifice with one or more mesh patches. Because of the fairly high early recurrence rate (approximately 7% after 8 months) [7], occasional plug migration, and plug-related pain, this technique has largely been abandoned.

The third method, first described by Toy and Smoot [11,12] in 1991, involves the intra-abdominal placement of an onlay polytetrafluoroethylene (PTFE) patch over the deep ring and inguinal floor without peritoneal dissection. This technique has

---

Table 3-3. Differential diagnosis of inguinal hernia

Hydrocele (communicating or noncommunicating)	Epididymitis
Varicocele	Epidermal cyst
Cord lipoma	Hidradenitis suppurativa
Musculoskeletal pain ("groin pull")	Perirectal abscess
Athletic pubalgia	Gastroenteritis
Urinary tract infection	Diverticulitis
Prostatitis	Intra-abdominal abscess
Femoral aneurysm or pseudoaneurysm	Colorectal carcinoma
Inguinal adenopathy	Tubal pregnancy
Hematoma/seroma from previous exploration	Pelvic inflammatory disease
Appendicitis	Psoas abscess
Testicular carcinoma	Rectus sheath hematoma
	Ovarian torsion
	Undescended testis
	Spermatocele

the advantage of simplicity and short operative time, but it is believed that its limited identification of detailed groin anatomy will lead to a high early recurrence rate and intraperitoneal mesh placement may cause adhesive complications [13]. Various modifications of this method are still in use.

The fourth method or "anatomic repair" consists of floor repair via laparoscopic suturing and reinforcement with mesh and was first described by Gazayerli [14] in 1992. Although theoretically attractive, the procedure is technically difficult and has not gained widespread acceptance.

The most widely used technique as of this writing is the laparoscopic TAPP placement of prosthetic mesh first described by Dion and Morin [16] in 1992 and preferred by numerous institutions including our own [5,16–21]. This procedure is the laparoscopic equivalent of the open anterior preperitoneal mesh repair described extensively by Nyhus [22–28]. The results with open preperitoneal mesh repair over the past two decades have been excellent, with recurrence rates in large series ranging from 1.4% to 1.7% [22,29]. Furthermore, these experiences have revealed that the often talked about risk of mesh infection or migration is rare (<1%). Thus, these studies appear to provide a precedent for the laparoscopic preperitoneal repair.

Finally, the sixth approach, the extraperitoneal or TEP placement of mesh, was first described by McKernan and Laws [30] in 1992 and, more recently, by other groups [31–33]. It is essentially identical to the TAPP procedure with the exception that the procedure is performed entirely in the preperitoneal space and has the theoretical advantage of not entering the peritoneum proper. Because these last two methods, the TAPP and TEP, have become the most routinely performed laparoscopic repairs, their detailed descriptions follow.

Figures 3-3 through 3-23 depict the surgical technique for inguinal herniorrhaphy.

Set-up

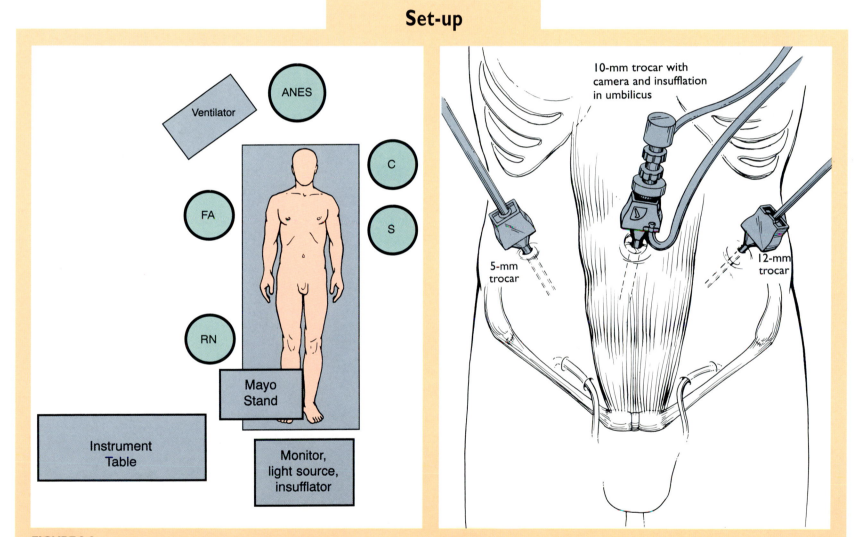

FIGURE 3-3.

Operative set-up for laparoscopic left inguinal herniorrhaphy. A single dose of antibiotic is administered before surgery. General anesthesia is preferred for comfort during pneumoperitoneum, although spinal anesthesia and an abdominal-wall lifting device (Laprolift; Origin Medsystems, Menlo Park, CA) can be used. Urinary and orogastric catheters are placed for decompression. The arms are tucked. Both the camera operator (C) and operating surgeon (S) stand on the hernia side while the optional first assistant (FA) stands on the contralateral side (the camera may also be operated by the FA if desirable). This sidedness is a matter of personal preference, however, and there is no need to switch positions to repair the second side of a bilateral hernia. Only one video monitor is required; it should be placed at the foot.

FIGURE 3-4.

Trocar and sheath placement for laparoscopic left inguinal herniorrhaphy. Three trocars are routinely used. The camera is placed via a 10-mm midline sheath at the umbilicus. A 12-mm trocar is placed on the hernia side and a 5-mm trocar on the contralateral side, both lateral to the rectus at the level of the umbilicus. Care is taken to avoid the epigastric vessels. The 5/12-mm trocar combination may be converted to 12/12 mm if bilateral herniorrhaphy is planned.

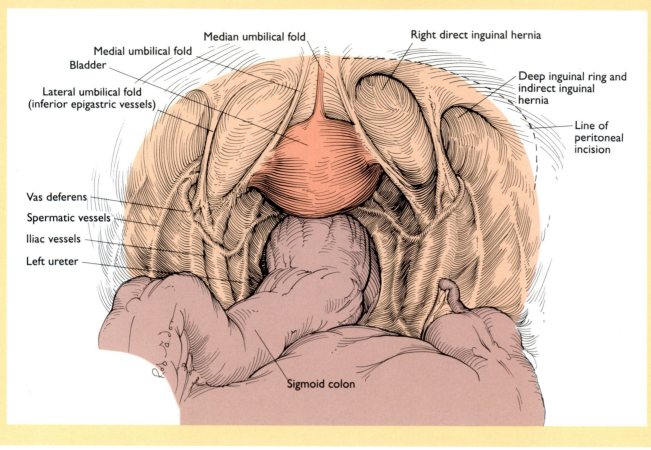

Median umbilical fold

Medial umbilical fold
Bladder

Lateral umbilical fold
(inferior epigastric vessels)

Right direct inguinal hernia

Deep inguinal ring and
indirect inguinal
hernia

Line of
peritoneal
incision

Vas deferens

Spermatic vessels

Iliac vessels

Left ureter

Sigmoid colon

FIGURE 3-5.
Initial view after laparoscopic insertion. The following structures should be identified: median and medial umbilical folds, bladder, lateral umbilical fold (overlying epigastric vessels), vas deferens, spermatic vessels, iliac vessels, and direct and indirect inguinal hernias. The *dashed line* represents the planned peritoneal incision.

Procedure

FIGURE 3-6.
Incision of peritoneum. The incision is begun at, but not medial to, the medial umbilical fold, and is extended laterally past the lateral umbilical fold on the arch of the transversus abdominis toward the anterior superior iliac spine.

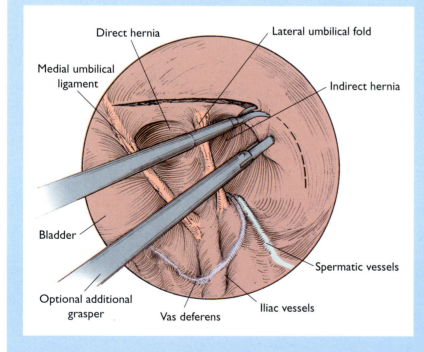

Direct hernia

Medial umbilical
ligament

Lateral umbilical fold

Indirect hernia

Bladder

Optional additional
grasper

Vas deferens

Iliac vessels

Spermatic vessels

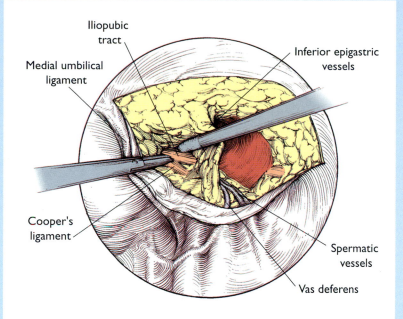

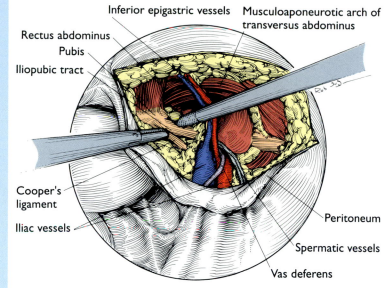

FIGURE 3-7.

Dissection of the inguinal floor. After peritoneal incision and reduction of the hernia sacs, further dissection is required to mobilize the peritoneal flap and identify the floor and relevant structures. Most, if not all, of this dissection should be performed bluntly. As in open herniorrhaphy, the cord should be skeletonized to completely identify and reduce any indirect component. Cooper's ligament should be cleaned of its overlying preperitoneal fat for complete identification. Laterally, the dissection is continued along the musculoaponeurotic arch of the transversus abdominis to the level of the anterior superior iliac spine. Occasionally, the dissection of the hernia sacs and related structures may be facilitated by external manipulation.

FIGURE 3-8.

Completed dissection of the inguinal floor before mesh insertion. Note that the complete dissection of pubis and Cooper's ligament as well as musculoaponeurotic arch of transversus abdominis a full 2 cm above and lateral to the internal inguinal ring.

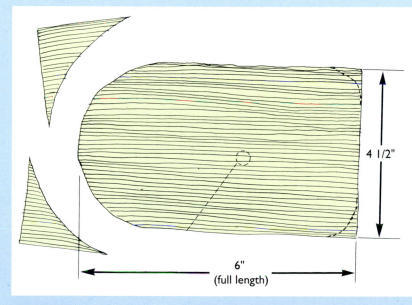

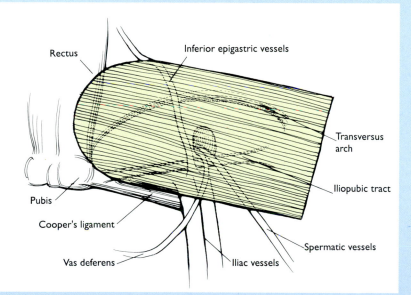

FIGURE 3-9.

Preparation of mesh. A 4½ × 6 inch polypropylene mesh is delivered to the field and modified as shown. The only required modification is rounding of the medial corners to facilitate positioning. Rounding of the lateral corners and creation of a "buttonhole" for the cord structures are optional modifications (*dashed lines*).

Procedure

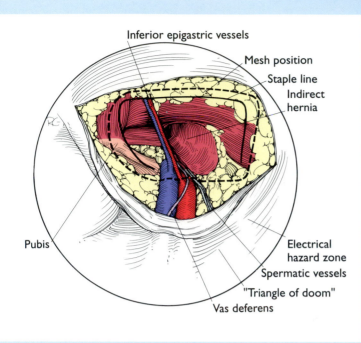

FIGURE 3-10.

Planned location of mesh and staple line on the right side. The mesh will cover the defects of any direct, indirect, and femoral hernias. The staple line courses clockwise from the 7 o'clock to the 4 o'clock position on the mesh. Leaving the inferolateral portion of the mesh unstapled avoids injury to the "triangle of doom" and electrical hazard zone.

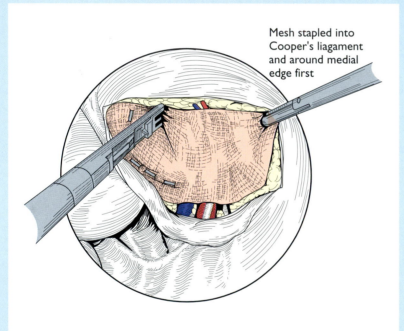

FIGURE 3-11.

Fixation of mesh to the right inguinal floor. The mesh is rolled from squared edge to rounded edge, delivered through the 12-mm sheath, placed near Cooper's ligament, and unrolled laterally. Stapling is begun medially by using an endoscopic stapling device (Multifire Endohernia Stapler; Autosuture, Norwalk, CT). The usual progression of stapling is clockwise: Cooper's ligament, pubis, lateral edge of rectus, medial musculoaponeurotic arch, and lateral musculoaponeurotic arch. As the mesh covers the epigastric vessels, care must be exercised to avoid their injury during stapling.

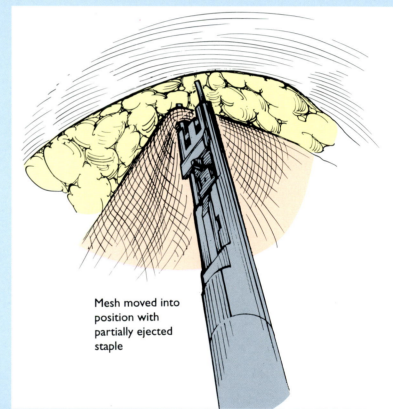

FIGURE 3-12.

Endoscopic stapling. Stapling of the mesh is facilitated by hooking the mesh with one spike of a partially delivered staple, delivering the mesh to the desired location, applying adequate pressure, and firing.

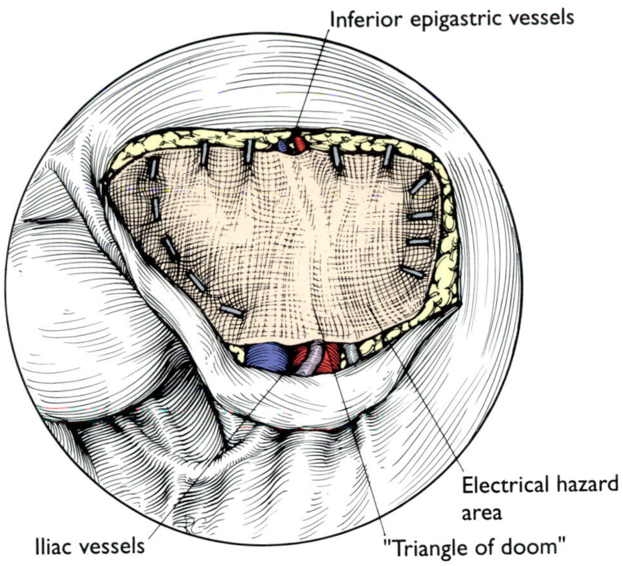

Procedure

FIGURE 3-13.

Completed right inguinal hernia repair. Note the absence of staples inferolaterally in the area of the "triangle of doom" and electrical hazard zone.

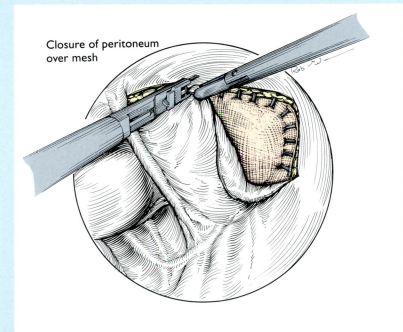

FIGURE 3-14.

Closure of the peritoneal flap. After irrigation and checks for hemostasis, the peritoneum is closed over the mesh with staples. Approximately eight staples are required. For bilateral repairs, closure is obviously deferred until completion of both repairs.

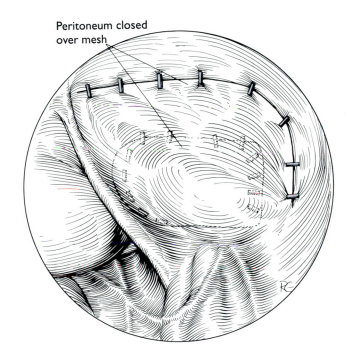

FIGURE 3-15.

Completed peritoneal flap closure.

Alternative Procedure

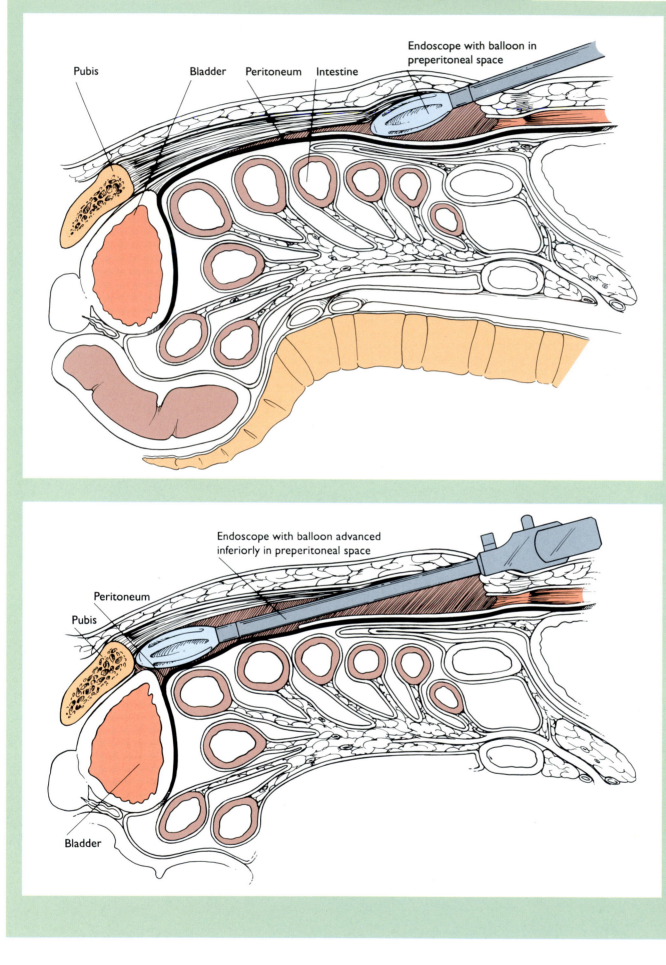

Pubis   Bladder   Peritoneum   Intestine   Endoscope with balloon in preperitoneal space

Endoscope with balloon advanced inferiorly in preperitoneal space

Peritoneum

Pubis

Bladder

FIGURE 3-16.

Alternative technique: the totally extraperitoned placement (TEP) repair. Some surgeons have advocated that laparoscopic inguinal herniorrhaphy be performed entirely within the preperitoneal space without entrance into the peritoneum. A specially designed laparoscope–cannula system with a blunt tip and inflatable balloon device (Origin Medsystems, Inc., Menlo Park, CA; and General Surgical Innovations, Portola Valley, CA) is inserted preperitoneally in the midline at the umbilicus as seen in this sagittal section.

FIGURE 3-17.

Advancement of the blunt tip to the pubis. The blunt-tip trocar is advanced in the preperitoneal space to the level of the pubis.

Alternative Procedure

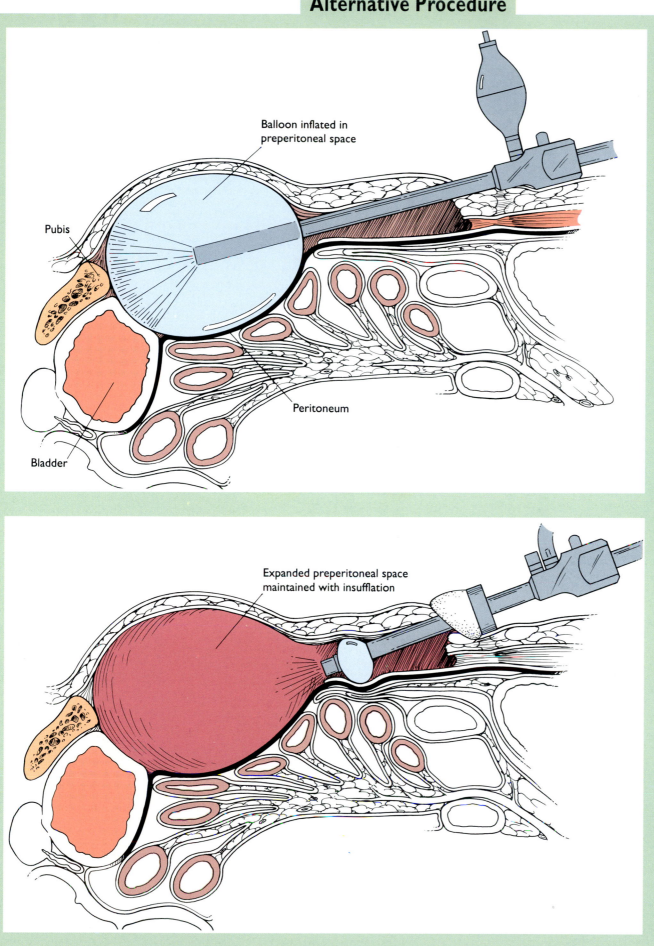

Balloon inflated in preperitoneal space

Pubis

Peritoneum

Bladder

Expanded preperitoneal space maintained with insufflation

FIGURE 3-18.
Inflation of the preperitoneal balloon. Under laparoscopic visualization, the balloon is insufflated with air, creating an operative field from the potential preperitoneal space.

FIGURE 3-19.
The preperitoneal operative field. Deflation of the balloon and exchange of trocars leave an operative field for herniorrhaphy.

Alternative Procedure

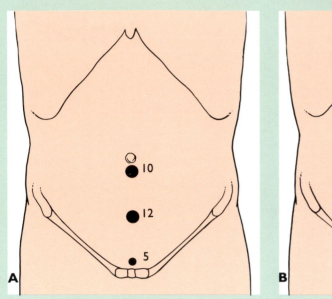

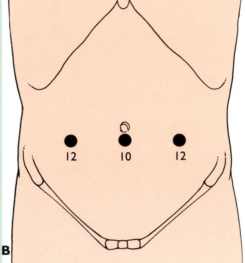

FIGURE 3-20.

Trocar placement. **A** and **B**, The remaining trocars can be placed in two configurations as shown. The authors prefer configuration B, if possible, although this can be accomplished only with favorable anatomy and the creation of a large preperitoneal operative field.

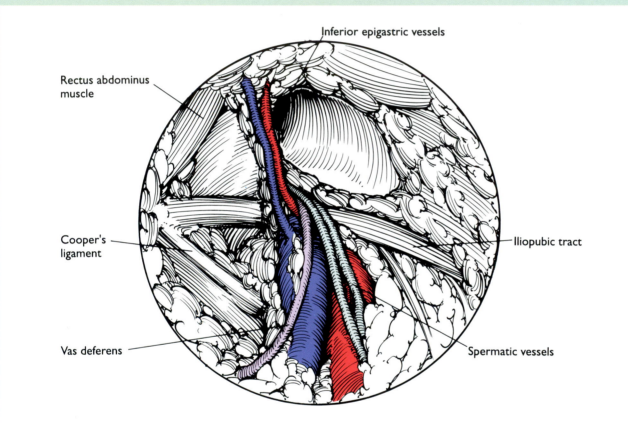

Inferior epigastric vessels

Rectus abdominus muscle

Cooper's ligament

Vas deferens

Iliopubic tract

Spermatic vessels

FIGURE 3-21.

The operative field. After additional trocar placement and blunt dissection, the operative field should be identical to that seen with transabdominal approach.

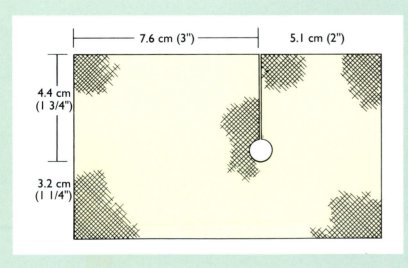

FIGURE 3-22.

Preparation of the mesh. The mesh is delivered to the field and prepared as shown. For this approach, it is helpful to create a buttonhole for the spermatic cord to traverse because there is limited operative space inferiorly. Frequently, a 6 × 6 inch piece of mesh is used and fashioned in a similar manner.

Alternative Procedure

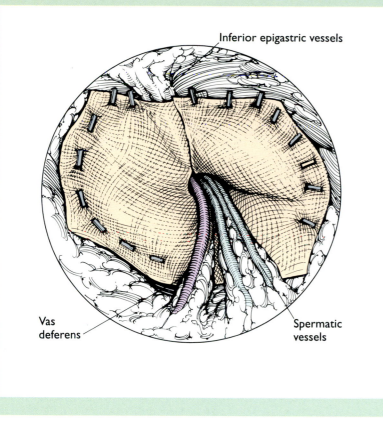

Inferior epigastric vessels

Vas deferens

Spermatic vessels

FIGURE 3-23.

Completed repair. The position of the mesh is identical to that used for the transabdominal preperitoneal placement (TAPP) approach.

Results

Laparoscopic inguinal herniorrhaphy is routinely performed on an outpatient basis. As indicated earlier, many studies have compared conventional open hernia repair with TAAP or TEP laparoscopic methods. In a randomized multicenter trial, Liem and coworkers [34] studied 507 patients treated by open repair and 487 patients treated by extraperitoneal laparoscopic repair between 1994 and 1995. Median duration of follow-up was 607 days. Patients in the laparoscopic group had significantly faster resumption of normal activities and return to work (6 compared with 10 days and 14 compared with 21 days; $P< 0.001$ for both comparisons). The recurrence rate was 6% in the open group and 3% in the laparoscopic group ($P= 0.05$).

Liebl and coworkers reported on 2700 TAPP procedures performed between 1993 and 1997 [35]. Seventeen percent of these were for recurrent inguinal hernias. Follow-up time was 20 months. The recurrence rate for this procedure was 1.03% with the most common cause in 39.3% attributed to the mesh being too small. The initial recurrence rate using a 12×8 cm mesh was 3.8% and decreased to 0.2% after using a 15×10 cm mesh size.

The second most common cause of recurrence in this series was an insufficient overlapping of the incised mesh for reconstructing a new deep inguinal ring. This problem can essentially be eliminated by implanting a nonincised mesh and performing adequate peritoneal mobilization. The most common site of recurrence was the medial compartment of Hesselbach's triangle. The overall reported complication rate was 4.6%.

Sayad and coworkers [36] reviewed all major articles on laparoscopic inguinal herniorrhaphy published from 1993 to 1996; these articles reported on a total of 11,222 hernia repairs. The most frequently performed procedure was the TAPP procedure, followed by the TEP procedure. The overall recurrence rate was 2.7%. A total of 1534 complications were reported: The most frequent were hematoma/seroma (456 cases), neuralgia (199 cases), urinary retention (150 cases), and chronic pain (39 cases).

Another advantage of the laparoscopic approach is the potential for identification of a contralateral inguinal hernia that can be repaired during the same operation. In conclusion, laparoscopic inguinal herniorrhaphy is a safe and effective procedure. The primary indications include bilateral and recurrent inguinal hernias.

References

1. Rutkow IM, Robbins AW: Demographic, classificatory, and socioeconomic aspects of hernia repairs in the United States. *Surg Clin North Am* 1993, 73:413N426.

2. Wagh PV, Read RC: Defective collagen synthesis in inguinal herniation. *Am J Surg* 1972, 124:819.

3. Pott PA, ed.: *A Treatise on Ruptures.* London: C. Hitch and L. Hawes; 1756.

4. Ger R, Monroe K, Duvivier R, Mishrick A: Management of indirect inguinal hernias by laparoscopic closure of the neck of the sac. *Am J Surg* 1990, 159:370–373.

5. MacFayden BV Jr, Arregui ME, Corbitt JD Jr, *et al.*: Complications of laparoscopic herniorrhaphy. *Surg Endosc* 1993, 7:155–158.

6. Schultz L, Graber J, Pietrafitta J, Hickok D: Laser laparoscopic herniorrhaphy: a clinical trial preliminary results. *J Laparoendosc Surg* 1990, 1:41–45.

7. Hawasli A: Laparoscopic inguinal herniorrhaphy: classification and 1 year experience. *J Laparoendosc Surg* 1992, 2:137–143.

8. Nolen M, Melichar R, Jennings WC, McGee JM: Use of a Marlex fan in the repair of direct and indirect hernias by laparoscopy. *J Laparoendosc Surg* 1992, 2:61–64.

9. Hawasli A: Laparoscopic inguinal herniorrhaphy: the mushroom plug repair. *Surg Laparosc Endosc* 1992, 2:111–116.

10. Seid AS, Deutsch H, Jacobson A: Laparoscopic herniorrhaphy. *Surg Laparosc Endosc* 1992, 2:59–60.

11. Toy FK, Smoot RT Jr: Laparoscopic hernioplasty update. *J Laparoendosc Surg* 1992, 2:197–205.

12. Toy FK, Smoot RT Jr: Toy-Smoot laparoscopic hernioplasty. *Surg Laparosc Endosc* 1991, 1:151–155.

13. Fitzgibbons RJ Jr, Salerno GM, Filipi CJ, *et al.*: A laparoscopic intraperitoneal onlay mesh technique for the repair of an indirect inguinal hernia. *Ann Surg* 1994, 219:144–156.

14. Gazayerli MM: Anatomical laparoscopic hernia repair of direct or indirect inguinal hernias using the transversalis fascia and iliopubic tract. *Surg Laparosc Endosc* 1992, 2:49–52.

15. Dion YM, Morin J: Laparoscopic inguinal herniorrhaphy. *Can J Surg* 1992; 35:209–212.

16. Winchester DJ, Dawes LG, Modelski DD, *et al.*: Laparoscopic inguinal hernia repair. A preliminary experience. *Arch Surg* 1993, 128:781–784.

17. Stoker DL, Spiegelhalter DJ, Singh R, Wellwood JM: Laparoscopic versus open inguinal hernia repair: randomized prospective trial. *Lancet* 1994, 343:1243–1245.

18. Soper NJ, Brunt LM, Kerbl K: Laparoscopic general surgery. *N Engl J Med* 1994, 330:409–419.

19. Dion YM: Laparoscopic inguinal herniorrhaphy: an individualized approach. *Surg Laparosc Endosc* 1993, 3:451–455.

20. Corbitt JD Jr: Transabdominal preperitoneal herniorrhaphy. *Surg Laparosc Endosc* 1993, 3:328–332.

21. Fitzgibbons RJ, Camps J, Coronet DA, *et al.*: Laparoscopic inguinal herniorrhaphy: results of a multicenter trial. *Ann Surg* 1995, 221:3–13.

22. Nyhus LM, Pollak R, Bombeck CT, Donahue PE: The preperitoneal approach and prosthetic buttress repair for recurrent hernia: the evolution of a technique. *Ann Surg* 1988, 208:733–737.

23. Nyhus LM, Klein MS, Rogers FB: Inguinal hernia. *Curr Probl Surg* 1991, 28:401–450.

24. Nyhus LM: Iliopubic tract repair of inguinal and femoral hernia: the posterior (preperitoneal) approach. *Surg Clin North Am* 1993, 73:487–499.

25. Nyhus LM, Klein MS, Rogers FB, Kowalczyk S: Inguinal hernia repairs: types, patient care. *Association of Operating Room Nurses Journal* 1990, 52:292–304.

26. Nyhus LM, Couden RE, Harkins HN: Clinical experiences with preperitoneal hernial repair for all types of hernia of the groin. *Am J Surg* 1960, 100:234.

27. Nyhus LM: The recurrent groin hernia: therapeutic solutions. *World J Surg* 1989, 13:541–544.

28. Nyhus LM: An anatomical reappraisal of the posterior inguinal wall: special consideration of the iliopubic tract and its relation to groin hernia. *Surg Clin North Am* 1964, 44:1305–1312.

29. Stoppa RE, Warlaumont CR: The preperitoneal approach and prosthetic repair of groin hernia. In *Hernia*, 3rd ed. Edited by Nyhus LM, Condon RE. Philadelphia: J.B. Lippincott; 1989:199.

30. McKernan JB, Laws HL: Laparoscopic preperitoneal prosthetic repair of inguinal hernias. *Surg Rounds* 1992, July:597–607.

31. Fromont G, Leroy J: Laparoskopischer Leistenhernienerschluss durch subperitoneale Protheseneinlage (Operation nach Stoppa) [in German]. (Laparoscopic repair of inguinal hernia by subperitoneal prosthesis implantation [Stoppa operation]). *Chirurg* 1993, 64:338–340.

32. Ferzli GS, Massad A, Albert P: Extraperitoneal endoscopic inguinal hernia repair. *J Laparoendosc Surg* 1992, 2:281–286.

33. Voeller GR, Mangiante EC Jr, Wilson C: Totally preperitoneal laparoscopic inguinal herniorrhaphy using balloon dissection. *Surg Rounds* 1995, March:107–112.

34. Liem MS, van der Graaf y, van Steensel CJ, *et al.*: Comparison of conventional anterior surgery and laparoscopic surgery for inguinal-hernia repair. *N Engl J Med* 1997, 336:1541–1547.

35. Liebl BJ, Schmedt CJ, Schwartz J, *et al.*: A single institution's experience with transperitoneal laparoscopic hernia repair. *Am J Surg* 1998, 175:446–452.

36. Sayad P, Hallak A, Ferzli G: Laparoscopic herniorrhaphy: review of complications and recurrence. *J Laparoendosc Adv Surg Tech* 1998, 8:3–10.

37. Franco P, ed.: *Petit Traitée Contenant une des Parties Principalles de Chirurgie, Laquelle les Chirurgiens Herniéeres Excercent* [in French]. Lyon: Antoine Vincent; 1556.

38. Richter AG, ed.: *Abhandlung von den Brüuchen* [in German]. Göttingen: J.C. Dieterich; 1778.

39. Gimbernat A, ed.: *Nuevo Méetodo de Operar en la Hernia Crural* [in Spanish]. Madrid: vda. Ibarra; 1793.

40. Cooper AP, ed.: *The Anatomy and Surgical Treatment of Inguinal and Congenital Hernia.* London: Cox; 1804.

41. Cooper AP, ed.: *The Anatomy and Surgical Treatment of Crural and Umbilical Hernia.* London: Longman; 1807.

42. Hesselbach FK, ed.: *Nueste anatomisch-pathologische Untersuchungen über den Ursprung und das Fortschreiten der Leisten-und Schenkel-br\üche* [in German]. Würzburg:Baumgärtner; 1814.

43. Hesselbach FK, ed.: *Anatomisch-Chirurgische Abhandlung über den Ursprung der Leistenbrüche* [in German]. Würzburg: Baumgärtner; 1806.

44. Scarpa A, ed.: *Sull'ernia del revineo.* Pavia: P. Bizzoni; 1821.

45. Scarpa A: *A Treatise on Hernia.* Translated by John Henry Wishart. Edinburgh: Longman, Hurst, Rees *et al*; 1814.

46. Marcy HO: A new use of carbolized catgut ligatures. *Boston Med Surg J* 1871, 85:315.

47. Marcy HO: The radical cure of hernia by the antiseptic use of the carbolized catgut ligature. *Trans Am Med Assoc* 1878, 29:295–305.

48. Bassini E: Nuovo metodo per la cura radicale dell'ernia. *Atti Cong Assoc Med Ital* 1889, 2:179.

49. Halsted WS: The radical cure of hernia. *Bull Johns Hopkins Hosp* 1889, 1:12.

50. Lothaissen G. Zur radikaloperation der schenkelhernien. *Zentralbl Chir* 1898, 25:548.

51. Anson BJ, McVay CB: The anatomy of the inguinal and hypogastric regions of the abdominal wall. *Anat Rec* 1938, 70:211–225.

52. McVay CB: Inguinal and femoral hernioplasty: anatomic repair. *Arch Surg* 1948, 57:524–530.

53. Cheatle GI: An operation for the radical cure of inguinal and femoral hernia. *BMJ* 1920, 2:68–69.

54. Henry AK: Operation for femoral hernia by a midline extraperitoneal approach; with a preliminary note on the use of this route for reducible inguinal hernia. *Lancet* 1936, 1:531–533.

55. Stoppa R, Petit J, Henry X: Unsutured Dacron prosthesis in groin hernias. *Int Surg* 1975, 60:411–412.

56. Shearburn EW, Myers RN: Shouldice repair for inguinal hernia. *Surgery* 1969, 66:450–459.

57. Lichtenstein IL, ed.: *Hernia Repair Without Disability.* St. Louis: C.V. Mosby; 1970.

58. Lichtenstein IL, Shulman AG, Amid PK, Montllor MM: The tension-free hernioplasty. *Am J Surg* 1989, 157:188–193.

59. Spaw AT, Ennis BW, Spaw LP: Laparoscopic hernia repair: the anatomic basis. *J Laparoendosc Surg* 1991, 1:269–277.

60. McKernan JB: Laparoscopic extraperitoneal repair of inguinofemoral herniation. *Endosc Surg Allied Technol* 1993, 1:198–203.

61. McKernan JB: Laparoscopic extraperitoneal inguinal hernia repair. *Curr Tech Gen Surg* 1994, 3:1–7.

Laparoscopic Ventral Herniorrhaphy

Paul J. Chai
Edward G. Chekan

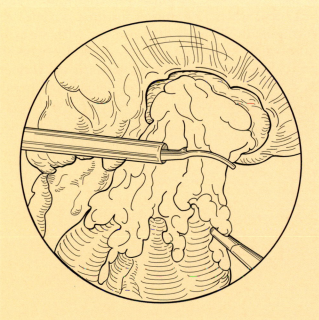

$\mathcal{V}$entral hernia is defined as any defect through the anterior abdominal wall. The three main types of ventral hernias are diastases recti, epigastric hernias, and incisional hernias. Diastasis recti is an innocuous condition caused by the spreading apart of the medial borders of the rectus muscle over time, with a diffuse bulge of the thinned-out linea alba in between. This type of hernia is usually asymptomatic and does not require surgical repair. Epigastric hernias are usually associated with obesity or pregnancy but can occur spontaneously. They are typically small defects in the fascia that frequently contain a small amount of incarcerated adipose tissue with resulting pain. Incisional hernias result from the failure of laparotomy closure; their reported incidence is 5% to 11% [1,2]. Patients with obesity, wound infection, malnutrition, or long-term steroid use have an increased incidence of incisional hernias.

Anatomy

The abdominal wall is composed of nine layers: skin, subcutaneous tissue, Scarpa's fascia, external oblique muscle, internal oblique muscle, transversus abdominus muscle, transversalis fascia, extraperitoneal adipose tissue, and peritoneum. The linea alba, which is an aponeurosis of all abdominal-wall muscle groups, defines the abdominal midline. The superior portion of the abdomen contains a strong posterior rectus sheath composed of internal oblique muscle fascia, transversus abdominus muscle fascia, and transversalis fascia; it also contains an anterior rectus sheath composed of both external and internal oblique aponeurosis. The inferior portion of the abdomen lacks this strong posterior rectus sheath. In the inferior portion, the fascia of the external and internal oblique muscles lie anterior to the rectus muscle and the posterior sheath consists of a thin layer of transversalis fascia.

Pathophysiology

The incidence of primary wound dehiscence can increase because of wound infection, patient obesity, poor nutrition, or medical therapy (eg, long-term steroid use) that impair wound healing. In a retrospective literature review of more than 320,000 cases reported during a 34-year period, Poole [3] found that mechanical factors such as wound infection, abdominal distention, and coughing appeared more responsible for wound disruption than systemic factors, such as malnutrition or long-term steroid treatment [3].

Wound infection is the most common causative factor in the development of incisional hernias. Infection interferes with the normal healing process, resulting in less collagen formation and collagen cross-linking in the wound. Antibiotic prophylaxis as well as meticulous surgical technique (eg, gentle handling, hemostasis) can help reduce the incidence of postoperative wound infection.

The importance of the technique used for abdominal closure (continuous vs. interrupted) as a risk factor for ventral hernia formation has long been debated. In a randomized study of 571 patients, Richards and Balch [4] compared both methods and found no significant difference in the rate of ventral hernia.

Presentation

Patients typically present with a painless mass at a previous laparotomy site. The mass often bulges with increased abdominal pressure (caused by coughing or the Valsalva maneuver) and should be reducible with gentle pressure. Computed tomography is sometimes necessary for diagnosis in severely obese patients or in patients with vague abdominal symptoms.

Patients who present with a symptomatic mass (ie, pain or signs of obstruction) may have an incarcerated or strangulated hernia. Most patients who present with incarceration are aware of their hernias as previously reducible ones. Strangulated hernias occur when a portion of intestine becomes ischemic from entrapment. Patients may present with signs of intestinal ischemia or obstruction (nausea, vomiting, or severe abdominal pain). The overlying area may be associated with erythema and tenderness. An incarcerated or strangulated hernia should be repaired immediately.

Surgical Technique

Figures 4-1 through 4-5 depict the surgical technique for laparoscopic ventral herniorrhaphy. Laparoscopic ventral hernia repair is best performed with the patient under general anesthesia. The bladder is decompressed with a Foley catheter, and the stomach is decompressed with a nasogastric tube. The patient is placed in the supine position (Fig. 4-1), and a Hasson trocar is placed via the open technique in the lower midline. The abdomen is then insufflated with CO_2 gas and the 30° laparoscope is placed into the abdomen. The abdominal cavity is then explored, with notation made of the hernia defect, severity of abdominal adhesions, and potential sites for additional trocar placement. Additional trocars are then placed under direct vision as far laterally as possible—usually one 11-mm trocar in the left lower quadrant and two 5-mm trocars on the right side. Abdominal-wall adhesions are taken down with endograspers and endoshears (Fig. 4-2), and the visceral contents are reduced from the hernia sac. The hernia sac is kept intact if possible.

The mesh is sized extracorporally over the hernia defect. The mesh should be sized to circumferentially cover the hernia defect by at least 2 to 3 cm. Drawing an outline of the hernia defect on the abdomen may help with mesh sizing. Orientation of the patch should be clearly marked before it is introduced into the abdominal cavity. The mesh can be introduced via the 11-mm trocar and then spread out in the peritoneal cavity.

If polypropylene mesh is chosen for the repair, the mesh can be secured over the hernia defect to the anterior abdominal wall (Fig. 4-3) by using only a laparoscopic stapling device, such as the Endotacker device (US Surgical Corp., Norwalk, CT). Care should be taken to position omentum between bowel and mesh after completion of the repair (Fig. 4-4).

If expanded polytetrafluoroethylene mesh (Gore-Tex) is chosen for the repair, staple fixation should be accompanied by transfascial suturing because of the slower tissue in-growth with this material. The patch is first secured in all four corners by using transabdominal suture fixation. Nonabsorbable suture is placed at the corners of the mesh before introduction into the peritoneal cavity. Small skin incisions (about 2 mm long) are made with an 11-blade scalpel, through which an endoscopic suture passer is inserted through the abdominal wall. The corner sutures are then grasped with the suture passer, pulled through the abdominal wall, and tied (Fig. 4-5). Several additional sutures can be placed evenly around the periphery of the mesh, and endoscopic staples are used to further secure the edges of the mesh in between the sutures.

After completion of the repair, trocars are removed and the pneumoperitoneum is evacuated. Trocar sites 10 mm or larger require fascial closure. The skin incisions are approximated byusing sutures and Steri-Strips, and a sterile dressing is applied.

Set-up

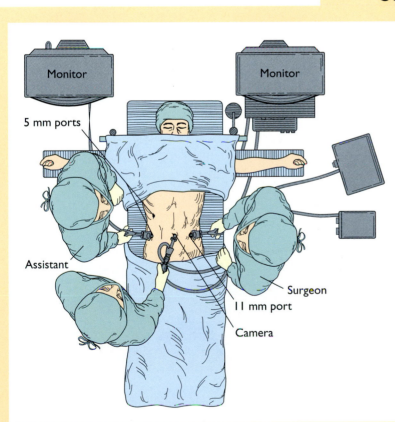

FIGURE 4-1.

Set-up for laparoscopic ventral herniorrhaphy.

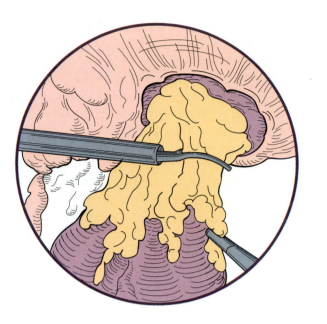

FIGURE 4-2.

Adhesions are taken down using the endoshears, with countertraction provided the nondominant hand using an endograsper. Electrocautery should be used as sparingly as possible.

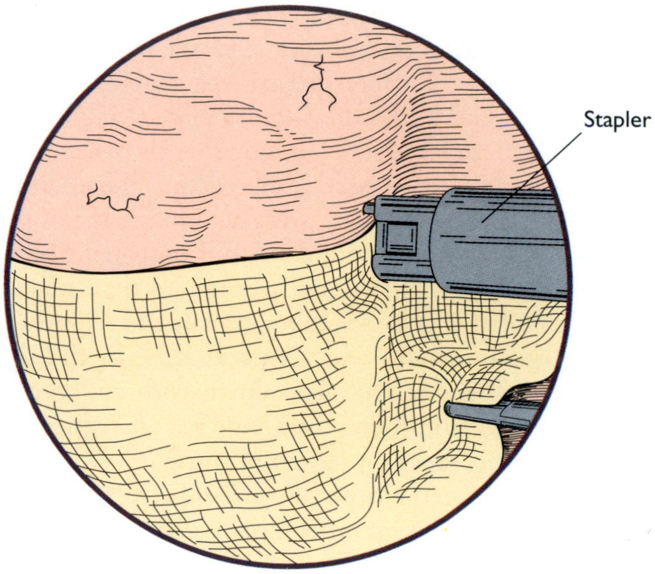

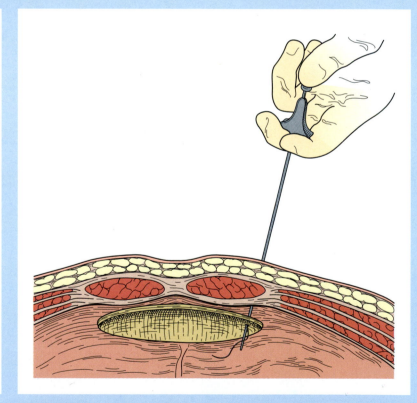

Stapler

FIGURE 4-3.

A laparoscopic stapling device is used to secure the mesh over the hernia defect to the anterior abdominal wall.

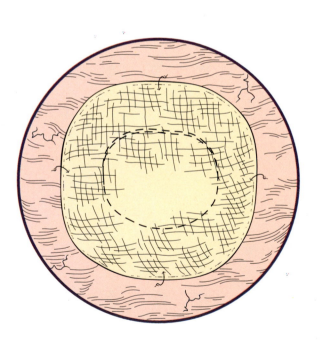

FIGURE 4-4.

Completed ventral herniorrhaphy.

FIGURE 4-5.

For hernia repair with Goretex mesh (W.L. Gore, Phoenix, AZ), corner sutures are grasped with an Endoclose (US Surgical Corp., Norwalk, CT), pulled through the abdominal wall, and tied.

Results

Long-term results for laparoscopic ventral hernia repair are not yet available. Short-term results, however, are very favorable in all published series. The mean follow-up period is 7 months for all reported cases, with a recurrence rate of approximately 3% [5–8]. Complications with laparoscopic repair are similar to those seen with the open approach— wound infection and seroma formation—with trends favoring the laparoscopic approach; incidence rates of 3% and 6%, respectively, have been reported [5]. The incidence of these complications is best minimized by not excising the hernia sac. Inadvertent bowel injury during takedown of adhesions or as a result of thermal injury from electrocautery has also been reported [6]. Use of electrocautery should therefore be minimized during dissection and lysis of adhesions.

In a retrospective study by Holzman and coworkers [6], laparoscopy demonstrated a trend toward shorter hospital stays and lower hospital costs , with no statistically significant difference in length of operation, compared with open repair. Laparoscopic repair of ventral hernias is clearly feasible, with results similar to those obtained with an open technique. Although long-term follow-up remains to be documented, shorter hospital stays and increased patient satisfaction should continue to make laparoscopic repair of ventral hernias an attractive option.

References

1. Mudge M, Heghes L: Incisional hernia: a 10 year prospective study of incidence and attitudes. *Br J Surg* 1985, 72:70–71.
2. Condon R: *Incisional Hernia*. Philadelphia: JB Lippincott; 1995.
3. Poole G: Mechanical factors in abdominal wound closure: the prevention of fascial dehiscence. *Surgery* 1985, 97:631–640.
4. Richards P, Balch C: Abdominal wound closure: a randomized prospective study of 571 patients comparing continuous versus interrupted suture techniques. *Ann Surg* 1983, 197:238–243.
5. Toy F, Bailey R, Carey S, *et al.*: Prospective multicenter study of laparoscopic ventral hernioplasty. *Surg Endosc* 1998, 12:955–959.
6. Holzman M, Purut C, Reintgen K, *et al.*: Laparoscopic ventral and incisional hernioplasty. *Surg Endosc* 1997, 11:32–35.
7. Park A, Gagner M, Pomp A: Laparoscopic repair of large incisional hernias. *Surg Laparosc Endosc* 1996, 6:132–138.
8. Saiz A, Paul D, Willis I, *et al.*: The use of T-bars in laparoscopic ventral hernia repair. *J Laparoendosc Surg* 1996, 6:109–112.

Laparoscopic Antireflux Procedures

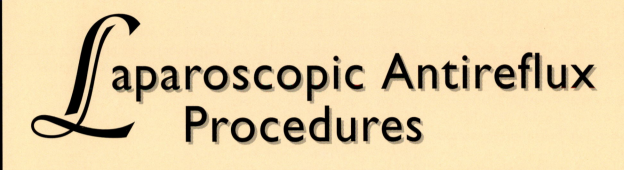

B. Zane Atkins
Theodore N. Pappas

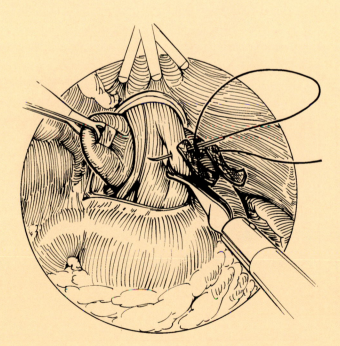

The term gastroesophageal reflux disease (GERD) has been introduced to represent a wide spectrum of damage to the oropharynx, larynx, respiratory tissue, and esophagus that is clinically recognized by heartburn.

In 1951, Allison [1] coined the term *reflux esophagitis* and described the relationship between hiatal hernia and reflux esophagitis. In 1956, Rudolph Nissen introduced fundoplication as a simple operative correction of reflux esophagitis [2]. The operation was performed over a large esophageal bougie through a left subcostal incision or a lower left thoracotomy (Figures 5-1 through 5-3.) Nissen's technique involved mobilization of the abdominal segment of the esophagus and the lesser curvature of the stomach by division of the gastrohepatic ligament. Coincident with Nissen's description, the Belsey Mark IV gastropexy was described (Figures 5-4 through 5-6). The Belsey Mark IV repair is performed through a left sixth interspace thoracotomy to create a 240° fundic wrap [3]. In 1963, Toupet [4] modified the Nissen fundoplication to create a posterior 270° fundic wrap (Figure 5-7).

In 1991, Geagea [5] completed the first Nissen fundoplication using exclusively laparoscopic techniques in a 43-year-old woman with severe reflux esophagitis. This procedure demonstrated the ability to fashion the 360° fundus wrap by use of laparoscopic methods. Soon after, Dallemagne and coworkers [6] reported the first series of 12 patients undergoing laparoscopic fundoplication. Although three patients required conversion to open laparotomy because of complications encountered during the laparoscopic procedure, the remaining nine patients were successfully managed by laparoscopic Nissen fundoplication and reported complete symptom relief after surgery. This report was succeeded by that of Bittner and coworkers [7], who obtained relief of reflux symptoms in 96% of 35 patients with GERD symptoms by use of laparoscopic Nissen fundoplication.

In 1993, Cuschieri and coworkers [8] described the successful completion of a partial fundoplication similar to the open Toupet procedure with its 270° posterior fundus wrap by laparoscopic methods. Partial fundoplications have since been favored in patients with GERD who also have evidence of decreased esophageal motility [9].

Laparoscopic fundoplication is now an established alternative for patients with GERD. The laparoscopic technique avoids many of the disadvantages of the traditional approach, such as a large abdominal incision, associated postoperative discomfort, and prolonged recovery periods.

Anatomy

The esophagus comprises the cervical, thoracic, and abdominal segments. The cervical esophagus originates at the caudal border of the cricoid cartilage and the lower margin of the cricopharyngeus muscle at the level of the sixth cervical vertebral body. The esophagus extends caudally through the superior and posterior mediastina of the thorax. It passes through the esophageal hiatus of the diaphragm to join the cardia of the stomach at the level of the tenth thoracic vertebra. The accompanying structures on its course through the hiatus are the anterior and posterior vagal

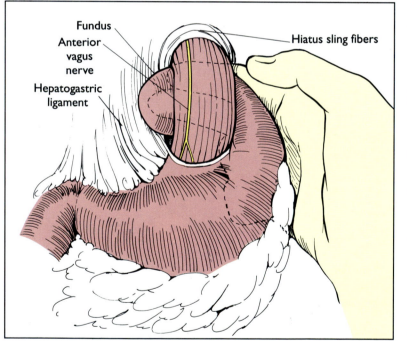

FIGURE 5-1.

Technique of Nissen fundoplication. Through a left subcostal laparotomy or a lower thoracotomy, the lower esophagus and upper portion of the stomach have been mobilized. The anterior fundic wall is brought around the esophagus. The short gastric vessels are not routinely divided.

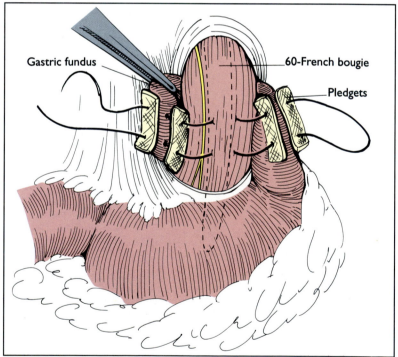

FIGURE 5-2.

Construction of the Nissen fundoplication. A 60-French bougie is passed across the gastroesophageal junction. Seromuscular heavy nonabsorbable sutures are used to approximate the adjacent layers of gastric fundus and incorporating the anterior wall of the esophagus. Pledgets at each tissue interface, buttressed with a horizontal mattress suture, hold the wrap. Interrupted sutures can also be used for the construction.

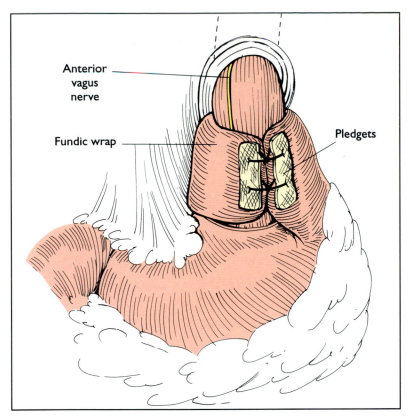

FIGURE 5-3.

Completed 360° Nissen fundoplication. Fundoplication should be 2 cm long and loose enough that one finger can easily be inserted between the plication and the esophagus with a bougie in place ("floppy Nissen"). Anterior and posterior vagus nerves are included in the wrap. Two interrupted heavy silk sutures are in place to stabilize the fundoplication.

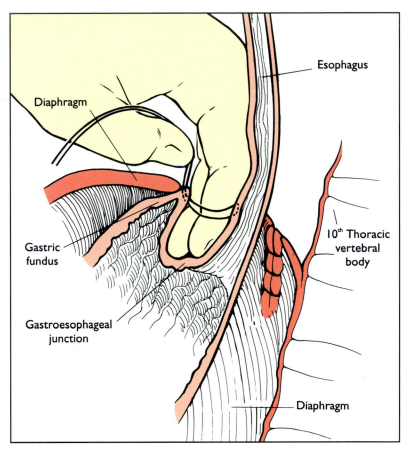

FIGURE 5-4.

Belsey Mark IV operation. Through a left sixth interspace posterolateral thoracotomy, the lower part of the esophagus and the hiatus are exposed. The esophagus is completely mobilized to the level of the lung root and the cardia. The upper part of the stomach is mobilized and brought through the hiatus into the left chest. The sutures in the crus posteriorly have been placed and tied to close the hiatus. The construction of a 240° partial fundoplication is started by placing the first row of three mattress sutures between the fundus of the stomach and esophagus, 2 cm above the gastroesophageal junction.

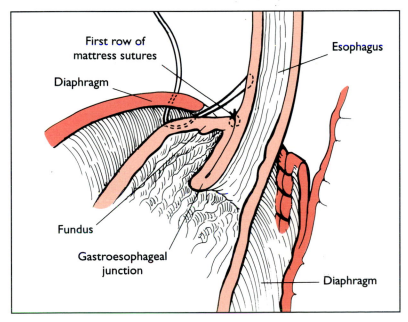

FIGURE 5-5.

Belsey Mark IV operation. After completion of the first row of mattress sutures, a second row of three mattress sutures is placed through the diaphragm, fundus, and esophagus. In this illustration, the first suture is in place.

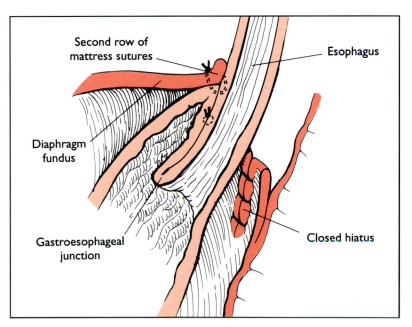

FIGURE 5-6.

Completed Belsey Mark IV operation. Sagittal section of repair. The second row of mattress sutures joining diaphragm, stomach, and esophagus are tied after the reconstruction has been placed beneath the diaphragm.

trunks (Figure 5-8). In its short abdominal portion (25 to 30 cm long), the esophagus lies on the diaphragm with the esophageal impression of the left lobe of the liver applied to its anterior aspect. The length of the intra-abdominal segment in the normal state averages 1.5 to 2 cm.

The lower esophagus segment is subdivided into the supradiaphragmatic portion, inferior esophageal constriction, vestibule, and cardia. This segment is supplied by an ascending branch of the left gastric artery. Venous drainage of this segment enters the coronary vein and pericardial venous plexus below the diaphragm. Preganglionic fibers of the vagus nerve synapse with ganglion cells in the myenteric plexus of the esophagus. Sympathetic innervation occurs from the thoracic ganglia.

The anatomy and physiology of the gastroesophageal junction and of the esophageal hiatus are essential to the understanding of reflux mechanisms and antireflux procedures. The muscle fibers surrounding the esophagus and creating the hiatus are mainly from the right crus of the diaphragm (Figure 5-8). In addition, several layers separating the thoracic and the abdominal cavity support the esophageal hiatus. The most important structure is the phrenoesophageal membrane, a condensation of endoabdominal and endothoracic fascia. This membrane anchors the esophagus within the hiatus (Figure 5-9). In most individuals, this membrane inserts 3.3 cm above the junction of the tubular esophagus with the stomach. The gastroesophageal junction is ill-defined because the internal junction does not coincide with the external junction. Gahagan [10] describes this region as follows: "the external junction, the termination of the tube, the esophagus and the beginning of a pouch, the stomach, lies 1 cm below the internal junction, the mucosal boundary."

Pathophysiology, Presentation, and Differential Diagnosis

Although there is no anatomical lower esophageal sphincter in humans, a physiologic sphincter mechanism exists and extends

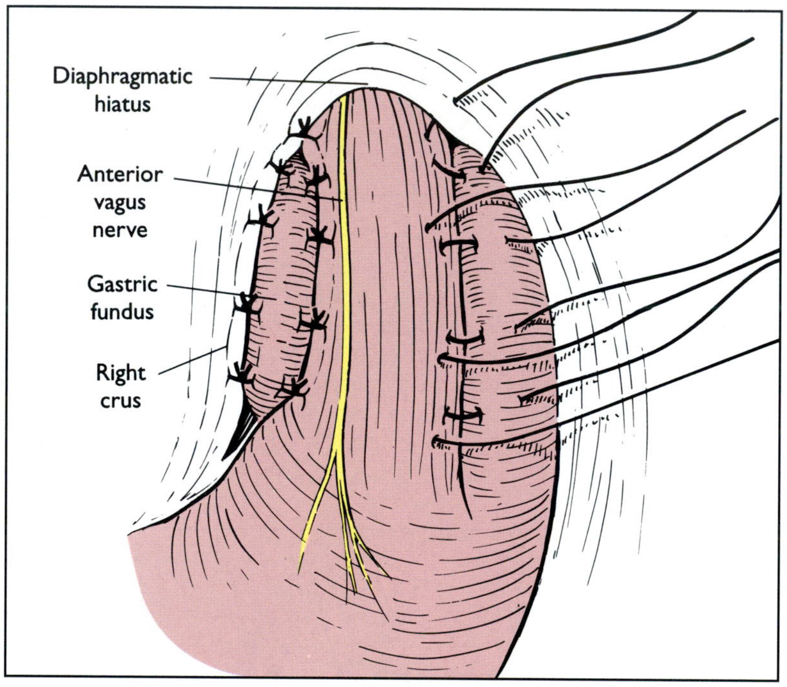

FIGURE 5-7.

The technique of the 270° Toupet fundoplication. The wrap is fixed to the crura posteriorly and anchored with seromuscular interrupted sutures anteriorly to the esophagus.

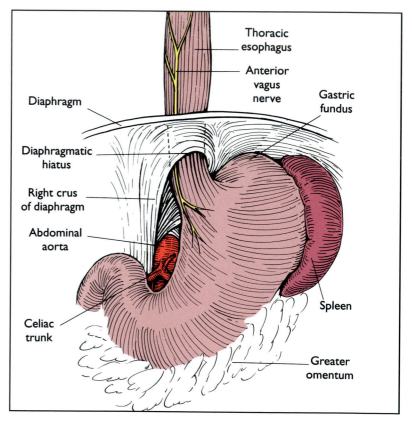

FIGURE 5-8.

Anatomy of the diaphragmatic hiatus and the abdominal segment of the esophagus. In most persons, the diaphragmatic hiatus is a sling of muscle fibers that arises from the right crus of the diaphragm.

over the terminal 1 to 4 cm of the esophagus. Manometrically, this specialized segment represents a zone of high pressure called the lower esophageal sphincter (LES). In the resting state, the LES is contracted and its mean pressure is 13 mm Hg. The overall length of the LES is 3.6 cm on average, 2 cm as the intra-abdominal portion and the remainder in the thoracic cavity. Gastroesophageal reflux is controlled by the following mechanisms: intrinsic muscle tone of the LES, intra-abdominal esophageal segment, abrupt opening of the narrow swallowing tube into dilated gastric pouch (La Place law), and normal gastric emptying. The functional state of the LES determines the development of GERD. Patients with LES pressure less than 5 mm Hg or an abdominal portion smaller than 1 cm present with GERD in 90% of cases [11].

Hiebert and Belsey's [12] observations clearly showed that pathologic reflux and hiatal hernia were separate entities. Approximately 80% of patients with GERD have a radiographically demonstrable axial hernia. When radiographic

maneuvers are applied to diagnose a hiatal hernia, only about 5% of such individuals have pathologic gastroesophageal reflux. Presumably, this is because the phrenoesophageal membrane insertion still leaves an adequate segment of distal esophagus exposed to abdominal pressure. Reflux is prevented when there is a 10-cm water column abdominothoracic pressure difference [13].

Although delayed gastric emptying has a strong correlation with severe reflux and esophagitis, it is not known whether the gastric emptying delay proceeds the pathologic reflux or whether esophageal inflammation from reflux esophagitis causes vagal nerve dysfunction and inhibits gastric emptying [14].

Twenty-four–hour intraesophageal pH monitoring documents that normal individuals have physiologic reflux after meals. Seven percent experience heartburn every day, and 36% of healthy individuals experience heartburn once a month. Pathologic degrees of reflux are diagnosed when reflux becomes prolonged or occurs throughout the day or at night.

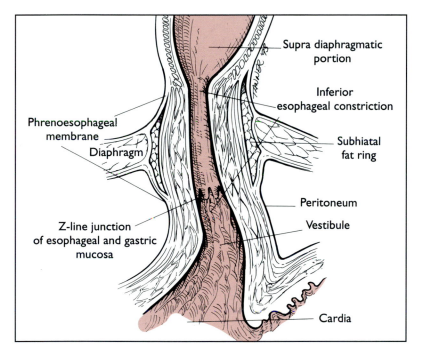

FIGURE 5-9.

Anatomy of the lower esophagus and the esophagogastric junction. The precise location of the gastroesophageal junction is difficult to define because the internal junction, the mucosal boundary (Z-line), does not coincide with the external junction.

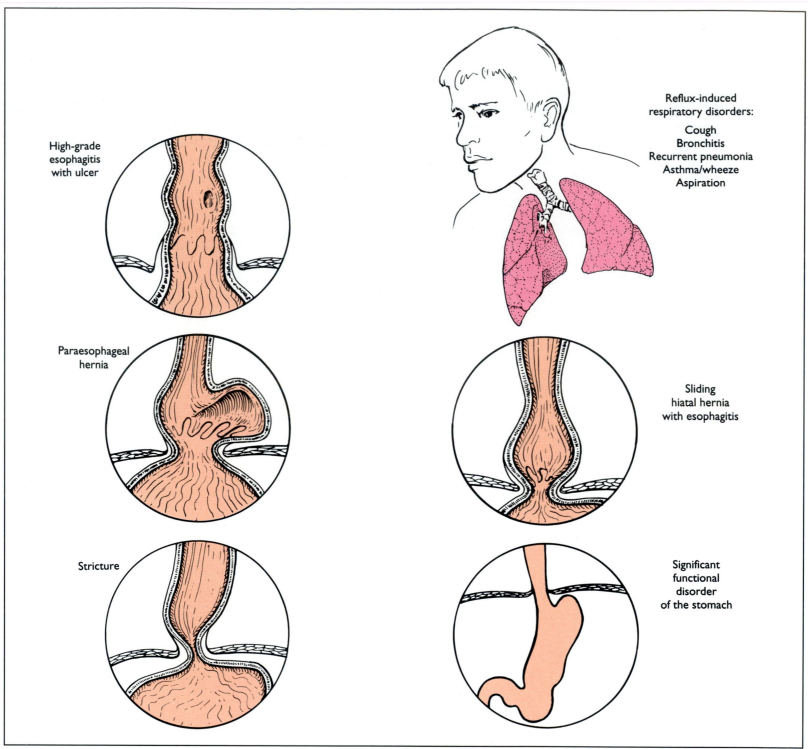

High-grade
esophagitis
with ulcer

Reflux-induced
respiratory disorders:

Cough
Bronchitis
Recurrent pneumonia
Asthma/wheeze
Aspiration

Paraesophageal
hernia

Sliding
hiatal hernia
with esophagitis

Stricture

Significant
functional
disorder
of the stomach

FIGURE 5-10.

Manifestations of gastroesophageal reflux disease and indications for surgery.

Esophagitis as a complication of reflux develops when gastric acid or pancreaticobiliary secretions reach the esophagus with increased frequency and protective esophageal mechanisms fail. An important aspect in the protection against the noxious effects of gastroesophageal reflux is coordinated peristaltic clearing and secondary peristalsis of the esophagus that is triggered by distention or irritation of the mucosa of the distal esophagus. When abnormal reflux occurs, the damage to the esophageal mucosa may range from none to the development of a severe peptic stricture (Figure 5-10). The degree of damage to the esophagus is graded as I (erythema of the mucosa without ulcerations), II (ulcerations), III (chronic ulcerations with fibrosis), and IV (stricture) [15]. Table 5-1 summarizes the symptoms and complications in patients who present with symptomatic GERD. The most common differential diagnoses, such as cholelithiasis, peptic ulcer disease, gastritis, esophageal motor disease, and angina pectoris are demonstrated in Figure 5-11.

Table 5-1. Symptoms and complications in patients with symptomatic gastroesophageal reflux disease*	
Symptoms or complications	**Patients, %**
Heartburn	85
Dysphagia	37
Stricture	19
Regurgitation	23
Nausea or vomiting	21
Cough	47
Bronchitis	35
Pneumonitis	16
Asthma or wheeze	16
Hemoptysis	13
Aspiration	8

*This table demonstrates the incidence and clinical features of reflux disease drawn from reports of 2178 patients [20,21]. Heartburn, dysphagia, and regurgitation are the classic esophageal symptoms. The complications of reflux disease are high-grade esophagitis, stricture, and Barrett's esophagus.

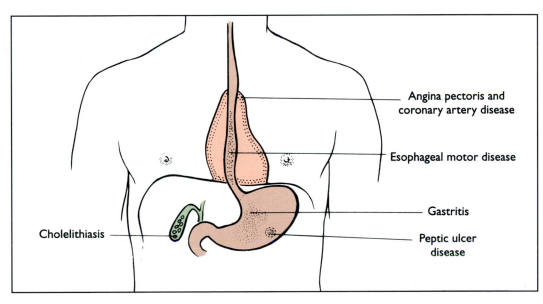

FIGURE 5-11.

The most important alternative diagnoses in patients with gastroesophageal reflux disease.

Diagnostic studies to define GERD and to evaluate patients for laparoscopic Nissen fundoplication include manometery of the esophagus, 24-hour pH monitoring, and esophagogastroduodenoscopy with biopsies (Figure 5-12). A mechanical sphincter defect is defined by a resting pressure less than 6 mm Hg or less than 2 cm in length [14].

The indications for laparoscopic Nissen fundoplication are identical to those for the open antireflux procedures. Primary indications for surgery are failure of medical management; need for long-term omeprazole treatment; or complications of GERD, such as high-grade esophagitis, stricture, or Barrett's esophagus (Figures 5-10 and 5-13).

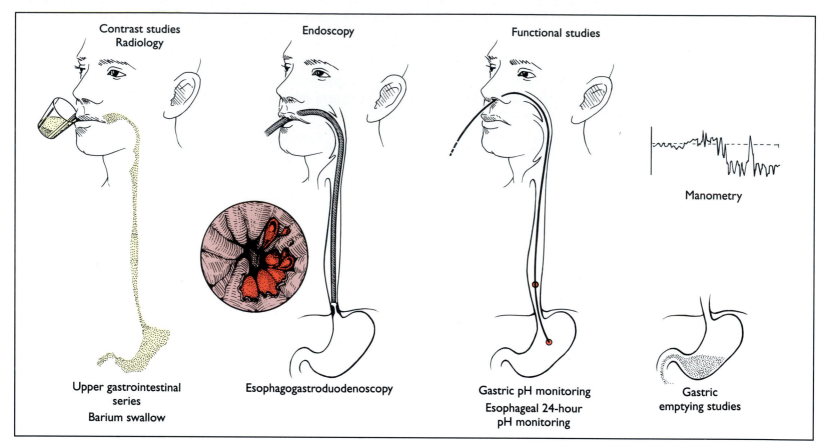

Contrast studies
Radiology

Endoscopy

Functional studies

Manometry

Upper gastrointestinal series
Barium swallow

Esophagogastroduodenoscopy

Gastric pH monitoring
Esophageal 24-hour pH monitoring

Gastric emptying studies

FIGURE 5-12.

Diagnostic studies in patients with gastroesophageal reflux disease.

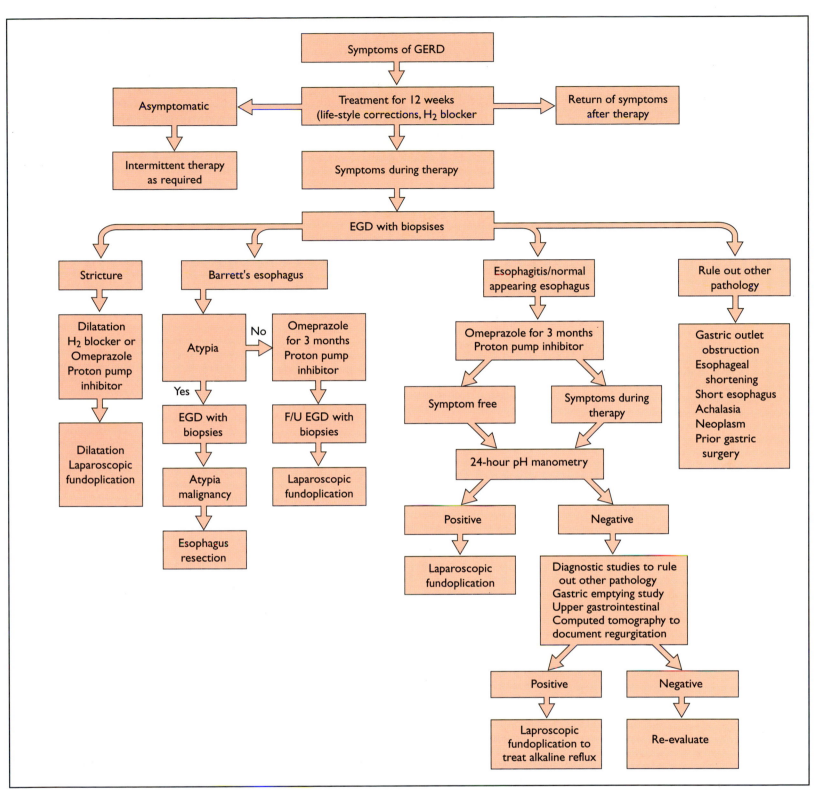

FIGURE 5-13.

Algorithm for the approach to patients with gastroesophageal reflux disease (GERD). Patients who initially present with dysphagia in their symptom complex should undergo upper endoscopy immediately to evaluate the obstructive cause. Every patient who is considered for laparoscopic fundoplication should undergo 24-hour pH study and manometry to exclude esophageal motility disorder. Diabetic patients should also be studied by gastric emptying studies to evaluate the gastric motility. EGD—esophagogastroduodenoscopy; F/U—follow-up; pH—24-hour pH study; R/O—rule out.

Surgical Technique

The Nissen fundoplication wrap, which is done laparoscopically, is identical to the wrap created by the open technique (Figures 5-14 to 5-19). For the laparoscopic construction of the fundoplication, pledgets can be used between the esophagus and stomach, as described by DeMeester and coworkers [13] in 1986. A "floppy Nissen" wrap of approximately 2 to 3 cm is created over a 58- to 60-French bougie to parallel the open technique as close as possible (Figures 5-20 to 5-26; Figure 5-27 illustrates an alter-native set-up). The short gastric vessels are selectively if ligated mobilization of the gastric fundus is required. Crural repair or approximation is not routinely undertaken. Anterior and posterior vagus nerves are included in the wrap. The Hasson cannula is used in all patients with a history of previous abdominal surgery. The partial laparoscopic fundoplication (Toupet) is approached in a manner similar to that presented in Figures 5-14 through 5-21. Completion of the 270° wrap is shown as an alternative procedure in Figure 5-28.

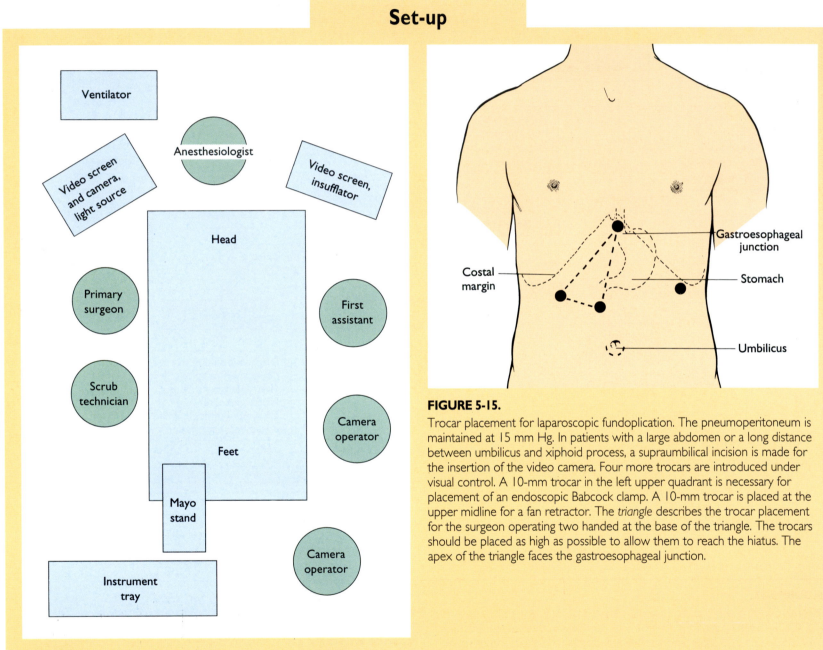

Set-up

FIGURE 5-14.

Operative set-up for laparoscopic fundoplication. Foley and nasogastric catheters are placed after induction of general anesthesia. The patient is then placed in the 30° Trendelenburg position with the arms tucked at the sides (optional). A pneumoperitoneum is established with a Veress needle inserted into the peritoneal cavity through a 1-cm infraumbilical incision. In patients with previous abdominal surgery, or as routine the open technique is used and an approximately 2.5-cm incision is made for the introduction of the Hasson cannula. A 10-mm sheath is used for the insertion of the video camera.

FIGURE 5-15.

Trocar placement for laparoscopic fundoplication. The pneumoperitoneum is maintained at 15 mm Hg. In patients with a large abdomen or a long distance between umbilicus and xiphoid process, a supraumbilical incision is made for the insertion of the video camera. Four more trocars are introduced under visual control. A 10-mm trocar in the left upper quadrant is necessary for placement of an endoscopic Babcock clamp. A 10-mm trocar is placed at the upper midline for a fan retractor. The *triangle* describes the trocar placement for the surgeon operating two handed at the base of the triangle. The trocars should be placed as high as possible to allow them to reach the hiatus. The apex of the triangle faces the gastroesophageal junction.

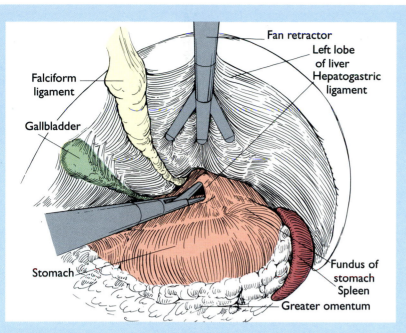

FIGURE 5-16.

The view as seen from the 10-mm trocar at the umbilicus. The fan retractor elevates the left lobe of the liver. The hepatogastric ligament is sharply dissected for the mobilization of the gastroesophageal junction.

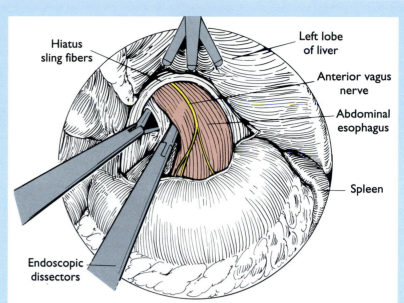

FIGURE 5-17.

The hepatogastric ligament is opened. The right crus of the diaphragm is then mobilized from the gastroesophageal junction. Care is taken to accurately distinguish the crus from the esophagus. Moving the nasogastric tube in the esophagus while the gastroesophageal junction is viewed helps to define the anatomy.

FIGURE 5-18.

With the esophagus retracted to the patient's right, the left diaphragmatic crus is dissected, and the space between this side of the esophagus and crura is opened bluntly. With the esophagus retracted upward, the retroesophageal space is dissected under direct vision. Care is taken not to enter the pleural space. At this point closure can be done as shown by other authors.

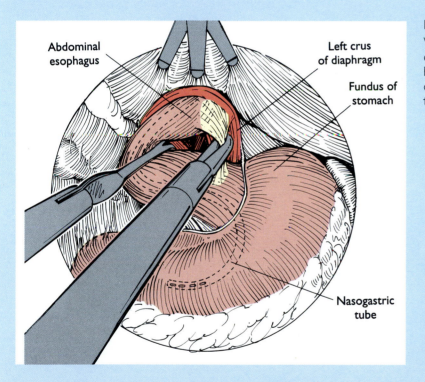

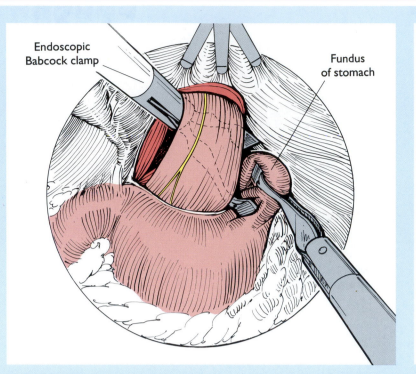

FIGURE 5-19.

An endoscopic Babcock clamp is placed from the most lateral right trocar and is passed behind the gastroesophageal junction. The placement of instruments in this area is done under direct vision. The fundus of the stomach is grasped with a second Babcock clamp from the left side and passed behind the gastroesophageal junction. The nasogastric tube is replaced with a 58- or 60-French bougie.

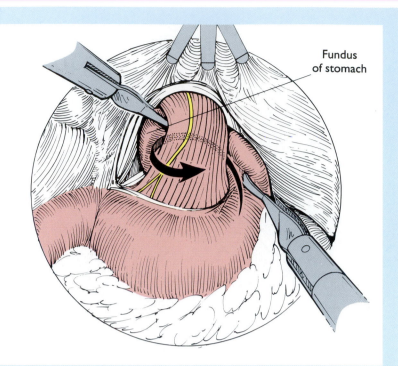

FIGURE 5-20.

The right endoscopic Babcock clamp is gently pulling the fundus of the stomach across the back of the gastroesophageal junction. With the same segment of stomach that was being passed around the back of the esophagus, the 360° wrap is created.

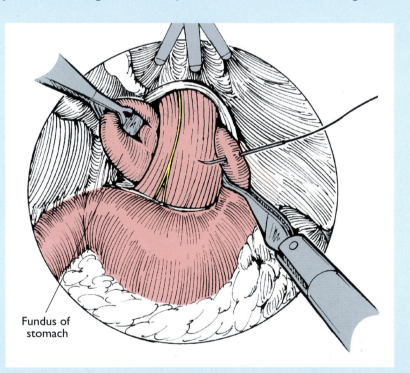

FIGURE 5-21.

Seromuscular sutures of 2-0 nonabsorbable material are used at each interface of stomach and esophagus. The anterior and posterior vagus nerves are included in the wrap.

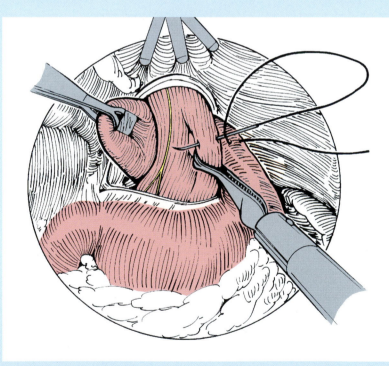

FIGURE 5-22.

At first the superior suture is placed, usually from the patient's left to the right side. Seromuscular stitches are performed.

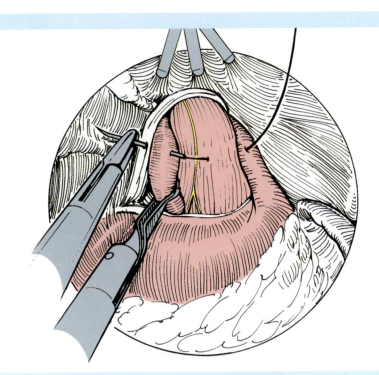

FIGURE 5-23.

The suture is passed from the left side through the stomach, esophagus, and stomach in a seromuscular fashion.

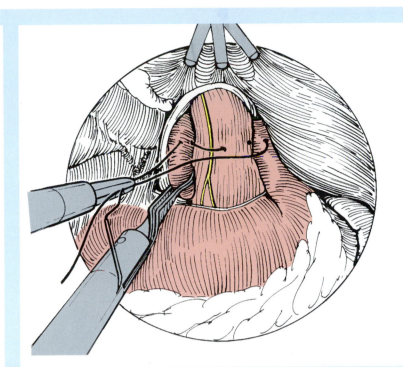

FIGURE 5-24.

The suture is then brought out through the same 10-mm trocar through which it was introduced. An extracorporal knot is tied, which is introduced into the peritoneal cavity and slid down with a pusher bar.

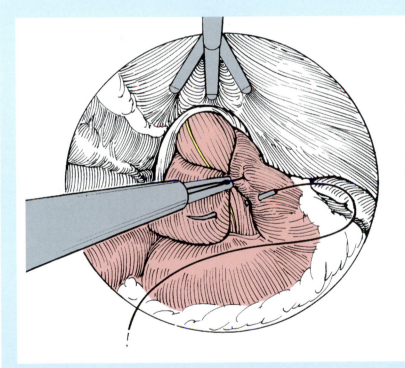

FIGURE 5-25.

A second suture is placed inferior to the previous one, approximately 1 to 1.5 cm apart, using an identical technique.

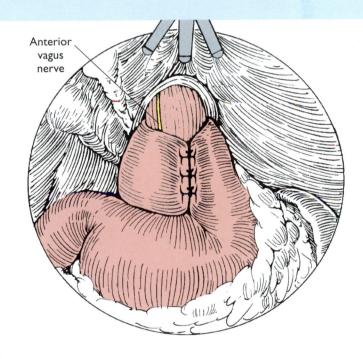

FIGURE 5-26.

The complete 360° wrap is demonstrated. The length of the wrap is approximately 2 cm and, as demonstrated above, created over a large bougie to create a loose "floppy Nissen." Trocars are then removed, the pneumoperitoneum released, the incisions closed with interrupted number 1 polyglactin sutures, and incision dressings applied.

Alternative Set-up

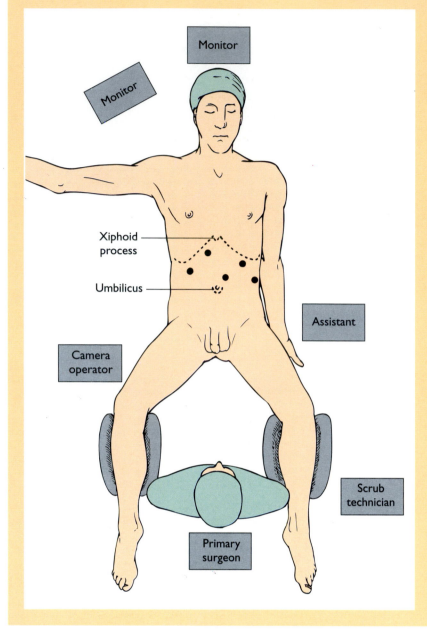

Monitor

Monitor

Xiphoid
process

Umbilicus

Assistant

Camera
operator

Scrub
technician

Primary
surgeon

FIGURE 5-27.

Alternative set-up. The surgeon is positioned between the legs of the patient. The patient is in lithotomy and reverse (20° to 30°) Trendelenburg position. Five trocars are placed high in the epigastrium. The video camera is introduced through the left upper quadrant trocar.

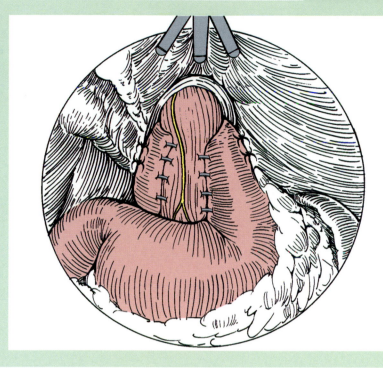

FIGURE 5-28.

Alternative laparoscopic antireflux procedure: Toupet fundoplication. Similar to the open Toupet procedure, this procedure results in a 270° posterior wrap with the anterior vagus nerve excluded from the wrap.

Results

Several reports have described the results of early laparoscopic fundoplication compared with those of open Nissen fundoplication. Peters and coworkers [18] compared 81 patients who underwent either open Nissen fundoplication or laparoscopic Nissen fundoplication. In 84% of patients in each group, GERD symptoms were relieved after surgery. However, laparoscopic fundoplication decreased in-hospital days from 9.2 to 4.7 days. In addition, laparoscopic fundoplication provided an increased LES tone compared with the open procedure (20.9 mm Hg compared with 12.1 mm Hg). In a separate study, Viljakka and coworkers [19] compared the long-term results of open and laparoscopic fundoplications at one institution. They noted a decreased morbidity rate in patients who had laparoscopic fundoplication compared with those who had open procedures; this decrease was primarily attributable to decreased incidence of wound infections and ventral hernias.

Hunter and colleagues [9] recently reported the results of laparoscopic Nissen and laparoscopic Toupet fundoplications in 300 patients with GERD between 1991 and 1995. Before operation, 98% of patients had abnormal results on 24-hour esophageal pH studies. On esophageal motility study, 17% had decreased motility and 2% had aperistalsis. Fifty-one percent of patients had erosive esophagitis according to esophagogastroduodenoscopy. The most frequent indication for operative manipulation was failure of medical therapy to alleviate GERD symptoms. During the operation, surgery for three patients was converted to an open procedure because of adhesive disease, and surgery for one patient was converted because of a markedly enlarged liver. After surgery, minor complications were encountered in 6% and major complications were seen in 2%. Median follow-up was 17 months. At 1 year, 93% of patients did not have typical GERD symptoms, such as heartburn. Atypical symptoms, including respiratory symptoms, were relieved in 87% and were not improved in 13%.

Table 5-2. Clinical assessment of operative results*

Assessment	Patients, %
Mortality	0.2
Conversion to open	5.8
Operative complications	4.2
Reflux control	97
Early dysphagia	20
Late dysphagia	5.5
Persistent dysphagia requiring surgery	0.9

*In-hospital and follow-up outcome (0–36 months) of the 2453 patients with symptomatic gastroesophageal reflux disease who were explored laparoscopically for Nissen fundoplication. Mean hospital stay was 3.7 days.

In 1997, Perdikis and coworkers [20] reviewed the existing world literature of 23 early reports of laparoscopic Nissen fundoplication with short-term follow-up. Nearly 2500 patients were included in the cumulative review. Surgery was converted to an open procedure in 5.8% of patients for a variety of reasons, including difficulty in exposure, gastroesophageal perforation, and excessive bleeding. The mortality rate was 0.2% because of missed esophageal perforation, missed duodenal perforation, postoperative myocardial infarction, and ischemic bowel. Ninety-seven percent of patients reported relief of reflux symptoms, and 5.5% reported late dysphagia. The clinical assessment of patients in this study is shown in Table 5-2.

Comparison of laparoscopic Nissen fundoplication with the laparoscopic Toupet procedure has shown differing results. Bell and coworkers [21] prospectively compared 11 patients undergoing Nissen fundoplication with 11 patients having Toupet fundoplication for severe GERD. The presence of such side effects as gas bloating, persistent dysphagia, and odynophagia significantly increased after complete fundoplication, whereas those repaired with the Toupet procedure had none of these side effects. Both groups were free of reflux symptoms at 12-month follow-up. Similarly, Coster and coworkers [22] noticed an earlier resumption of normal diet by patients treated with laparoscopic Toupet fundoplication in their study comparing laparoscopic Nissen and laparoscopic Toupet fundoplication. Not all reports comparing laparoscopic Nissen fundoplication with laparoscopic Toupet fundoplication have shown such clear advantages of the Toupet procedure over the Nissen procedure. For instance, Jobe and coworkers [23] studied 100 consecutive patients who underwent laparoscopic Toupet fundoplication for medically refractory GERD. Follow-up at 22 months detected abnormal 24-hour pH studies in 90% of patients who returned with dysphagia and in 39% of asymptomatic patients. Although the authors concluded that these data indicated a high incidence of recurrent reflux, a randomized trial with longer-term follow-up comparing complete with partial fundoplication is needed.

In conclusion, laparoscopic Nissen fundoplication can be performed safely and is an effective antireflux procedure. It has the same good results as open fundoplication procedures. The best results are obtained in carefully selected patients who present predominantly with regurgitation and heartburn. As in many other laparoscopic procedures, a shorter hospital stay and an earlier return to baseline activities are recognized. Total costs are lower than those the standard technique because of a decreased hospital stay and an earlier return to work [22]. Furthermore, laparoscopic Toupet fundoplication appears preferable in patients with esophageal dysmotility and GERD. Patients with normal esophageal motility may be best managed with laparoscopic Nissen fundoplication, but further investigation with long-term follow-up is needed.

References

1. Allison PR: Reflux esophagitis, sliding hiatal hernia and the anatomy of repair. *Surg Gynecol Obstet* 1951, 92:419–431.

2. Nissen R: Eine einfache Operation zur Beeinflussung der Refluxoesophagitis. *Schweiz Med Wochenschr* 1956, 86:590–592.

3. Baue AE, Belsey RHR: The treatment of sliding hiatus hernia and reflux esophagitis by the Mark IV technique. *Surgery* 1967, 62:396–406.

4. Toupet AM: Technique d'oesophago-gastroplastic avec phreno-gastropexie appliquee dans le cure radicale des herniers hiatales et comme complement de l'operation de Heller dans les cardiospasmes. *Academie de Chirurgie* 1963, 89:394–399.

5. Geagea T: Laparoscopic Nissen's fundal plication is feasible. *Can J Surg* 1991, 34:313.

6. Dallemagne B, Weerts JM, Jehaes C, *et al.*: Laparoscopic Nissen fundoplication: preliminary report. *Surg Laparosc Endosc* 1991, 3:138–143.

7. Bittner HB, Meyers WC, Brazer SR, Pappas TN: Laparoscopic Nissen fundoplication: operative results and short-term follow-up. *Am J Surg* 1994, in press.

8. Cuschieri A, Hunter J, Wolfe B, *et al.*: Multicenter prospective evaluation of laparoscopic antireflux surgery: preliminary report. *Surg Endosc* 1993, 7:505–510.

9. Hunter JG, Trus TL, Branum GD, *et al.*: A physiologic approach to laparoscopic fundoplication for gastroesophageal reflux disease. *Ann Surg* 1996, 223:673–687.

10. Gahagan T: The function of the musculature of the esophagus and stomach in the esophagogastric sphincter mechanism. *Surg Gynecol Obstet* 1962, 114:293–303.

11. Stein HJ, DeMeester TR: Who benefits from antireflux surgery. *World J Surg* 1992, 16:313–319.

12. Hiebert CA, Belsey RHR: Incompetency of the gastric cardia without radiologic evidence of hiatal hernia. *J Thoracic Cardiovasc* 1961, 42:352–362.

13. DeMeester TR, Wernly JA, Bryant GH, *et al.*: Clinical and in vitro analysis of determinants of gastroesophageal competence. *Am J Surg* 1979, 137:39–46.

14. Skinner DB: Pathophysiology of gastroesophageal reflux. *Ann Surg* 1985, 202:546–556.

15. Ismail-Beigi F, Horton PF, Pope CE II: Histologic consequences of gastroesophageal reflux in man. *Gastroenterology* 1970, 58:163–170.

16. Stein HJ, Barlow AP, DeMeester TR, Hinder RA: Complications of gastroesophageal reflux disease: role of the lower esophageal sphinchter, esophageal acid and acid/alkaline exposure, and duodenogastric reflux. *Ann Surg* 1992, 216:35–43.

17. DeMeester TR, Bonavina L, Albertucci M: Nissen fundoplication for gastroesophageal reflux disease: evaluation of primary repair in 100 consecutive patients. *Ann Surg* 1986, 204:9–20.

18. Peters JH, Heimbucher J, Kauer WK, *et al.*: Clinical and physiologic comparison of laparoscopic and open Nissen fundoplication. *J Am Coll Surg* 1995, 180:385–393.

19. Viljakka MT, Loustarinen ME, Isolauri JO: Complications of open and laparoscopic antireflux surgery: 32 year audit at a teaching hospital. *J Am Coll Surg* 1997, 185:446–450.

20. Perdikis G, Hinder RA, Lund RL, *et al.*: Laparscopic Nissen fundoplication: where do we stand? *Surg Laparosc Endosc* 1997, 7:17–21.

21. Bell RCW, Hanna P, Powers B, *et al.*: Clinical manometric results of laparoscopic partial (Toupet) and complete (Rosetti-Nissen) fundoplication. *Surg Endosc* 1996, 10:724–728.

22. Coster DD, Bower WH, Wilson VT, *et al.*: Laparoscopic partial fundoplication vs. laparoscopic Nissen-Rosetti fundoplication. *Surg Endosc* 1997, 11:625–631.

23. Jobe BA, Wallace J, Hansen PD, *et al.*: Evaluation of laparoscopic Toupet fundoplications as a primary repair for all patients with medically resistant gastroesophageal reflux. *Surg Endosc* 1997, 11:1080–1083.

Laparoscopic Heller Myotomy for Esophageal Achalasia

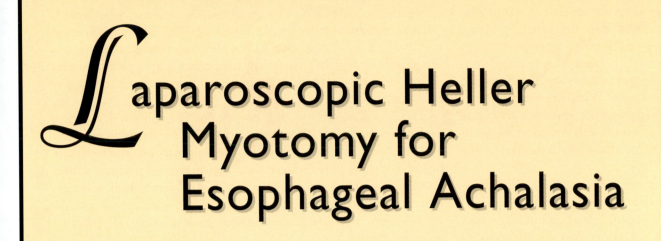

Thomas Z. Hayward III
Steve Eubanks

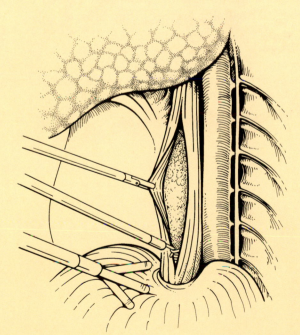

Achalasia is a rare condition of unknown cause that affects about 1 in 100,000 persons [1]. The term *achalasia* means "failure to relax" and is an apt description of the syndrome caused by the incomplete relaxation of the lower esophageal sphincter (LES) [2]. This inability of the LES to relax, coupled with the absence of peristalsis in the body of the esophagus, creates a functional obstruction in the distal esophagus that leads to symptoms.

The surgical treatment of achalasia, first described by Heller in 1914, initially consisted of two myotomies on opposite sides of the esophagus via a laparotomy [3]. Later, the original technique was modified to the single anterior myotomy performed through a laparotomy or thoracotomy. With the emergence of minimally invasive surgery, the laparoscopic approach to Heller myotomy was preferred in Europe and South America; surgeons in the United States, Great Britain, and Canada preferred the thorascopic approach [4].

As minimally invasive techniques have evolved, the laparoscopic approach has become increasingly popular. This is because parallel dissection to the esophagus is technically easier to perform, an adequate-length myotomy (despite earlier concerns) can easily be obtained, an antireflux procedure can be added to the operation, and conversion to an open procedure can be performed easily should it become necessary. Other benefits are perioperative management simplified by elimination of the double-lumen endotracheal tube, left lateral decubitus positioning, intraoperative collapse of the left lung, and chest tube management issues. Finally, the initial dissection and the anatomy are similar to those for the more commonly performed laparoscopic Nissen fundoplication; as a result, the learning curve for laparoscopic Heller myotomy is substantially reduced and the clinical skills needed for this infrequently performed procedure can be adequately maintained.

Anatomy

The esophagus is a muscular tube, 25 cm long, that lacks a serosal layer and is lined with squamous epithelium. The upper 5% of the muscular wall of the esophagus is composed of striated muscle; the middle 35% to 40% is a mixture of striated and smooth muscle; and the lower 50% to 60% consists of smooth muscle only. The inner esophageal muscular layer is circular and runs from the upper esophageal sphincter around the level of C5-C6 to the LES. The outer muscular layer is longitudinal and begins below the cricopharyngeus muscle, where it runs uniformly throughout the remainder of the esophagus (Fig. 6-1).

The blood supply of the esophagus is segmental and has limited overlap; this creates the possibility of devascularization and ischemia. Most notably for the laparoscopic surgeon, the blood supply for the chest portion of the esophagus comes from the aorta, intercostal arteries, and bronchial arteries, whereas the blood supply to the short intra-abdominal portion comes from the left gastric, short gastric, and left inferior phrenic arteries.

Physiology

The basic purpose of the esophagus is to serve as a conduit for food transport, a function initiated by swallowing (Fig. 6-2). Both excitatory and inhibitory ganglionic neurons are dysfunctional during achalasia. An absence or degeneration of the ganglion cells of the myenteric plexus of Auerbach is a constant finding [5]. The inhibitory ganglionic neurons, probably nitric oxide (with or without vasoactive intestinal polypeptide), mediate LES relaxation and the proximal-to-distal migration of the esophageal peristaltic wave [6] (Fig. 6-3).

FIGURE 6-1.

Anatomy of the diaphragmatic hiatus and the abdominal segment of the esophagus. The diaphragmatic hiatus is a sling of muscle fibers that arises from the right crus of the diaphragm in the majority of individuals.

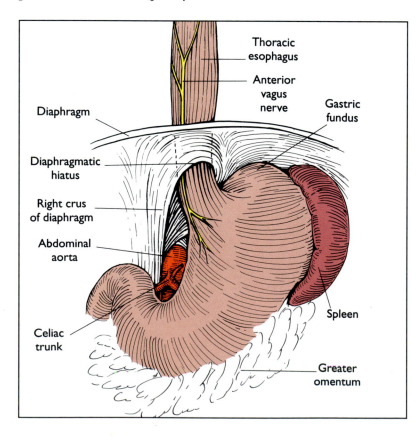

Thoracic esophagus

Anterior vagus nerve

Gastric fundus

Diaphragm

Diaphragmatic hiatus

Right crus of diaphragm

Abdominal aorta

Celiac trunk

Spleen

Greater omentum

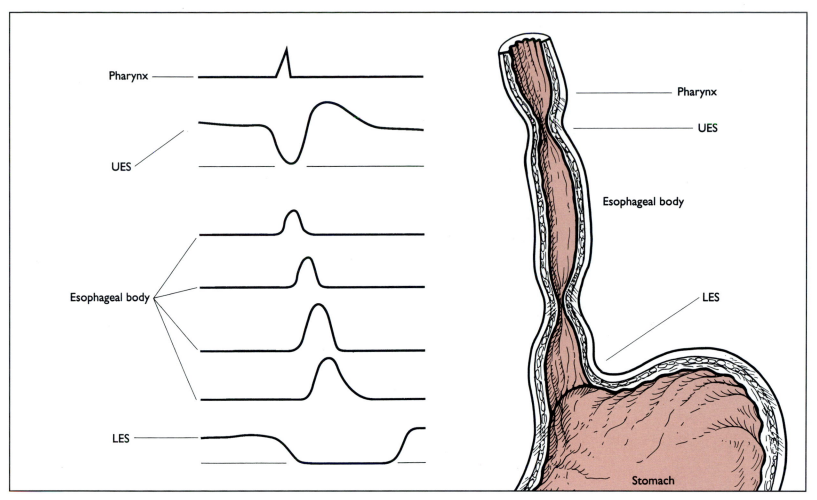

FIGURE 6-2.

Manometric evaluation of peristalsis. With deglutition, relaxation of the upper esophageal sphincter (UES) is followed by segmental contractions of the body of the esophagus that are propagated distally. The lower esophageal sphincter (LES) normally relaxes to allow passage of the food bolus into the stomach.

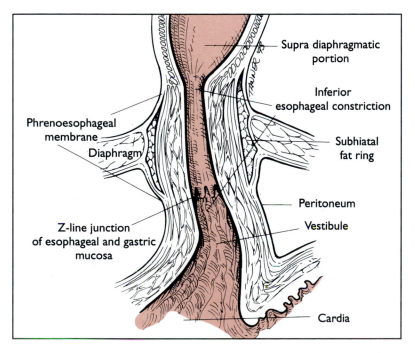

FIGURE 6-3.

Anatomy of the lower esophagus and the esophagogastric junction. The precise location of the gastroesophageal junction is difficult to define since the internal junction, the mucosal boundary (Z-line), does not coincide with the external junction.

Clinical Findings

Symptoms

The primary symptoms of achalasia are dysphagia and chest pain with progressive intolerance for both solids and liquids. In the early stages of the disease, this can be overcome by certain maneuvers performed while eating: drinking liquids with meals, sitting straight up, raising the hands above the head, standing, or jumping. However, the onset of achalasia can be insidious and can be mistaken for other disease processes unless a complete preoperative evaluation takes place.

Imaging Studies

A barium esophagram can show aperistalsis, minimal LES opening with the characteristic "bird beak" appearance, and, in advance cases, varying degrees of esophageal dilatation and tortuosity. Fluoroscopic examination may show the weak or absent peristatic waves that are the hallmarks of achalasia. Computed tomography or esophageal Doppler ultrasonography can differentiate achalasia from pseudo-achalasia, identify the cause of pseudo-achalasia, and assist with tumor staging and operative plan (Fig. 6-4).

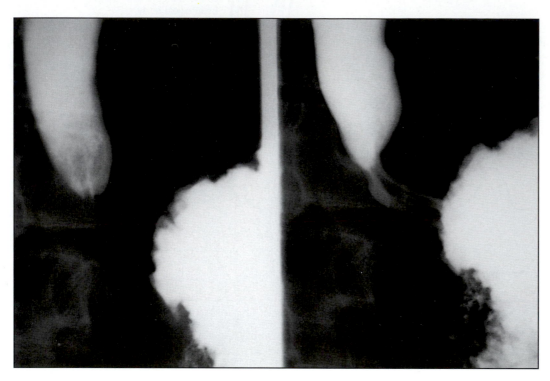

FIGURE 6-4.

Barium esophagogram in a patient with achalasia demonstrating the typical bird's beak deformity.

Endoscopy

Endoscopy should be performed on all patients for two reasons. First, tumor-related pseudo-achalasia, which accounts for 5% of cases, can have clinically and radiographically identical presentations. Endoscopy enables the differential diagnosis of these conditions. Second, endoscopy can rule out the presence of food or yeast in the distal esophagus; this is important because these conditions can easily be treated, resulting in decreased risk for aspiration or operative contamination.

Manometry

Manometry is the most sensitive diagnostic method for achalasia because it demonstrates the functional abnormality of the esophagus. It also allows differentiation from other functional diseases of the esophagus that have similar clinical presentations: scleroderma, tumors (benign and malignant), and strictures. The classic triad of manographic findings are weak or absent peristaltic curves, increased resting LES pressure (30 to 40 mm Hg), and inadequate relaxation of the LES in response to swallowing (Fig. 6-5).

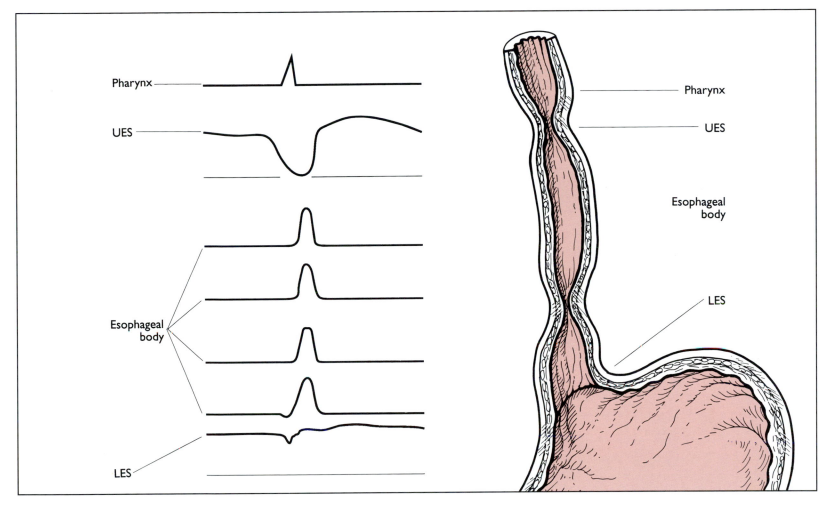

FIGURE 6-5.

Manometric evaluation of the esophagus in a patient with achalasia. Pertinent findings include absence of propulsive peristalsis in the body of the esophagus (note simultaneous contractions), elevated resting lower esophageal sphincter (LES) pressure, and absence of LES relaxation.

Surgical Technique

Figures 6-6 through 6-13 depict the surgical technique for laparoscopic Heller myotomy.

Set-up

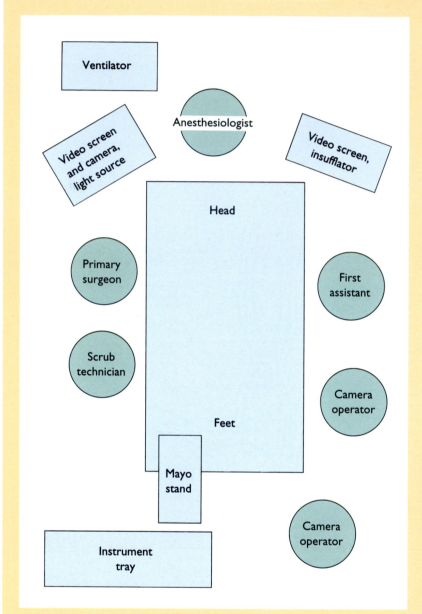

FIGURE 6-6.

Operative setup for laparoscopic Heller myotomy. Preoperative therapy with broad-spectrum antibiotics (such as cefazolin) is given intravenously in case the esophageal mucosa is violated during the procedure. In addition, a Foley catheter is placed for patient monitoring. Instruments for a laparotomy must be available and opened in case conversion to an open procedure is required.

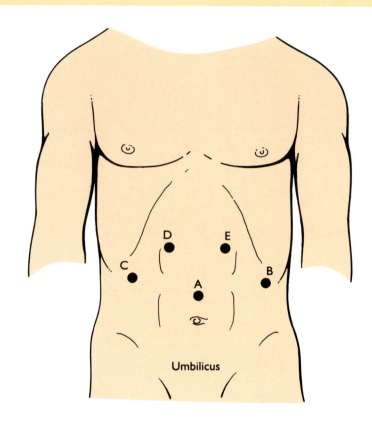

FIGURE 6-7.

The patient is positioned supine on the operating table. The legs can be placed in stirrups if the surgeon prefers to operate from between the patient's legs. An endoscope is passed into the stomach. After induction of the pneumoperitoneum, four or five 10-mm trocars are inserted into the abdominal cavity as follows: 1) *A* is placed 3 to 4 cm above the umbilicus and is used for the telescope; 2) *B* is placed in the left upper quadrant at the anterior axillary line and is used for retraction of the stomach. 3) *C* and *D* are placed in the right upper quadrant and are used for retraction of the liver (*C*) and for counteraction on the myotomy (*D*); 4) *E* is placed in the left upper quadrant and is used by the operator for the dissection.

Set-up

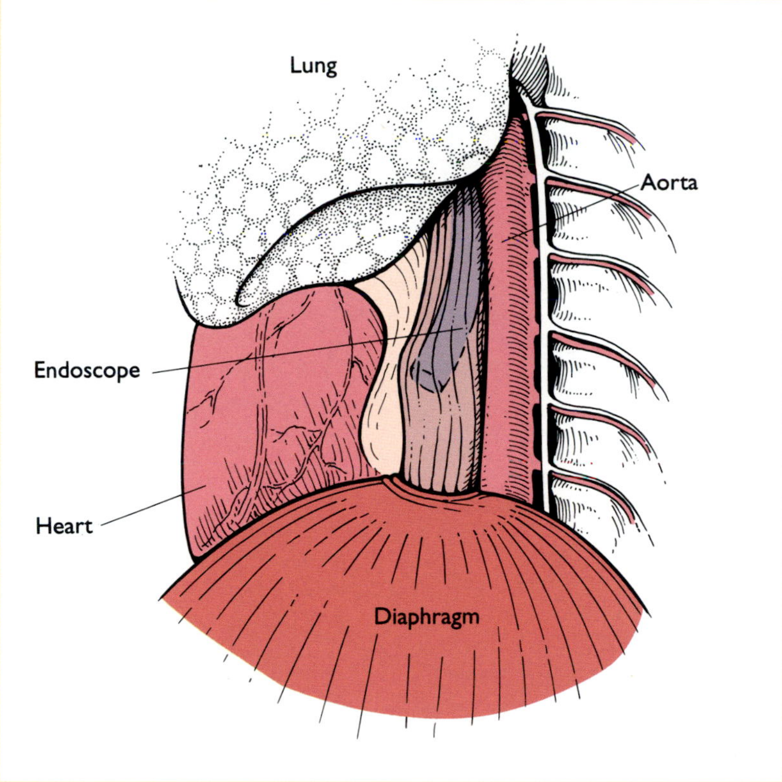

FIGURE 6-8.

After induction of anesthesia a fiberoptic endoscope is inserted into the esophagus. Intraoperative endoscopy, which can be performed by a gastroenterology medicine colleague or a member of the surgical team, facilitates the operation by providing internal illumination to help identify the esophageal layers. In addition, endoscopy establishes the length of the narrowing, allows immediate evaluation of the adequacy of the myotomy, and helps to confirm the integrity of the mucosa at the end of the procedure.

Procedure

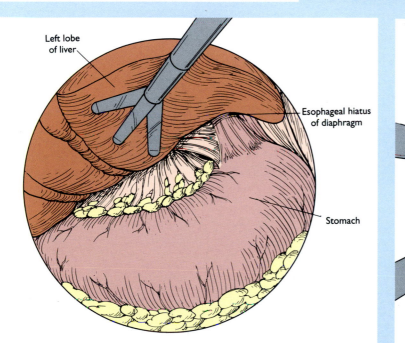

FIGURE 6-9.

An expandable retractor is used to elevate the left lobe of the liver; doing so exposes the hepatogastric ligament, which is then sharply dissected. The use of a 30° or 45° telescope improves the operative view throughout all aspects of this procedure.

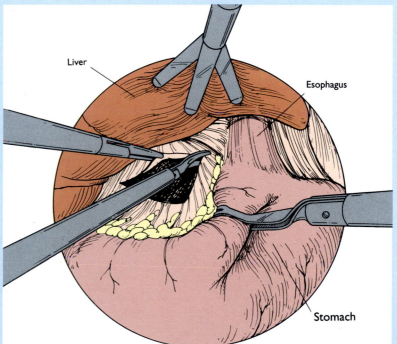

FIGURE 6-10.

Mobilization of the hepatogastric ligament facilitates dissection of the gastroesophageal junction, and the assistant's use of an endoscopic Babcock clamp to pull the stomach inferiorly and laterally significantly improves the operative view. The phrenoesophageal ligament is then divided by using both sharp and blunt dissection, with care taken not to injure the vagus nerve or its branches. A low threshold for mobilizing the fundus of the stomach by detaching it from the short gastrics should be used to ensure that a partial fundoplication can be performed without tension.

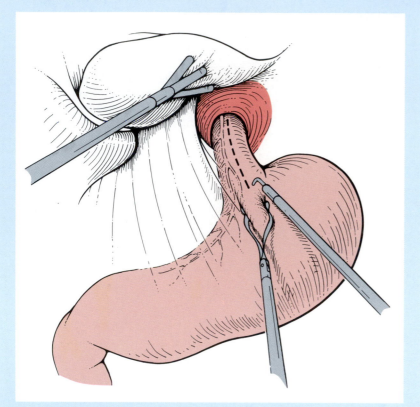

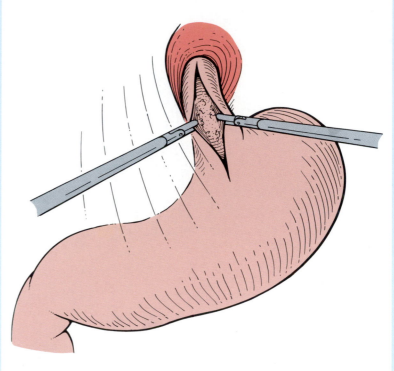

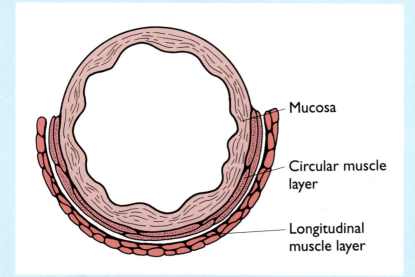

FIGURE 6-11.

The myotomy is started in the middle third of the exposed esophagus, lateral to the anterior vagus nerve. The longitudinal fibers are divided at a point midway between the inferior pulmonary vein and the diaphragm or a point 6 cm above the gastroesophageal junction. The incision is deepened until the circular muscle fibers are identified; at this point, the myotomy is extended upward and downward by using the hook cautery or bipolar scissors.

FIGURE 6-12.

Extending the myotomy to the cardioesophageal junction and completing the myotomy. The myotomy is then carried inferiorly across the sling muscles of the gastroesophageal junction 1 cm down onto the stomach or until the obstruction is relieved, as visualized by the simultaneous endoscopy. The muscularis is much more attenuated at the gastric fundus, and the underlying mucosa is more adherent; thus, the potential for iatrogenic injury in this area increases substantially.

FIGURE 6-13.

Cross-sectional anatomy of the esophagus after completion of the myotomy. The myotomy is completed when the edges of the muscularis are stripped away from the mucosa for 40% to 50% of the circumference of the esophagus. This avoids narrowing of the lower esophageal sphincter region during healing of the myotomy. Fundoplication is performed on any patient with esophageal dilation, young patients, or patients considered at increased risk for postoperative gastroesophageal reflux disease.

Mucosa

Circular muscle layer

Longitudinal muscle layer

Avoiding Pitfalls

To avoid pitfalls, the surgeon should obtain and maintain adequate exposure at all times. All esophageal attachments should be freed before the esophagus itself is dissected. Concomitant intra-operative endoscopy should be used to help determine the distal extent of the myotomy, facilitate dissection and division of the circular fibers, and improve the ability to detect and repair esophageal perforations should they occur.

Results

Definitive treatments of achalasia are dilatation and open Heller myotomy. Only one randomized, controlled trial has compared these two therapies [7]. The trial showed that 95% of the surgical group had almost complete resolution of symptoms compared with 51% of the dilatation group ($P < 0.01$) after 5 years of follow-up. Although surgery is more efficacious and dilatation is associated with a 3% esophageal perforation rate, dilatation has been the preferred treatment because of the morbidity associated with a thoracotomy [8].

Laparoscopic Heller myotomy for the treatment of achalasia is a safe and effective alternative to open procedures, with short hospital stays and convalescent periods (Table 6-1). The success of laparoscopic Heller myotomy may shift the hierarchy of treatment in favor of surgery once achalasia has been definitively diagnosed.

Table 6-1. Laparoscopic Heller myotomy literature summary

Study	Year	Procedure	Patients, n	Dysphagia, %	GERD, %	Morbidity, %	Duration of follow-up, mo
Ancona and coworkers [9]	1995	LHM/DF	17	6	0	0	7
Rosati and coworkers [10]	1995	LHM/DF	25	4	NR	4	12
Delgado and coworkers [11]	1996	LHM/DF	12	16	NR	1.6	3
Swanstrom and Pennings [12]	1995	LHM or THM	12	8	17	0	16
Holzman and coworkers [13]	1997	LHM + DF orTHM	10	20	10	20	7–39
Hunter and Richardson [4]	1997	LHM + DF or THM	40	10	5	7.5	12.5
Anselmino and coworkers [14]	1997	LHM + DF	43	11.6	5.7	NR	12

DF—Dor fundoplication; GERD—gastroesophageal reflux disease; LHM—laparoscopic Heller myotomy; NR—not recorded or mentioned in paper; THM—thorascopic Heller myotomy.

References

1. Howard P, Maher L, Pryde A, *et al.*: Five year prospective study of the incidence, clinical features and diagnosis of achalasia in Edinburgh. *Gut* 1992, 33:1011–1015.

2. Lendrum F: Anatomic features of the cardiac orifice of the stomach with special reference to cardiospasm. *Arch Intern Med* 1937, 59:474–511.

3. Heller E: Extramukose kerrkioplastic beim chronishen Kardiospasmus mit Dilatation des Oesophagus. *Mitt Grenzgeb Med Chir* 1914, 27:141–149.

4. Hunter JG, Richardson WS: Surgical management of achalasia. *Surg Clin North Am* 1997, 77:993–1015.

5. Csendes A, Smok G, Braghetto I, *et al.*: Gastroesophageal sphincter pressure and histologic changes in patients with achalasia of the esophagus. *Dig Dis Sci* 1985, 30:941–944.

6. Guelrud M, Rossiter A, Souney P, *et al.*: The effect of vasoactive intestinal polypeptide on the lower esophageal sphincter in achalasia. *Gastroenterology* 1992, 103:377–382.

7. Csendes A, Braghetto I, Henriquez A, *et al.*: Late results of a prospective randomized study comparing forceful dilation and oesophagomyotomy in patients with achalasia. *Gut* 1989, 30:299–304.

8. Spiess A, Kahrilas P: Treating achalasia from whalebone to laparoscope. *JAMA* 1998, 280:638–642.

9. Ancona E, Anselmino M, Zaninotto G, *et al.*: Esophageal achalasia: laparoscopic versus conventional open Heller-Dor operation. *Am J Surg* 1995, 170:265–270.

10. Rosati R, Fumagalli U, Bonavina L, *et al.*: Laparoscopic approach to esophageal achalasia. *Am J Surg* 1995, 169:424–427.

11. Delgado F, Bolufer JM, Martinez-Abad M, *et al.*: Laparoscopic treatment of esophageal achalasia. *Surg Laparosc Endosc* 1996, 6:83–90.

12. Swanstrom LL, Pennings J: Laparoscopic esophagomyotomy for achalasia. *Surg Endosc* 1995, 9:286–292.

13. Holzman MD, Sharp KW, Ladipo JK, *et al.*: Laparoscopic surgical treatment of achalasia. *AmJ Surg* 1997, 173:308–311.

14. Anselmino M, Zaninotto G, Costantini M, *et al.*: One-year follow-up after laparoscopic Heller-Dor operation for esophageal achalasia. *Surg Endosc* 1997, 11:3–7.

demonstrated [7]. However, the critically ill nature of these patients and the paucity of instrumentation designed specifically for laparoscopic procedures in neonates have precluded the use of laparoscopic techniques in this patient population.

Although the specific indications for endoscopic repair of diaphragmatic hernias are poorly defined, the indications for surgical intervention are essentially identical for both open and laparoscopic approaches. The congenital Morgagni-Larrey subcostosternal diaphragmatic hernia is uncommon (3% of all diaphragmatic hernias). Most lesions are identified by computed tomography after the patient reports pain, dyspnea, or intermittent bowel obstruction. Complications are rare but do occur, particularly in children [8], and diagnosis mandates surgical intervention. Several groups have reported effective laparoscopic repairs [9,10], with debate focusing on the efficacy of primary versus mesh repair and the extent of dissection. Generally, the hernia sac should be excised and the diaphragmatic repair should be tension free.

In general, patients with paraesophageal hernias report substernal chest pain and cough related to intermittent aspiration. All paraesophageal hernias should be reduced because of the risk for volvulus and subsequent incarceration. General principles of operative repair include reduction and resection of the hernia sac, anterior reapproximation of the crura to close the diaphragmatic defect, and gastropexy of the reduced stomach to prevent reherniation through the completed repair. Although a minority of patients with paraesophageal hernia have reflux disease, the decision to pursue laparoscopic reduction should not preclude a definitive antireflux procedure if preoperative endoscopy shows esophagitis. Vascular compromise of an incarcerated hernia should be approached as an open procedure, with preparation of the left side of the chest for possible resection of nonviable tissues that are not reducible via a transabdominal approach.

Sliding hiatal hernias do not require operative repair unless esophageal manometry and 24-hour pH studies show gastroesophageal reflux in the context of clinical symptoms. Laparoscopic details of various antireflux procedures are discussed elsewhere (*see* Chapter 5).

Traumatic diaphragmatic injury complicates 2% to 5% of blunt abdominal trauma and up to 1 in 5 patients with penetrating trauma to the intrathoracic abdomen [11]. Both laparoscopic [12] and thoracoscopic [11] approaches have been used to diagnose and treat traumatic injuries. Historically, the approach to traumatic hernias is determined by the likelihood of associated injuries and duration of disease: abdominal approaches should be used for acute injury because of the frequency of associated intraabdominal trauma, whereas thoracic approaches should be used for chronic herniations wherein the possibility of pleural adhesions complicates repair. However, Domene and coworkers [12] recently reported successful laparoscopic reduction and repair of a traumatic diaphragmatic hernia 3 years after the precipitating event.

Several technical aspects of the laparoscopic approach to diaphragmatic trauma deserve comment: 1) all patients should be intubated with a dual-lumen endotracheal tube and positioned for a thoracoabdominal incision in anticipation of thoracoscopy or thoracotomy, 2) a 30° laparoscope facilitates visualization of the subdiaphragmatic recess, 3) insufflation of the abdomen in a patient with diaphragmatic injuries can result in tension pneumothorax [13] and thus the possibility for emergency thoracostomy should be anticipated, and 4) tension-free repair of the diaphragmatic defect is aided by a reduction in pneumoperitoneum to less than 10 mm Hg. Minimally invasive approaches mandate a hemodynamic stability. Avulsed posterior-margin diaphragmatic defects require resuspension from the costal margin with interrupted mattress sutures encircling the rib and should be approached via open thoracotomy or laparotomy. Laparoscopic approaches have limited utility for right-sided diaphragmatic injuries.

Surgical Technique

Figures 7-2 through 7-15 depict the surgical technique for laparoscopic repair of diaphragmatic hernia.

Set-up

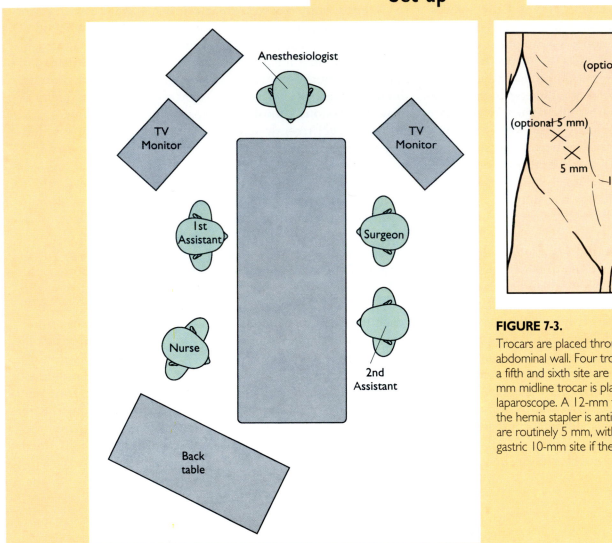

FIGURE 7-2.
The operating room set-up for the laparoscopic repair of a diaphragmatic hernia. The position of equipment and personnel is identical to that for laparoscopic Nissen fundoplication or laparoscopic cholecystectomy.

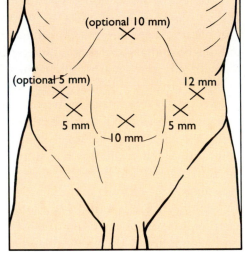

FIGURE 7-3.
Trocars are placed through the supraumbilical abdominal wall. Four trocar sites are routinely used; a fifth and sixth site are occasionally required. A 10-mm midline trocar is placed to allow access for the laparoscope. A 12-mm trocar is required if use of the hernia stapler is anticipated. The remaining sites are routinely 5 mm, with the exception of an epigastric 10-mm site if the liver retractor is needed.

Procedure

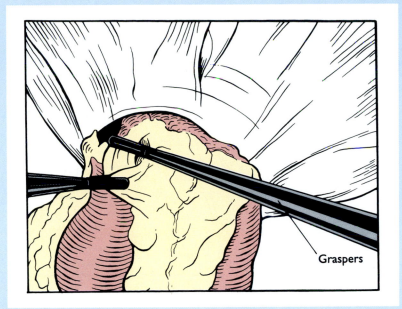

FIGURE 7-4.

The diaphragmatic defect is identified, and the contents of the hernia sac are reduced into the abdominal cavity. Atraumatic graspers are used to grasp the omentum and the antimesenteric surface of the bowel. Sharp dissection may be necessary if the incarcerated contents of the hernia adhere to the hernia sac.

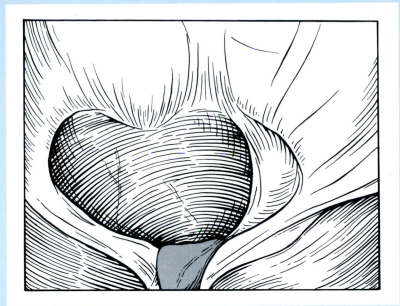

FIGURE 7-5.

The empty hernia sac is examined after reduction of the contents of the sac. A decision is made at this point regarding the need for dissection of the hernia sac in order to better delineate the edges of the defect.

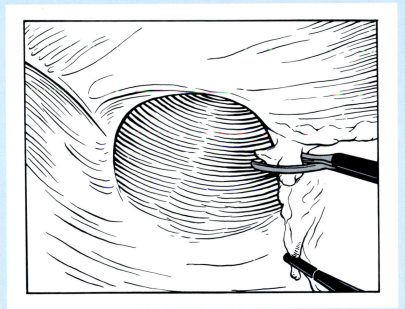

FIGURE 7-6.

The hernia sac is removed by using sharp dissection with the endoscopic scissors and cautery. Extreme caution must be exercised during this phase of the procedure to prevent the development of a tension pneumothorax. The proper tissue planes must be precisely identified to avoid inadvertent entry into the pericardium.

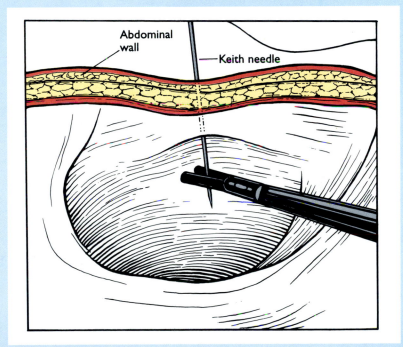

FIGURE 7-7.

A heavy monofilament suture on a Keith needle is passed through the anterior abdominal wall via a 2-mm skin incision. The needle is grasped intra-abdominally and passed through the edge of the diaphragm. An alternative method for repairing the diaphragmatic defect would include laparoscopic suturing or use of the hernia stapler to secure the edge of the diaphragmatic defect to the anterior abdominal wall. An extremely large hernia defect that cannot be approximated without excessive tension should be closed with prosthetic materials.

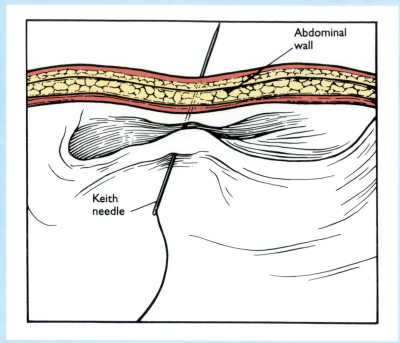

FIGURE 7-8.

Multiple horizontal mattress sutures are placed through the abdominal wall and edge of the hernia defect. Two or three mattress sutures are usually required to approximate these tissues.

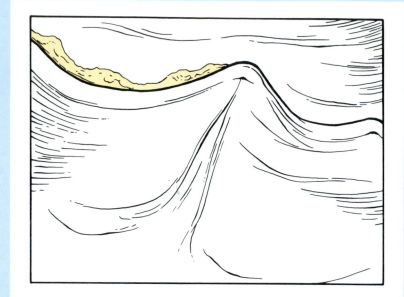

FIGURE 7-9.

The repaired hernia is demonstrated. The sutures are tied in a fashion that allows the knots to be buried underneath the skin at the fascia level.

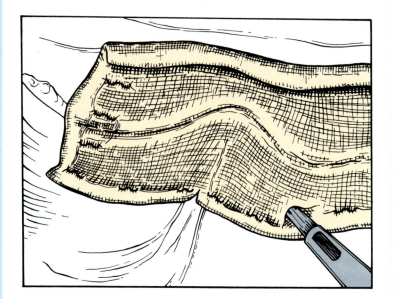

FIGURE 7-10.

The repaired hernia may be reinforced with the placement of synthetic mesh. This is secured circumferentially using a laparoscopic hernia stapler.

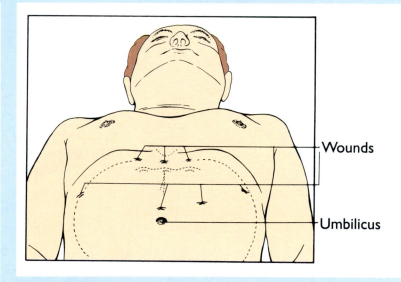

FIGURE 7-11.

The complete repair is demonstrated. The closed trocar sites and small counter incisions provide an excellent cosmetic result.

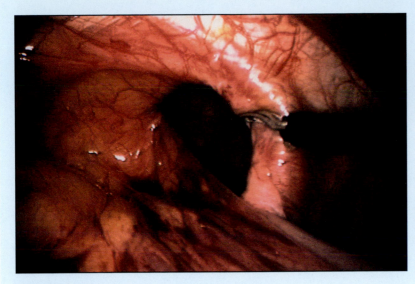

FIGURE 7-12.

The paraesophageal hernia is demonstrated with the previously incarcerated stomach reduced into the abdominal cavity. Releasing the graspers caused the stomach to quickly return to the thoracic portion of the hernia. This demonstrates the need to divide the adhesions between the gastric surface and the hernia sac. This is accomplished by using the laparoscopic scissors with cautery to maintain excellent hemostasis.

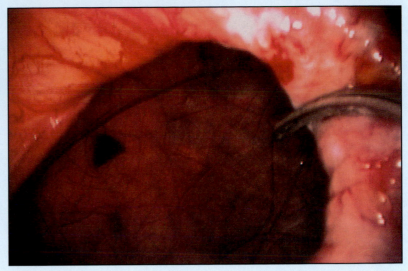

FIGURE 7-13.

The empty paraesophageal hernia sac is examined. The edges of this defect are clearly demarcated thus, there is no need for extensive dissection of the hernia sac. The edge of the sac along the diaphragmatic opening is divided-without removing the hernia sac. An attempt should be made to mobilize the esophagus at the gastroesophageal junction to allow elevation of the esophagus toward the anterior abdominal wall. This allows assessment of the posterior aspect of the hernia defect. The right and left crura should be approximated with interrupted or running sutures if this maneuver can be accomplished without excessive tension on the tissue.

FIGURE 7-14.

The right and left crura are approximated with sutures as the esophagus is elevated with a Penrose drain. Care should be taken to avoid injury to the anterior or posterior vagus nerves during this portion of the procedure.

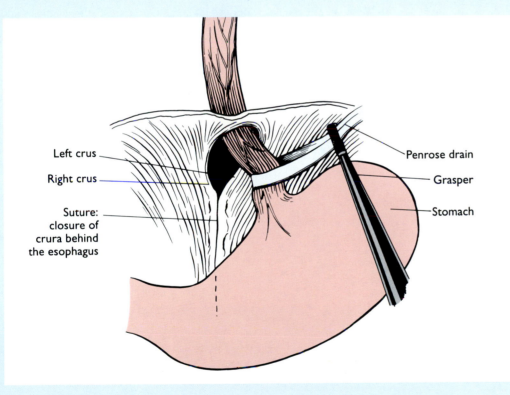

Left crus

Right crus

Suture: closure of crura behind the esophagus

Penrose drain

Grasper

Stomach

Procedure

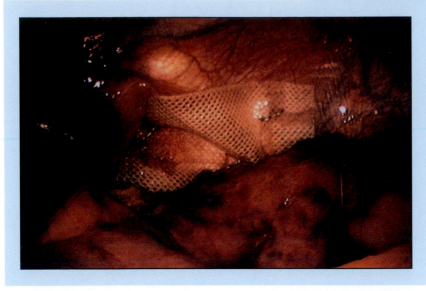

FIGURE 7-15.

Repair of the paraesophageal hernia using mesh may be required when the defect is too large to be closed by suture approximation of the crura. The mesh should be fashioned to fit over the esophagus at the gastroesophageal junction. The mesh is secured to the diaphragm by using the laparoscopic hernia stapler. The stomach should be fixed intra-abdominally either by suturing of the greater curvature of the fundus to the diaphragm (as shown) or by placement of a gastrostomy tube.

References

1. Morgagni GB: Seats and causes of diseases. Zellts 54. *Monograph on Hernia of the Diaphragm*; 1769.
2. Thomas TV: Subcostal diaphragmatic hernia. *J Thorac Cardiovasc Surg* 1972, 63:278.
3. Harrington SW: Various types of diaphragmatic hernias treated surgically: report of 430 cases. *Surg Gynecol Obstet* 1948, 86:735.
4. Bochdalek: *Einige Betrachtungen uber die Entstehung des angeborenen Zwerchfellbruches. Als Beitrag zur pathologischen Anatomie der Hernien. Vierteljahrschrift fur die praktische Heilkunde.* 1948; 19:89–97.
5. Skinner D: Hiatal hernia and gastroesophageal reflux. In *Textbook of Surgery*, 14th ed. Edited by Sabiston DC. Philadelphia: W.B. Saunders Company; 1991:704–715.
6. Skandalakis LJ, Colborn GL, Skandalakis JE: Surgical anatomy of the diaphragm. In: *Mastery of Surgery*, edn 3. Edited by Nykus LM, Baker RJ, Fischer JE: Boston: Little, Brown; 1997:649–670.
7. Harrison MR, Adzick NS, Flake A, *et al.*: Correction of congenital diaphragmatic hernia in utero: VI. Hard earned lessons. *J Pediatr Surg* 1993, 28:1411–1417.
8. Kimmestiel FM, Holgersen LO, Hilfer C: Retrosternal (Morgagni) hernia with small bowel obstruction secondary to a Richter's incarceration. *J Pediatr Surg* 1987, 22:998–1000.
9. Newman L, Eubanks S. Bridges M, Lucas G: Laparoscopic diagnosis and treatment of Morgagni hernia. *Surg Laparosc Endosc* 1995, 5:27–31.
10. Bortul M, Calligaris L, Gheller P: Laparoscopic repair of a Morgagni-Larrey hernia. *J Laparoendosc Adv Surg Tech* 1998, 8:309–313.
11. Koehler RH, Smith RS: Thoracoscopic repair of missed diaphragmatic injury in penetrating trauma: case report. *J TraumaI 1994, 36:424N427.*
12. Domene C, Volpe P, Santo M, *et al.*: Laparoscopic treatment of traumatic diaphragmatic hernia. *J Laparoendosc Adv Surg Tech* 1998, 8:225–229.
13. Ivatury RR, Simon RJ, Weksler B, *et al.*: Laparoscopy in the evaluation of the intrathoracic abdomen after penetrating trauma. *J Trauma* 1992, 33:101–108.

Laparoscopic Repair of Perforated Ulcer and Vagotomy

Ashish S. Shah
Theodore N. Pappas

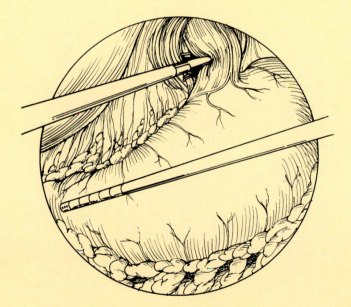

Peptic ulcer disease is primarily an affliction of the 20th century, although it was first identified in 1799 [1]. As the disease became widespread in the early to mid 1900s, antiulcer operations were developed and refined. Truncal vagotomy was introduced by Dragstedt and Owens in 1943 [2]. When paired with a drainage procedure, it quickly superseded more extensive operations to become the mainstay of surgical therapy for peptic ulcer disease. This and other procedures soon made up a large proportion of elective abdominal surgery.

The discovery and widespread use of medical therapy have profoundly affected the management of peptic ulcer disease. In particular, therapy directed against *Helicobacter pylori* infection has improved ulcer cure rates and reduced recurrence rates [3]. Elective surgery is confined to patients with recurrent or resistant ulcer disease. Despite the decline in the number of elective operations performed for peptic ulcer disease, the number of operations performed for complications remains unchanged [4]. These patients are older and moribund and remain a surgical challenge.

Laparascopic approaches to peptic ulcer disease have flourished over the past decade. Among the array of operations performed for antiulcer surgery, vagotomy (paricularly highly selective vagotomy) and repair of duodenal perforation have been amenable to laparoscopic techniques. To date, these methods have been shown to improve postoperative recovery with outcomes similar to those seen with conventional surgery.

Anatomy

The right and left vagus nerves provide parasympathetic input to the stomach and the remaining gastrointestinal tract (Fig. 8-1). Closely approximating the outer wall of the esophagus near the diaphragmatic hiatus, the right and left trunks follow the direction of embryonic foregut rotation. Accordingly, the right vagus rotates to a posterior position while the left vagus curves anteriorly. Before reaching the gastroesophageal junction, the posterior trunk bifurcates, sending a branch to the celiac plexus. The anterior trunk

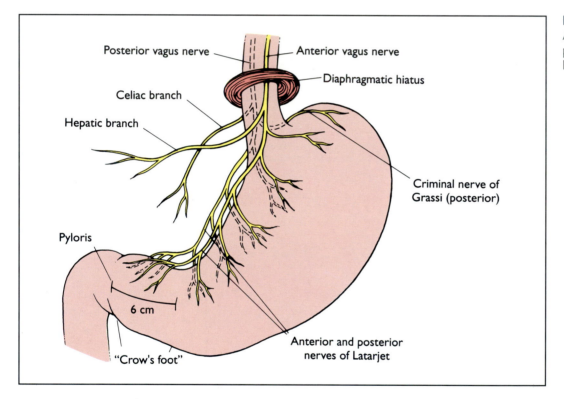

Posterior vagus nerve

Anterior vagus nerve

Diaphragmatic hiatus

Celiac branch

Hepatic branch

Criminal nerve of Grassi (posterior)

Pyloris

6 cm

Anterior and posterior nerves of Latarjet

"Crow's foot"

FIGURE 8-1.

Anatomy showing the right and left vagus nerves providing parasympathetic input to the stomach, liver, and celiac plexus.

also splits, forming a division that supplies the liver. The posterior and anterior gastric branches (nerves of Latarjet) then follow the lesser gastric curvature, where smaller branches enter the gastric wall. The primary nerves terminate in a "crow's foot," which innervates the pylorus and approximately 6 cm of distal stomach. Here, the vagus primarily affects gastric emptying.

Pathophysiology, Presentation, and Differential Diagnosis

The exact pathophysiologic mechanism of peptic ulcer formation is unknown, although there are a number of closely associated factors (Fig. 8-2). The normal physiology of gastric acid secretion is illustrated in Figure 8-3. Production of gastric acid by the parietal cell is affected by acetylcholine, histamine, and gastrin. Increased gastric acid and pepsin secretion are often present in patients with peptic ulcer disease. The markedly high acid levels are thought to be due to abnormal proliferation of oxyntic glands

[5]. It has become evident, however, that impairment of mucosal resistance may be just as important [6]. Alterations in blood flow, growth factor concentrations, bicarbonate production, mucus secretion, and prostaglandin synthesis can all damage the mucosal barrier. Nonsteroidal anti-inflammatory drugs (NSAIDs) may compromise mucosal defenses by inhibiting the synthesis of protective prostaglandins [7]. Table 8-1 outlines pharmacologic and other agents that are associated with peptic ulcer formation. Other factors, including altered gastric motility, genetic disposition, glucocorticoid use, cigarette smoking, and psychologic stress have undetermined roles in the pathogenesis of peptic ulcer disease [8]. In addition, interactions among ulcerogenic factors are highly complex and may vary among individuals. The therapeutic approach to peptic ulcer disease has been revolutionized by the identification of *H. pylori*. This gram-negative bacteria has been implicated in chronic gastric and duodenal ulcers, as well as ulcer recurrence. Eradication of the bacteria in patients with ulcer dramatically reduces the recurrence rate. Therefore, identification

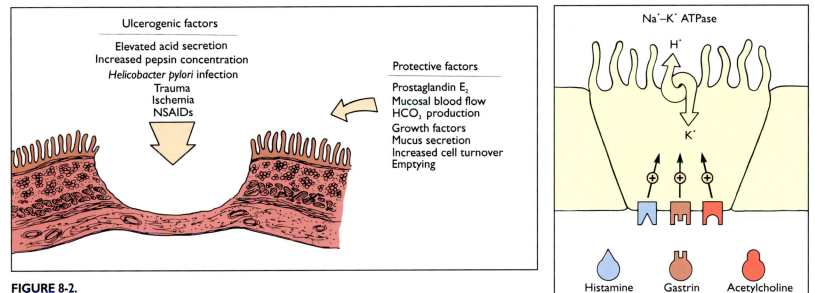

FIGURE 8-2.

Pathogenesis of peptic ulcer formation. NSAIDs—nonsteroidal anti-inflammatory drugs.

FIGURE 8-3.

Normal physiology of gastric acid secretion. Three separate pathways, mediated by histamine, gastrin, and acetylcholine, stimulate the parietal cell Na^+-K^+ adenosine triphosphatase (ATPase) to produce gastric acid.

and antimicrobial treatment play integral roles in the medical management of peptic ulcer disease [9,10].

Peptic ulcer disease commonly presents with pain, often described as a burning, gnawing, aching, or even hungry sensation. Pain will occur 1 to 3 hours after meals and may awaken the patient at night. The classic pattern of epigastric pain relieved by meals or antacids may not always be present. Also, some patients without pain have upper gastrointestinal endoscopy or radiologic contrast studies that reveal persistent ulceration of the duodenal bulb. Candidates for laparoscopic vagotomy are patients with persistent pain or documented ulceration refractory to medical therapy. These conditions may be due either to severe ulcer diathesis or noncompliance with medication.

Perforation is a persistent problem in peptic ulcer disease. Approximately 50% of perforations occur in the duodenum and are associated with the use of steriods and NSAIDs. Perforation commonly presents as acute abdominal pain and may be a cata-strophic event associated with hypotension, tachycardia, and tachypnea. The presence of diffuse abdominal tenderness and rigidity confirms the presence of peritoneal irritation. It is important to note, however, that more than 20% of patients are already hospitalized and that 50% have a significant medical illness at the time of presentation [3]. Thus, other causes of acute abdominal pain must be carefully considered. Because many of these patients are not candidates for definitive ulcer operations, laparoscopic repair of the ulcer may be well suited for this population.

The differential diagnosis for chronic epigastric pain in lieu of proven peptic ulcer disease includes gastric ulceration, gastritis, Zollinger-Ellison syndrome, pancreatitis, carcinoma of the stomach or pancreas, esophageal disease, symptomatic cholelithiasis, chronic cholecystitis, abdominal wall disorders, and angina from myocardial ischemia or pericarditis. Many other conditions cause abdominal symptoms that can mimic ulcer disease or its complications (Table 8-2).

Table 8-1. Ulcerogenic drugs and other associated factors

Ulcerogenic drugs		Other associated factors
NSAIDs:		Chronic gastritis
Diclofenac	Meclofenamic acid	Cigarette smoking
Etodolac	Nabumetone	Coffee
Fenoprofen	Naproxen	Ethanol
Flurbiprofen	Phenylbutazone	Glucocorticoids
Ibuprofen	Piroxicam	Lewis phenotype
Indomethacin	Sulindac	Male sex
Ketoprofen	Tenoxicam	Psychologic stress
Ketorolac	Tolmetin	Prior localized radiation therapy

NSAIDs—nonsteroidal anti-inflammatory drugs.

Table 8-2. Differential diagnosis of peptic ulcer disease

Upper gastrointestinal tract	Other intra-abdominal	Other
Esophagitis	Colonic carcinoma	Pneumonia
Gastric ulcer	Benign colonic diseases	Pleuritic pain
Gastritis	Mesenteric ischemia	Pulmonary embolus
Zollinger-Ellison syndrome	Infarction of liver or spleen	Costochondritis
Carcinoma of the stomach, pancreas, or esophagus	Bowel obstruction	Myocardial ischemia
Pancreatitis	Meckel's diverticulitis	Pericarditis
Gallbladder disease		Sickle cell crisis
		Abdominal wall disorders
		Renal pain
		Factitious abdominal pain

Surgical Technique

Laparoscopic vagatomy

Figures 8-4 through 8-24 depict the surgical technique for laparoscopic vagotomy.

Set-up

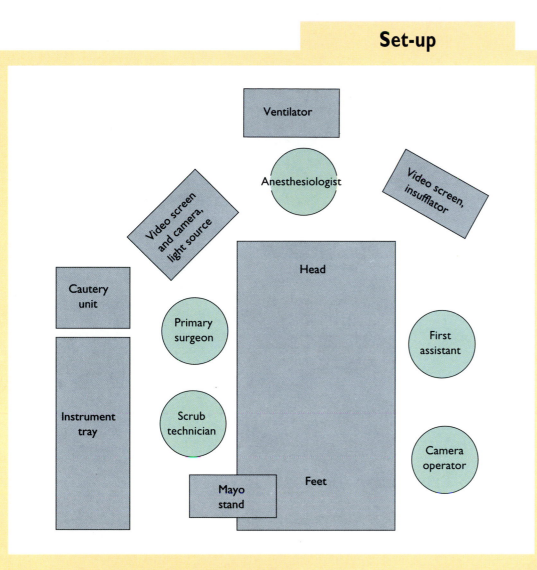

FIGURE 8-4.
Operative set-up for laparoscopic vagotomy. Antibiotics are administered at the time of induction of general anesthesia. Foley and nasogastric catheters are placed. The abdomen is prepared in the usual fashion.

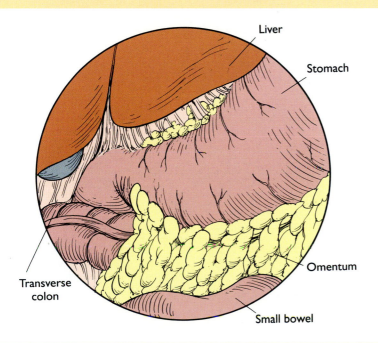

FIGURE 8-5.
The patient is first placed in the Trendelenburg position. A Veress needle or Hasson trocar is used to enter the peritoneal cavity for carbon dioxide insufflation to 12 to 15 mm Hg. The laparoscope is inserted through the 10-mm sheath placed above or below the umbilicus, and the abdominal contents are examined. In individuals with long abdomens, a better view of the hiatus is obtained with supraumbilical camera placement. The patient is then placed in reversed Trendelenburg position and the liver, gallbladder, small bowel, omentum, and stomach are identified.

Set-up

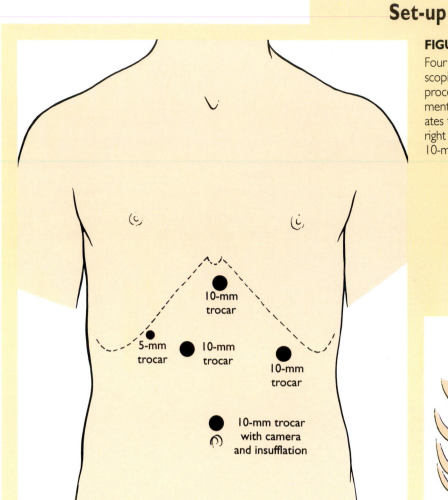

FIGURE 8-6.

Four additional trocars are placed in the upper abdomen under direct laparoscopic vision. A 10-mm trocar is placed in the upper midline near the xyphoid process and to the left of the falciform ligament. Through it, a retracting instrument is introduced for holding the liver away from the hiatus. The surgeon operates from two ports, a 5-mm and 10-mm port placed a few centimeters to the right of the midline. The first assistant operates from the left side through a 10-mm trocar placed in the left midclavicular line near the costal margin.

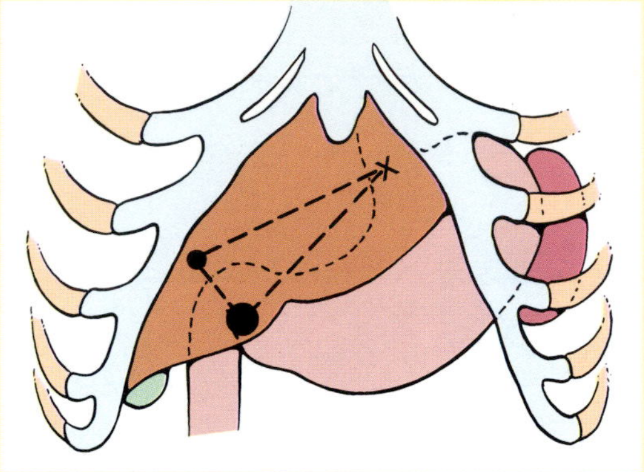

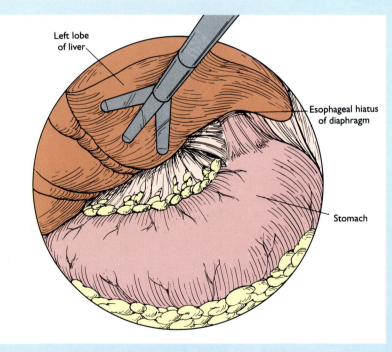

FIGURE 8-7.

The position of the primary surgeon's operating trocars. The 5- and 10-mm ports are located at the basal corners of an isosceles triangle. This hiatus represents the apex of the triangle. This set-up allows the surgeon to use both hands simultaneously.

Procedure

FIGURE 8-8.

The internal anatomy of the hiatal area is shown. A fan retractor is used to hold the left lobe of the liver away from the gastroesophageal junction. The assistant may use an endoscopic Babcock to pull the stomach inferiorly.

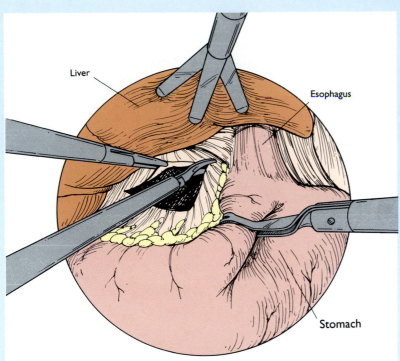

FIGURE 8-9.

Exposure of the hiatus. Endoscopic scissors or a small blunt grasper with electrocautery is used by the surgeon to divide the lesser omentum. The edges are retracted away, exposing the diaphragmatic hiatus.

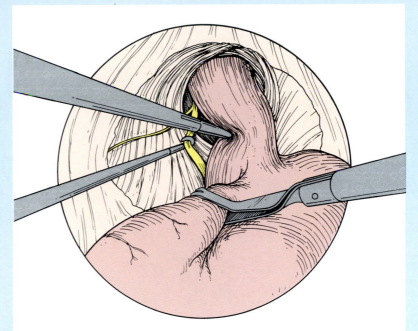

FIGURE 8-10.

Exposure of the posterior vagus is illustrated. After creation of a plane between the right crus of the diaphragm and the esophagus, the surgeon retracts the esophagus to the left with a blunt dissector. The posterior vagus is identified on the posterior surface of the esophagus at the inferior border of the hiatus. With the hook dissector in the other hand, the surgeon dissects and lifts the nerve away from surrounding structures.

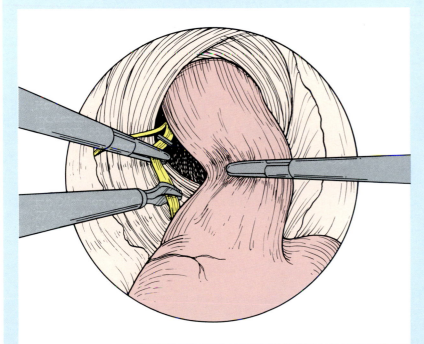

FIGURE 8-11.

The posterior vagus is grasped with endoscopic forceps and clipped superiorly and inferiorly with endoscopic clips. It should be clipped as high as possible in the hiatus to ensure division of the criminal nerve of Grassi.

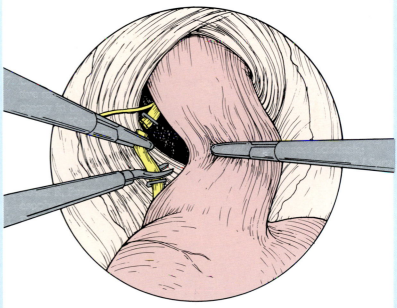

FIGURE 8-12.

Endoscopic scissors are used to remove the section between clips for pathologic confirmation. Before proceeding, the posterior esophagus is examined for any remaining vagal fibers.

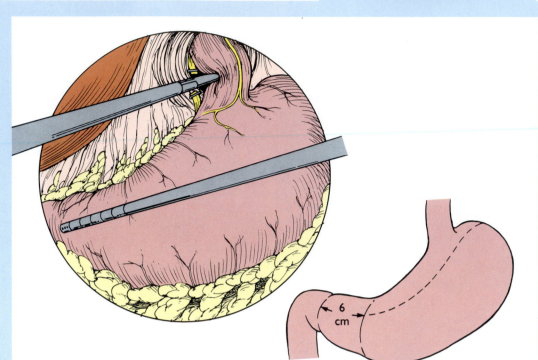

FIGURE 8-13.
Following posterior truncal vagotomy, anterior highly selective vagotomy is performed. Dissection of the branches of the anterior nerve of Latarjet is begun 6 cm from the pylorus, sparing the "crow's foot" innervation to the pylorus. This distance may be measured by placing 1-cm markings on an endoscopic suction/irrigation device before insertion into the abdomen. The 6-cm distance may then be measured and superficially marked on the stomach wall with the electrocautery.

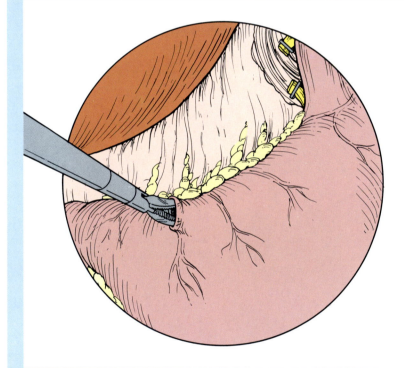

FIGURE 8-14.
Dissection of the anterior vagal branches is illustrated. The alligator forceps are used to dissect and isolate each anterior neurovascular bundle along the lesser curvature, as shown. Dissection is limited to areas on the stomach wall. Special care is taken to include the anterior fibers at the base of the esophagus.

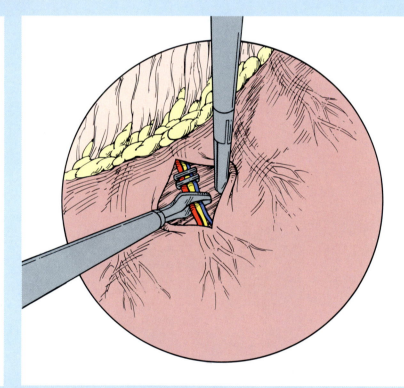

FIGURE 8-15.
Each neurovascular bundle along the line of dissection is doubly clipped. (A total of four clips are placed in each bundle.)

Procedure

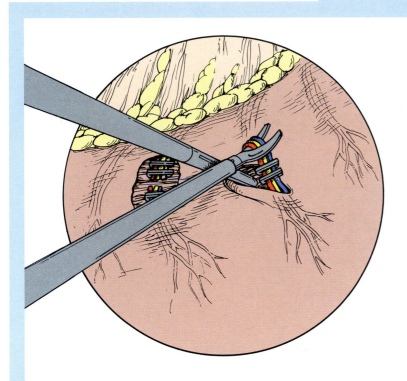

FIGURE 8-16.
Nerve branch, artery, and vein are sharply divided between clips.

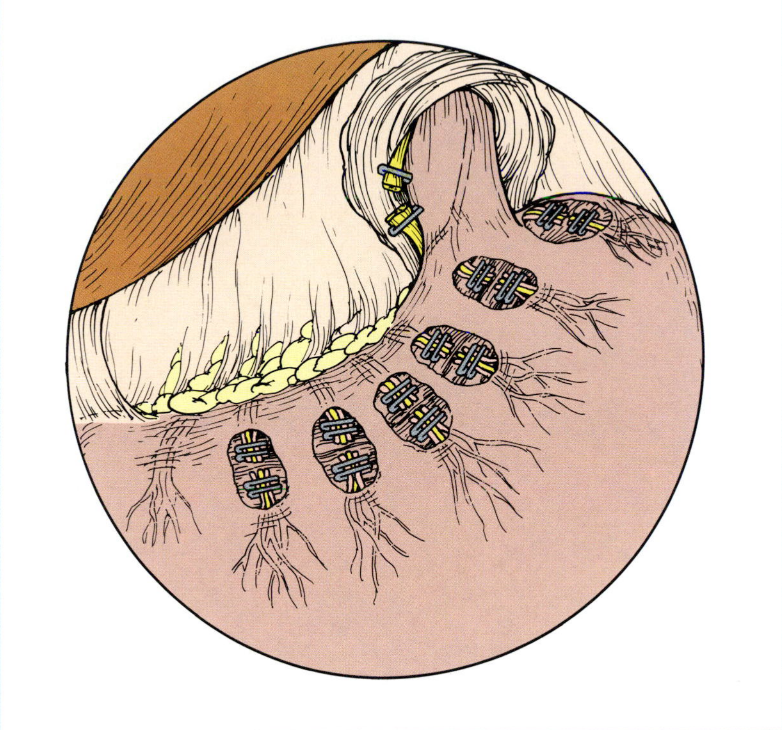

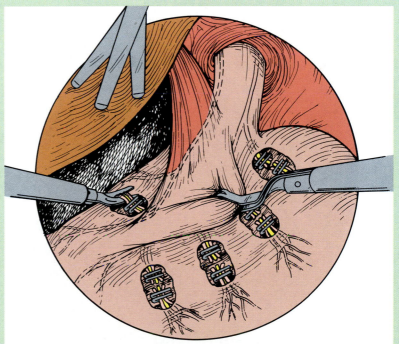

FIGURE 8-17.
The completed posterior truncal vagotomy and anterior highly selective vagotomy are illustrated.

Alternative Procedure

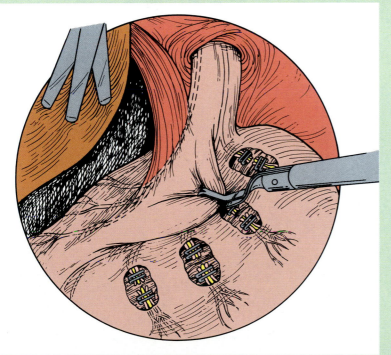

FIGURE 8-18.
When technically feasible, anterior and posterior highly selective vagotomy is a desirable alternative to posterior truncal vagotomy and anterior highly selective vagotomy. Retraction of the lesser curvature by the assistant gives the surgeon access to the posterior wall of the stomach.

FIGURE 8-19.
As with the anterior highly selective vagotomy, dissection is initiated 6 cm from the pylorus. Nerve branch, artery, and vein are isolated, clipped, and divided.

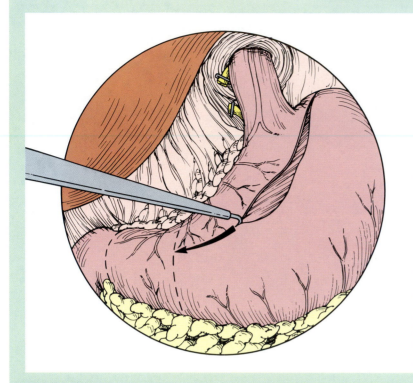

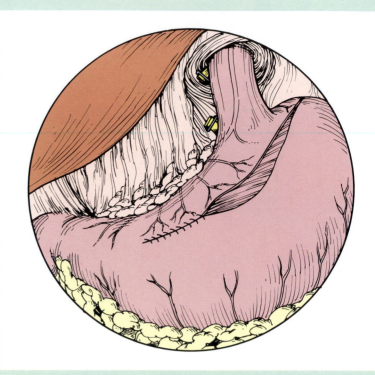

FIGURE 8-20.

Anterior lesser curvature seromyotomy is an alternative to anterior highly selective vagotomy. A hook electrocautery dissector or laser probe is used to perform a seromyotomy 1.5 cm from the lesser curvature, beginning at the gastroesophageal junction and ending 6 cm from the pylorus. Close-range direct laparoscopic vision is required.

FIGURE 8-21.

Homeostasis is facilitated by oversewing using running suture technique or by application of fibrin glue or other procoagulant materials. Intragastric methylene blue dye confirms the absence of perforation.

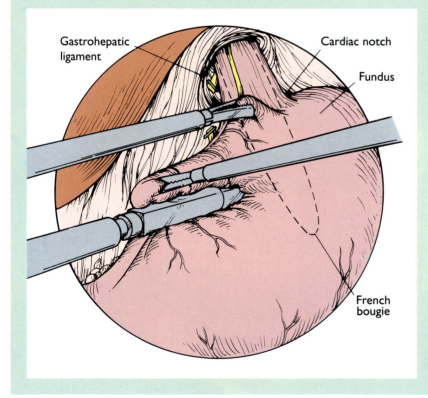

Gastrohepatic ligament

Cardiac notch

Fundus

French bougie

FIGURE 8-22.

Anterior highly selective vagotomy may alternatively be performed with a stapling device. After insertion of a bougie dilator through the gastroesophageal junction, the endoscopic stapling device is placed across a double full thickness of the anterior gastric wall.

Alternative Procedure

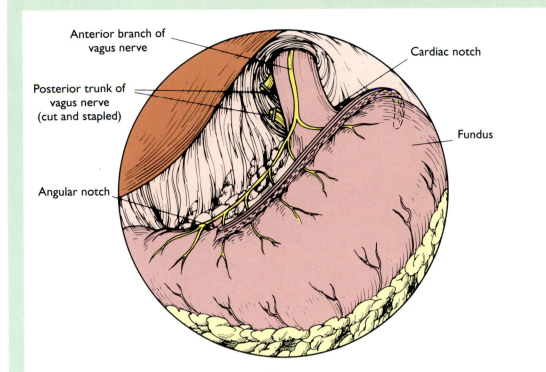

Anterior branch of vagus nerve

Posterior trunk of vagus nerve (cut and stapled)

Angular notch

Cardiac notch

Fundus

FIGURE 8-23.
Serial end-to-end stapling along the lesser curvature is used to complete the procedure.

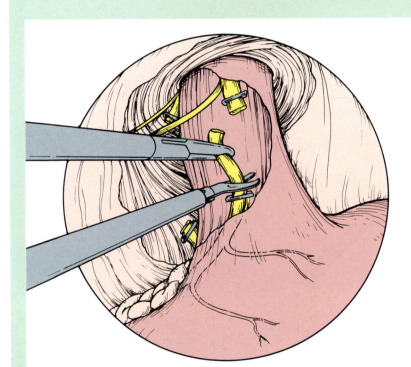

FIGURE 8-24.
Anterior and posterior truncal vagotomy with drainage is preferred for patients with obstruction. The anterior vagal trunk is dissected, clipped superiorly and inferiorly, and the interposing segment is removed for histologic section. The posterior truncal vagotomy is performed as previously described.

Laparoscopic repair of duodenal perforation

Figures 8-25 through 8-28 depict the surgical technique for laparoscopic repair of duodenal perforation.

Procedure

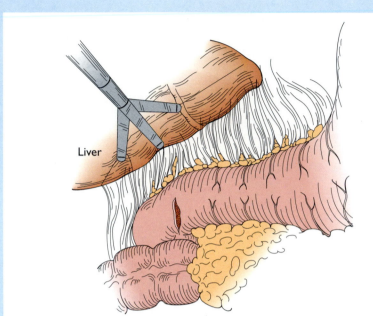

FIGURE 8-25.

Operative set up and exposure is the same for repair of perforation. After identification of relevant anatomy, the liver is retracted superiorly to expose the site of perforation. Any fibrin and tissue should also be debrided and irrigated from the anterior duodenum.

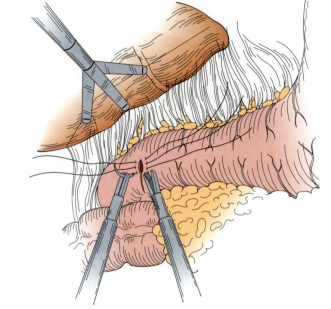

FIGURE 8-26.

To prevent further intraperitoneal soilage, attention is first turned to closure of the perforation. Three fine silk or polyglactin sutures are placed across the perforation, with the tails left long. The sutures are then tied to close the perforation. Care should be taken to take ample seromuscular bites of duodenum away from friable, ulcerated tissue.

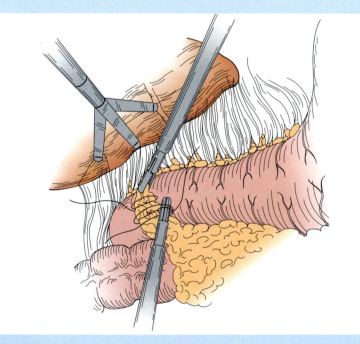

FIGURE 8-27.

A pedicle of greater omentem is placed across the perforation by using a grasper through the subxiphoid port and sutures tied over the onlay patch, using an intracorporeal suture technique. Alternatively, a laparoscopic endoclip may be used to tack the omentum to the doudenal wall. Care must be taken not to strangulate the omental patch.

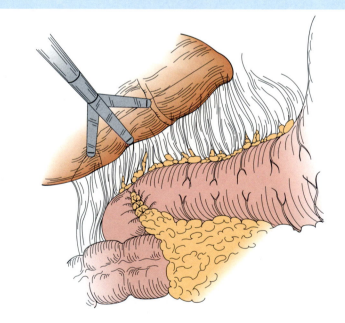

FIGURE 8-28.

Finished repair. After closure of the perforation, the abdominal cavity should be copiously irrigated. Special attention should be paid to the paracolic gutters and around the liver. No abdominal drains are placed.

Results

The use of laparoscopic vagotomy and particularly highly selective vagotomy has steadily increased over the past decade. Table 8-3 outlines series and case reports to date with short-term results. No operative deaths have been reported, and few operative morbidities have occurred. In all cases, the procedure was well tolerated and associated with a brief in-hospital postoperative recovery.

Highly selective vagotomy is the traditional operation of choice for uncomplicated intractable peptic ulcer disease. Compared with other procedures, it is associated with a lower incidence of side effects such as dumping syndrome. In recent studies, conventional highly selective vagotomy has been associated with a recurrence rate less than 10% in patients in whom medical therapy has failed [11]. Truncal vagotomy and antrectomy have much lower recurrence rates; however, the incidence of diarrhea and dumping is high. The acid-reducing efficacy of laparascopic highly selective vagotomy has been clearly demonstrated, and a number of studies have documented recurrence rates that are similar to those of open surgery. Conversion to an open procedure is rare, and complications are related to patients with delayed gastric emptying. Many of these patients have been succesfully treated by balloon dilatation or medical therapy. More compelling, however, is the consistent and significant reductions in hospital stay and overall recovery period [12]. Table 8-4 summarizes significant reports of laparoscopic duodenal perforation repair. Overall, the mortality in larger series' approaches 5% [13], thus demonstrating the feasibility of the laparoscopic approach. In patients without an ulcer history, an antiulcer operation is necessary at the time of repair, although one may be performed laparoscopically as described. Some studies have also reported the use of a vagotomy procedure for recurrent ulceration in a small number of these patients.

Over the past decade, laparoscopic methods have expanded to include treatment of complications of peptic ulcer disease. Both vagotomy for recurrent and resistant disease, as well as duodenal perforation, have been safely and effectively treated with laparoscopic intervention. The benefit of the approach appears to lie in improved postoperative recovery time and patient comfort. In addition, some investigators have argued that improved video imaging may improve precision in performing highly selective vagotomy. Further prospective studies will help explore and clarify the role of each of these treatment methods.

Table 8-3. Reported laparoscopic vagotomy cases

Study	Year	Total, n	HSV	PTAHS	PTASM	TBDP	Thor	TGJ	T	Decrease in acid secretion, %	Postoperative in-hospital days
Dallamagne and coworkers [12]	1994	35	35	—	—	—	—	—	—	77	3.6
Kum and Goh [14]	1992	12	—	6	2	3	—	—	—	12	4
Bailey and coworkers [15]	1991	1*	—	1	—	—	—	1	—	NR	2
Mouiel and Katkhouda [16]	1993	36	—	—	34	2	—	—	—	36	3–5
Laws and coworkers [17]	1992	4	—	—	—	—	4	—	—	NR	1–3
Chisholm and coworkers [18]	1992	1	—	—	—	—	1	—	—	NR	3
Murphy and McDermott [19]	1991	4	—	—	—	—	—	—	4	NR	NR
Nottle [20]	1991	1	—	1	—	—	—	—	—	NR	3
Katkhouda and coworkers [21]	1998	10	10	—	—	—	—	—	—	74	2
Frantzides and coworkers [22]	1997	11	11	—	—	—	—	—	—	NR	1.7
Autanz and coworkers [23]	1997	32	—	—	—	32	—	—	—	70	4.8
Nisii and coworkers [24]	1997	9	—	9	—	—	—	—	—	73	9
Wyman and coworkers [25]	1996	12	—	—	—	—	—	12	—	NR	6

*Performed with laparoscopic cholecystectomy.
HSV—highly selective vagotomy; NR—not reported; PTAHS—posterior truncal and anterior highly selective vagotomy; PTASM—posterior truncal vagotomy and anterior lesser curvature seromyotomy; T—truncal vagotomy without drainage; TBDP—truncal vagotomy with balloon dilation of the pylorus; TGJ—truncal vagotomy and gastrojejunostomy; Thor—thoracoscopic vagotomy.

Table 8-4. Reported cases of laparoscopic perforated ulcer repair

Study	Year	Total, n	Operative mortality, %	Length of in-hospital stay, d
Miserez and coworkers [26]	1996	18	5.5	10
So and coworkers [27]	1996	15	0	7
Druart and coworkers [13]	1997	100	5	9.3
Matsuda and coworkers [28]	1995	11	0	17
Thompson and coworkers [29]	1995	5	0	6.5

References

1. Wilbur DL: The history of disease of the stomach and duodenum with reference also to etiology. In *The Stomach and Duodenum.* Edited by Eusterman GB, Balfour DL. Philadelphia: W.B. Saunders; 1935.

2. Dragstedt LR, Owens RM, Jr: Supradiaphragmatic section of vagus nerves in treatment of duodenal ulcer. *Proc Soc Exp Biol Med* 1943, 53:152–154.

3. Pappas TN: The stomach and duodenum: historical aspects, anatomy, pathology, physiology, and peptic ulcer disease. In *Sabiston Textbook of Surgery.* 1997, 15:847–867.

4. Hamby LS, Zweng TN, Strodel WE. Perforated gastric and duodenal ulcer: an analysis of prognostic factors. *The American Surgeon* 1993, 59:319–324.

5. Mulholland MW, Debas HT: Chronic duodenal and gastric ulcer. *Surg Clin North Am* 1987, 67:489.

6. Szabo S: Gastroduodenal mucosal injury—acute and chronic: pathways, mediators, and mechanisms. *J Clin Gastroenterol* 1991, 13(suppl):S1–S8.

7. Selling JA, Hogan DL, Aly A, *et al.*: Indomethacin inhibits duodenal mucosal bicarbonate secretion and endogenous prostaglandin E_2 output in human subjects. *Ann Intern Med* 1987, 106:368–371.

8. Mertz HR, Walsh JH: Peptic ulcer pathophysiology. *Med Clin North Am* 1991, 75:799–814.

9. Hentschel E, Brandstäatter G, Dragosics B, *et al.*: Effect of ranitidine and amoxicillin plus metronidazole on the eradication of *Helicobacter pylori* and the recurrence of duodenal ulcer. *N Engl J Med* 1993, 328:308–312.

10. Walsh JH, Peterson WL: The treatment of Helicobacter pylori infection in the management of peptic ulcer disease. *New Engl J Med* 1995, 333:984–991.

11. Wilkinson JM, Hosie KB, *et al.*: Long-term results of highly selective vagotomy: a prospective study with implication for future laparoscopic surgery. *Br J Surg* 1994, 81:1469–1471.

12. Dallemange B, Weerts JM, *et al.*: Laparoscopic highly selective vagotomy. *Br J Surg* 1994, 81:554–556.

13. Druart ML, Van Hee R, *et al.*: Laparoscopic repair of perforated duodenal ulcer. A prospective multicenter clinical trail. *Surg Endosc* 1997, 11:1017–1020.

14. Kum CK, Goh P: Laparoscopic vagotomy: a new tool in the management of duodenal ulcer disease [letter]. *Br J Surg* 1992, 79(9):977.

15. Bailey RW, Flowers JL, Graham SM, *et al.*: Combined laparoscopic cholecystectomy and selective vagotomy. *Surg Laparosc Endosc* 1991, 1(1):45–49.

16. Mouiel J, Katkhouda N: Laparoscopic vagotomy for chronic duodenal ulcer disease. *World J Surg* 1993, 17:34–39.

17. Laws HL, Naughton MJ, McKernan BJ: Thoracoscopic vagectomy for recurrent peptic ulcer disease. *Surg Laparosc Endosc* 1992, 2(1):24–28.

18. Chisholm EM, Chung SCS, Sunderland GT, *et al.*: Thoracoscopic vagotomy: a new use for the laparoscope. *Br J Surg* 1992, 79:254.

19. Murphy JJ, McDermott EWM: Laparoscopic truncal vagotomy without drainage for the treatment of chronic duodenal ulcer. *Irish Med J* 1991/1992, 84(4):125–126.

20. Nottle PD: Laparoscopic vagotomy for chronic duodenal ulcer. *Med J Aust* 1991, 155(9):648.

21. Katkhouda N, Waldrep DJ, *et al.*: An improved technique for laparoscopic highly selective vagotomy using harmonic shears. *Surg Endosc* 1998, 12:1051–1054.

22. Franzitedes, *et al.*:Laparoscopic highly selective vagotomy. *J Laparoendosc Adv Surg Tech A* 1997, 7:143–146.

23. Autanz L, Ozman V, *et al.*: Video endoscopic truncal vagotomy without gastric drainage. *Surg Lap Endosc* 1997, Dec: 439–444.

24. Nisii H, Hirai T, *et al.*: Laparoscopic Hill's vagotomy by the abdominal wall lifiting method. *Surg Lap Endosc* 1997, 7:394–398.

25. Wyman A, Stuart RC, *et al.*: Laparoscopic truncal vagotomy and gasteroenterostomy for pyloric stenosis. *Am J Surg* 1996, 171:600–603.

26. Miserez A, Eypasch E, *et al.*: Laparoscopic and conventional closure of perforated peptic ulcer. A comparison. *Surg Endosc* 1996, 8:831–836.

27. So JB, Kum Ck, *et al.*: Comparison between laparoscopic and conventional omental patch repair for perforated duodenal ulcer. *Surg Endosc* 1996, 10:1060–1063.

28. Matsuda M, Nishiyama M, Hanai T, Saeki S, Watanabe T: Laparoscopic omental patch repair for perforated peptic ulcer. *Ann Surg* 1995, 221:236–240.

29. Thompson AR, Hall TJ, Anglin BA, Scott-Connor CE. Laparoscopic plication of perforated ulcer: results of a selective approach. *South Med J* 1995, 88:185–189.

*L*aparoscopic Ostomies

Lisa A. Clark
John P. Grant

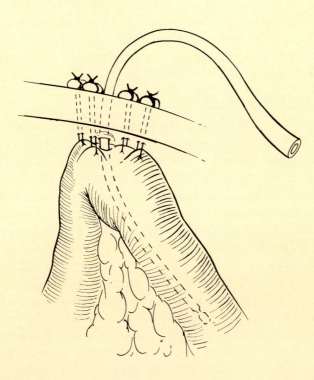

$\mathcal{D}$irect access to the alimentary track through the abdominal wall is desirable in a variety of clinical settings. In general, the goal is to provide access for nutritional support or to establish intestinal diversion. Laparoscopic techniques are now available to perform intestinal access, offering a minimally invasive approach for selected patients. In this chapter we discuss laparoscopic gastrostomy, jejunostomy, ileostomy, and colostomy.

Laparoscopic Gastrostomy and Jejunostomy

Access for prolonged enteral feeding in the debilitated patient is a common clinical necessity. It is important in these patients to minimize morbidity and cost while enhancing quality of life. Although oral feeding is optimal, the presence of an altered mental status, dysphagia, or obstruction often requires that artificial access be established into the stomach or jejunum. If access can be placed, enteral feeding has been shown to be effective and inexpensive and to require relatively simple care that can be provided in the hospital, nursing care facility, or home.

Indications for instituting long-term enteral feedings are summarized in Table 9-1. Several issues should be considered when choosing an anatomic site for long-term feeding access. Because the stomach serves as a reservoir for masticated food, dilutes hypertonic fluids, has a digestive role in the initial breakdown of food, and regulates efflux of food into the proximal duodenum, gastric feeding is advantageous over jejunal feeding. In contrast to jejunal access, gastrostomy tube placement allows intermittent bolus feeding, is more economical (because it usually requires less equipment), and allows safe administration of nearly all required medications. The jejunal route should be considered only for long-term feeding; when gastric access is contraindicated (such as in the presence of gastroparesis); in patients with small gastric remnants, gastric varices, or gastric carcinoma; and when there is a risk of aspiration. When jejunal feeding is indicated, steady infusion by use of a pump is preferable over bolus feeding to prevent diarrhea secondary to the "dumping" that occurs when hyperosmolar, carbohydrate-rich formulas are administered too rapidly into the small bowel. Feedings can usually be done cyclically over 12 to 14 hours per day. Great care must be exercised when medications are given directly into the jejunum to avoid clogging of the tube, prevent diarrhea from hyperosmolality, and assure absorption of the drug. Both a gastrostomy for decompression and a jejunostomy for feedings are sometimes required.

Placement of both gastrostomy and jejunostomy tubes has traditionally been done through a laparotomy incision. In 1980, Gauderer and coworkers [1] reported on a new method for gastrostomy tube placement, percutaneous endoscopic gastrostomy (PEG). This technique has been widely accepted because it does not require general anesthesia or a laparotomy and has been associated with few complications (major complications, 2.8%; minor complications, 6.0%) [2]. If jejunal access is required, a feeding tube can be advanced through the gastrostomy tube or via the nose as a nasojejunal tube. Unfortunately, patients with obstructing esophageal lesions or oral or esophageal trauma are not candidates for the percutaneous endoscopic approach. With the advent of laparoscopic surgery in the late 1980s, placement of gastrostomy and jejunostomy tubes by this method now offers an alternative to laparotomy when a PEG cannot or should not be done.

Anatomy

The stomach is the largest dilation of the foregut that comes to lie in the left upper quadrant anteriorly. It is generally divided into five regions: cardia, fundus, corpus, antrum, and pylorus. The proximal margin of the stomach is the functional lower esophageal sphincter, whereas the anatomic pyloric sphincter separates the stomach from the duodenum. The optimal site for gastrostomy placement is in the mid-corpus. The small intestine extends from the pylorus to the cecum and consists of the duodenum (20 cm), jejunum (100 to 110 cm), and ileum (150 to 160 cm). The proximal margin of the jejunum is at the ligament of Treitz. The optimal site for jejunostomy placement is 20 to 30 cm distal to the ligament of Treitz.

Surgical Technique

Laparoscopic placement of a gastrostomy or jejunostomy tube is usually performed under general anesthesia. Because abdominal insufflation need be only 8 to 10 mm Hg, use of local anesthesia with intravenous sedation is acceptable in selected patients. Patients are placed supine on the operating table. For placement of a gastrostomy tube, the patient is placed in the reverse Trendelenburg position. For placement of a jejunostomy tube, a mild Trendelenburg position is preferred. The open Hasson technique for placement of the initial infraumbilical trocar should be used liberally in all patients, especially those with a history of abdominal surgery, to avoid inadvertent perforation of adjacent viscera or injury to major vascular structures. A Foley catheter may be helpful in avoiding bladder injuries, especially with the low-midline trocar placement for laparoscopic jejunostomy. The remaining technical aspects of the procedure are summarized in the figures below.

Figures 9-1 through 9-4 depict the relevant anatomy and operative set-up for laparoscopic jejunostomy or gastrostomy.

Table 9-1. Indications for enteral feeding

Dysfunctional swallow/recurrent aspiration
Head and neck neoplasia
Benign and malignant esophageal obstruction
Severe facial trauma
Anorexia
Gastroparesis
Altered mental status
Esophageal trauma

Set-up

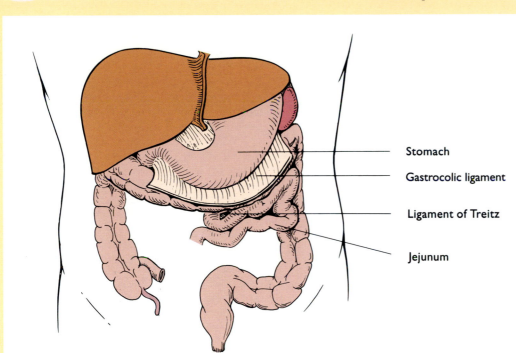

FIGURE 9-1.
Anatomy relevant to laparoscopic jejunostomy or gastrostomy tube placement. Identification of the ligament of Treitz for J-tube placement is essential, and the antrum adjacent to the pylorus should be avoided for G-tube placement.

Stomach

Gastrocolic ligament

Ligament of Treitz

Jejunum

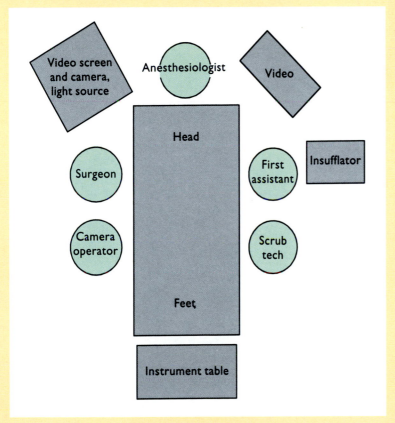

Video screen and camera, light source

Anesthesiologist

Video

Head

Surgeon

First assistant

Insufflator

Camera operator

Scrub tech

Feet

Instrument table

FIGURE 9-2.
Operative set-up for laparoscopic feeding tube placement. Foley and nasogastric catheters are routinely placed before initial trocar placement. Video monitors are oriented directly across from the surgeon and first assistant as illustrated.

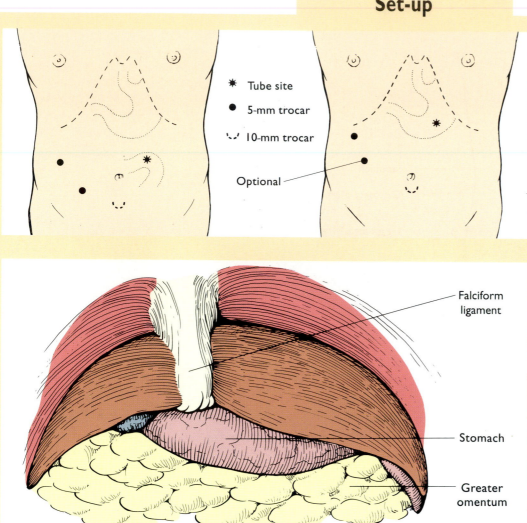

FIGURE 9-3.

Trocar positioning for jejunostomy (*left*) and gastrostomy (*right*) tube placement. Initially, the patient is placed in the Trendelenburg position, a 10-mm port is placed infraumbilically by using an open Hasson technique, the abdomen is insufflated to 10 mm Hg, and exploratory laparoscopy is performed with adhesiolysis as necessary. One or two additional 5-mm ports are then placed under direct vision in the labeled positions. The 10-mm trocar should be placed midway between the umbilicus and the pubis for jejunostomy and just below the umbilicus for gastroscopy.

FIGURE 9-4.

After insertion of the laparoscope, the inferior aspect of the stomach, greater omentum, gastrocolic ligament, and transverse colon are visualized. The anterior wall of the stomach is easily accessible with retraction inferiorly by the first assistant. Access to the proximal small bowel requires cephalad-anterior retraction of the greater omentum and transverse colon.

Figures 9-5 through 9-16 depict the surgical technique for laparoscopic jejunostomy.

Procedure

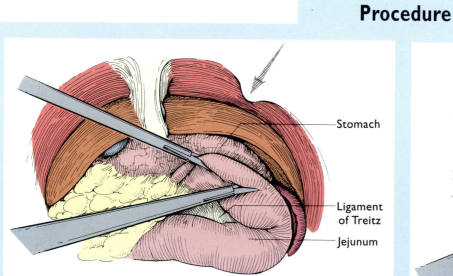

FIGURE 9-5.

Laparoscopic J-tube placement is initiated by running the bowel proximally to locate the ligament of Treitz. Positioning the patient in the reverse Trendelenburg position will facilitate this step. The site for tube placement is generally 10 to 20 cm from the ligament of Treitz. The loop of jejunum should approximate to the anterior abdominal wall in a tension-free manner. Extrinsic compression of the anterior abdominal wall in the left upper quadrant by the first assistant (*arrow*) is helpful in selecting the site for the tube tract.

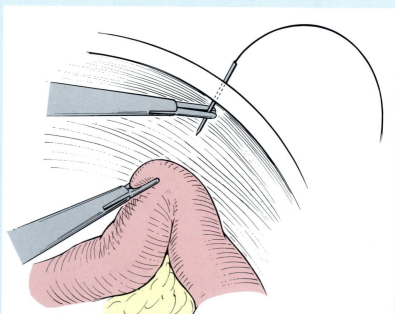

FIGURE 9-6.

Once the jejunostomy site is determined, the loop is held adjacent to the abdominal wall and a 3-0 silk on a Keith needle is placed transabdominally.

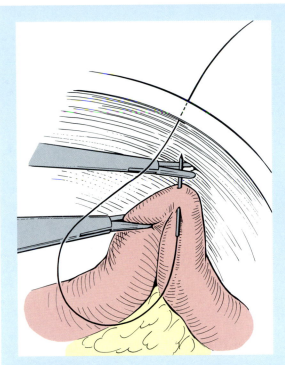

FIGURE 9-7.

This suture is mattressed through the seromuscular layers of the jejunal loop, and brought back through the abdominal wall.

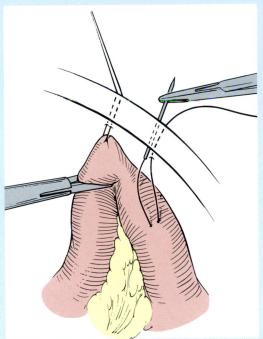

FIGURE 9-8.

A second seromuscular suture is placed in a similar manner. The tails of these sutures are temporally tagged with hemostats.

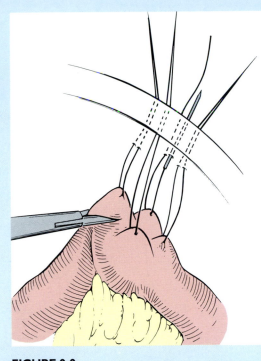

FIGURE 9-9.

The third and fourth seromuscular sutures are placed square to the others.

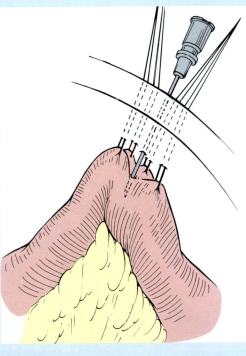

FIGURE 9-10.

A 16-G needle from an introducer kit is placed through the abdominal wall into the lumen of the jejunal loop within the boundaries of the seromuscular sutures.

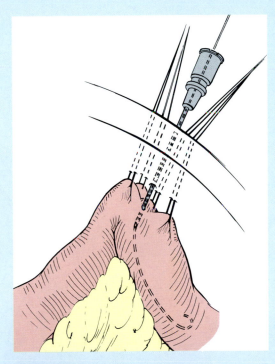

FIGURE 9-11.

A guidewire is then passed through the needle (Seldinger technique) and directed into the distal bowel for a distance of 10 to 15 cm.

Procedure

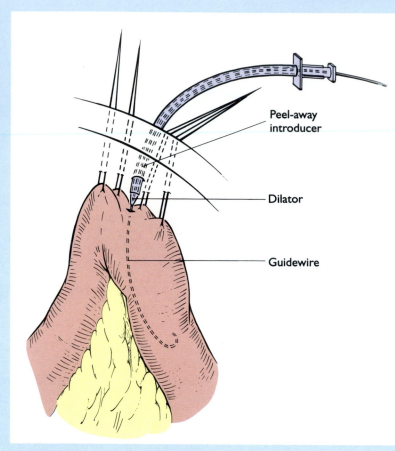

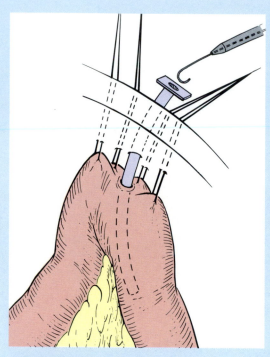

FIGURE 9-13.

The guidewire and dilator are removed leaving the peel-away introducer in place for subsequent jejunostomy tube placement.

FIGURE 9-12.

A 19-French dilator and peel-away introducer are placed over the guidewire and passed distally into the small bowel over the wire under direct vision. The jejunal loop may require traction by an assistant to facilitate this step.

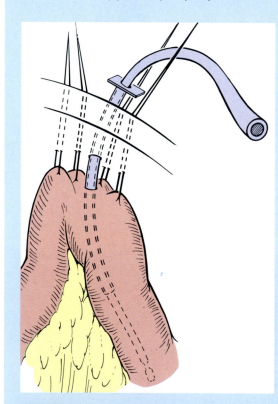

FIGURE 9-14.

A 12-French rubber Robinson catheter is passed through the peel-away introducer into the distal limb of the jejunostomy.

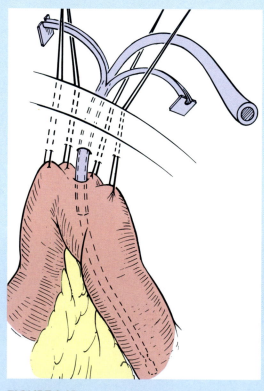

FIGURE 9-15.

The peel-away introducer is split and discarded leaving the jejunostomy tube correctly positioned.

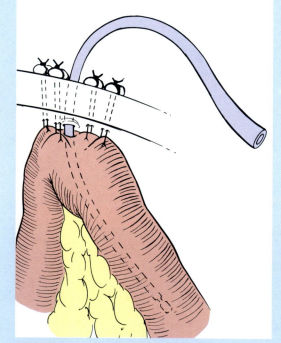

FIGURE 9-16.

The jejunal loop is approximated to the abdominal wall by the seromuscular sutures, and these sutures are secured over rubber bolsters at the skin level. An additional 3-0 nylon suture is placed to secure the jejunostomy tube to the skin.

Figures 9-17 through 9-25 depict the alternative method employing a commercial T-fastener kit.

Alternative Procedure

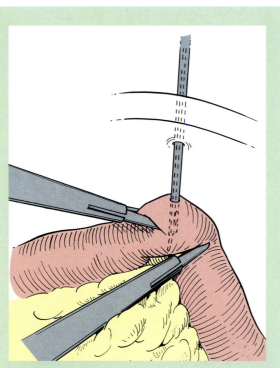

FIGURE 9-17.
After locating a suitable site for tube placement as above, a T-fastener applier is introduced through the abdominal wall into the bowel lumen and fired.

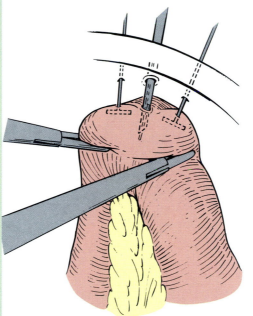

FIGURE 9-18.
The remaining T-fasteners are placed in a similar manner forming a square through which the jejunostomy tube will be placed.

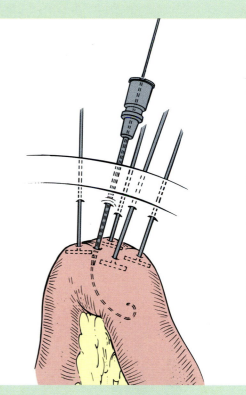

FIGURE 9-19.
A 16-G needle from an introducer kit is placed through the abdominal wall into the lumen of the jejunal loop within the boundaries of the T-fasteners, and a guidewire is passed distally through this needle.

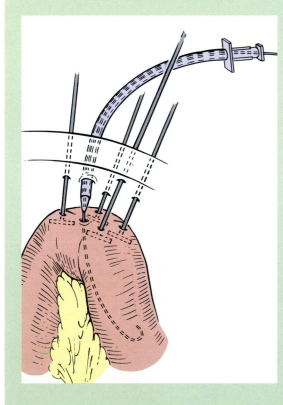

FIGURE 9-20.
Placement of a dilator and peel-away introducer over the guidewire follows, as above.

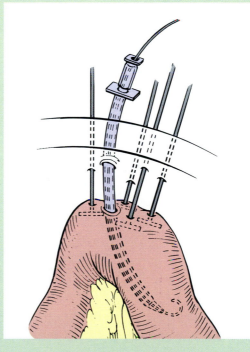

FIGURE 9-21.
Continued placement of a dilator and peel-away introducer.

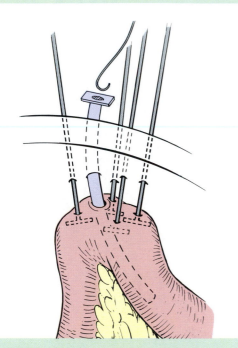

FIGURE 9-22.

The guidewire and dilator are withdrawn leaving the peel-away introducer in place for jejunostomy tube placement.

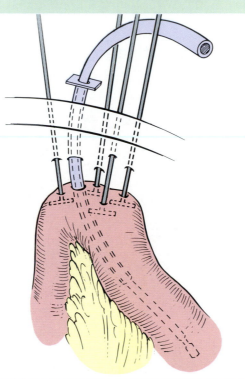

FIGURE 9-23.

A 12-French red rubber Robinson catheter is passed through the peel-away introducer into the distal limb of the jejunostomy.

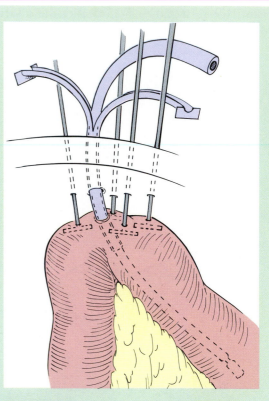

FIGURE 9-24.

The peel-away introducer is split and discarded leaving the jejunostomy tube correctly positioned.

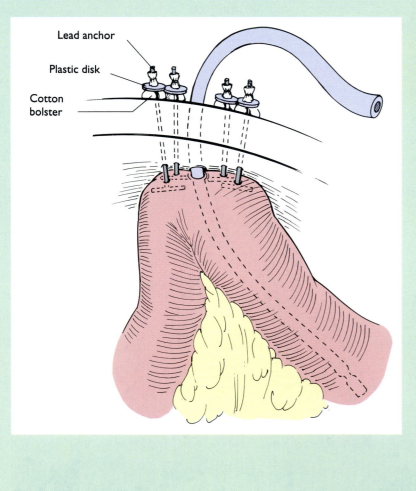

FIGURE 9-25.

The jejunal loop is approximated to the abdominal wall by placing lead anchors over plastic disks and cotton bolsters on the T-fasteners, following which the lead anchors are crimped. The extra length of the T-fasteners is cut back to the lead anchors. An additional 3-0 nylon suture is placed to secure the jejunostomy tube to the skin.

Lead anchor

Plastic disk

Cotton bolster

Figures 9-26 through 9-32 depict the surgical technique for laparoscopic gastrostomy.

Procedure

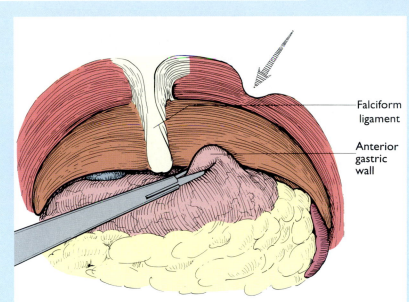

Falciform ligament

Anterior gastric wall

FIGURE 9-26.

Following initial laparoscopic exploration, air is insufflated into the stomach, if possible, to slightly distend it. A convenient area of the anterior gastric wall is chosen as the gastrostomy site and held in place with a grasper. A suitable skin exit site is located with the aid of blunt digital palpation (*arrow*) such that the gastrostomy site will not be under tension.

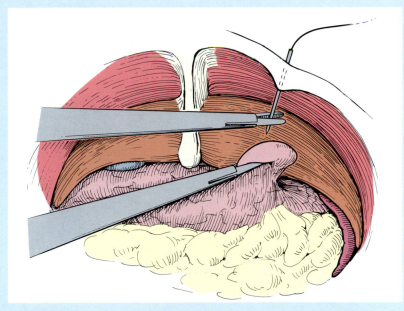

FIGURE 9-27.

Once the gastrostomy site is determined, a 3-0 silk suture on a Keith needle is placed transabdominally adjacent to the predetermined stoma site at the skin level. This suture is mattressed through the seromuscular layers of the gastric wall and brought back through the abdominal wall in a similar manner as the jejunostomy seromuscular sutures described previously.

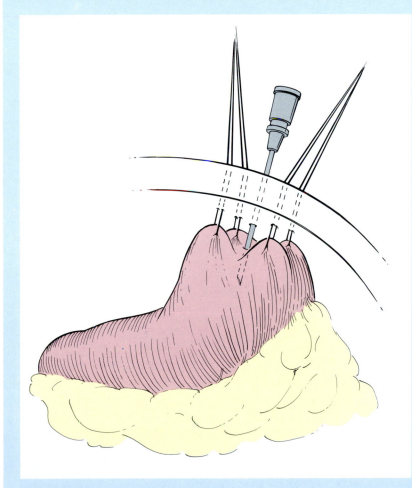

FIGURE 9-28.

A total of four gastric seromuscular sutures are placed oriented square to each other, and a 16-G needle from an introducer kit is placed into the gastric lumen.

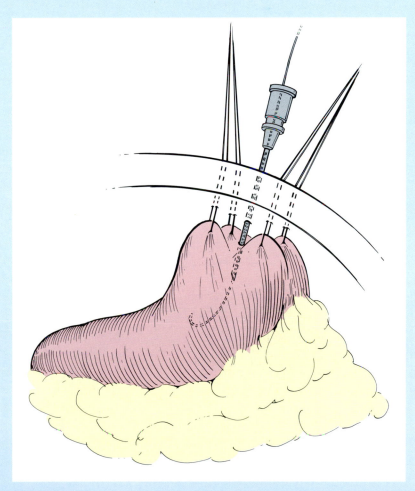

FIGURE 9-29.

A guidewire is placed through this needle into the gastric lumen, and the needle is withdrawn over the guidewire.

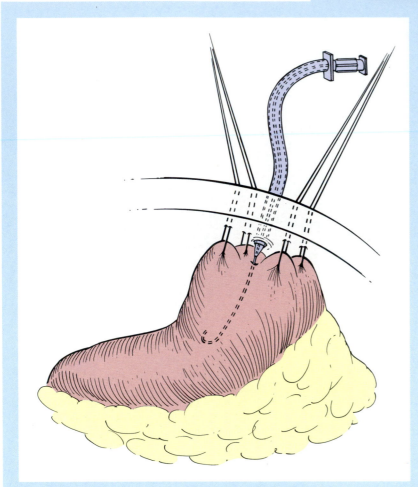

FIGURE 9-30.

An 18-French dilator and peel-away introducer are then placed over the guidewire into the gastric lumen dilating the tract to allow for subsequent tube placement. It may be necessary to incise the skin adjacent to the guidewire to facilitate placement.

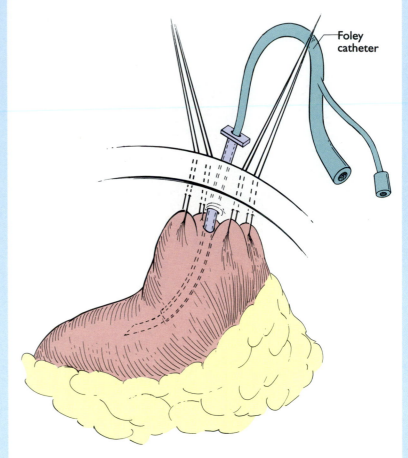

FIGURE 9-31.

A 16-French Foley urologic catheter is placed through the dilator into the gastric lumen.

FIGURE 9-32.

The catheter balloon is inflated and the serosa is approximated to the abdominal wall by placing traction on the previously placed sutures and Foley catheter. The sutures are secured over cotton bolsters at the skin level. An additional 3-0 nylon suture is placed to secure the gastrostomy tube to the skin.

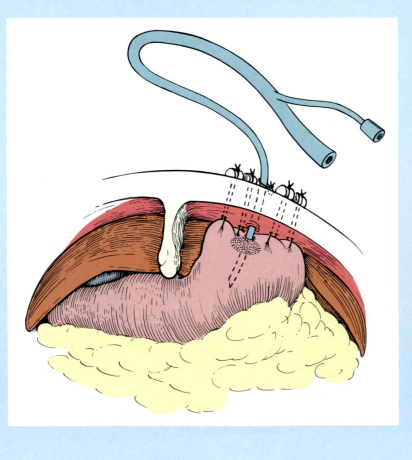

Figures 9-33 through 9-37 depict the alternative T-fastener method.

Alternative Procedure

FIGURE 9-33.

After locating a suitable site for tube placement as above and insufflating air into the stomach if possible, a T-fastener applier is introduced through the abdominal wall into the gastric lumen and fired. The antrum adjacent to the pylorus should be avoided to decrease the incidence of both distal tube migration and gastric outlet obstruction.

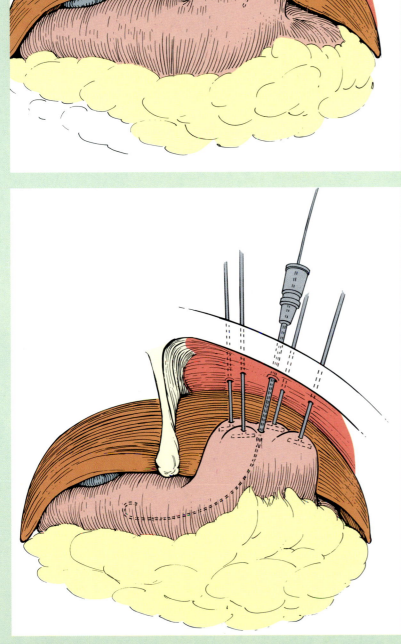

FIGURE 9-34.

The remaining T-fasteners are placed in a similar manner forming a square through which the gastrostomy tube will be placed. A 16-G needle from a Hickman introducer kit is placed through the abdominal wall into the gastric lumen within the boundaries of the T-fasteners, and a guidewire is passed distally through this needle.

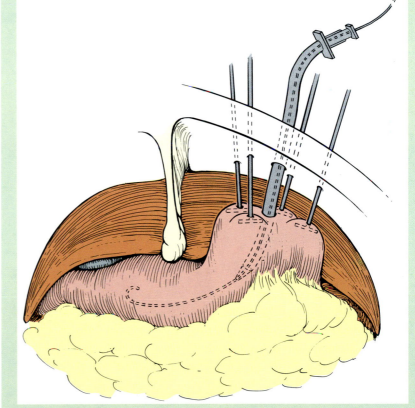

FIGURE 9-35.

The needle is withdrawn over the guidewire, and placement of a dilator and peel-away introducer follows, as above.

Alternative Procedure

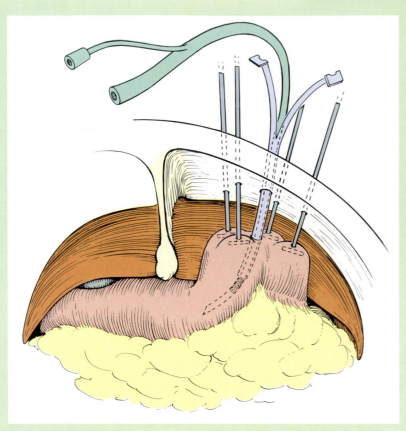

FIGURE 9-36.
The guidewire and dilator are withdrawn, and a 16-French Foley catheter is passed through the peel-away introducer into the gastric lumen. The Foley balloon is inflated with 10 mL of saline, and the peel-away introducer is split and discarded leaving the gastrostomy tube correctly positioned.

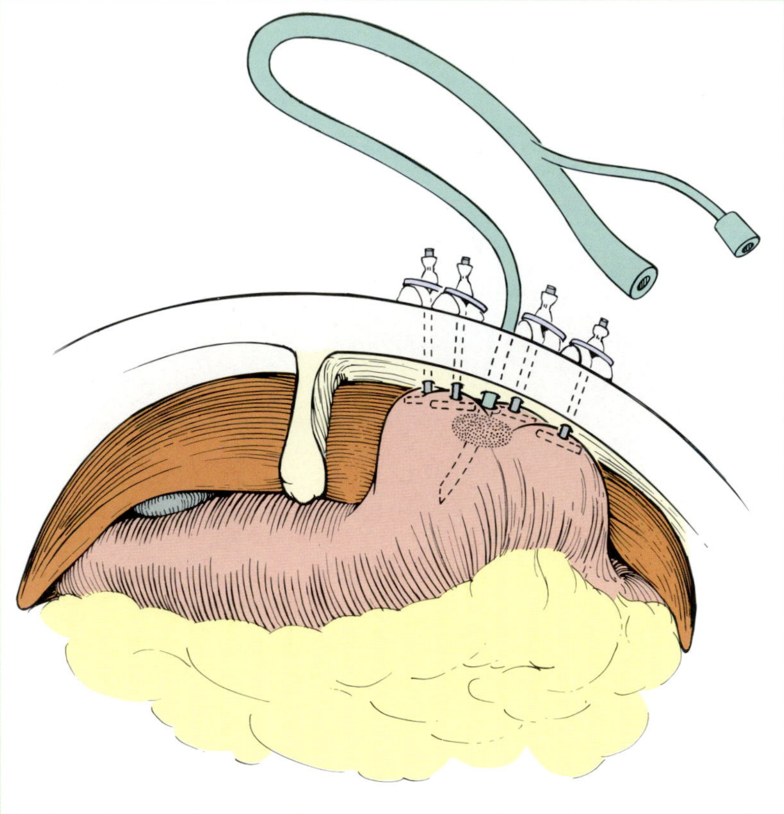

FIGURE 9-37.
The gastric serosa is approximated to the abdominal wall by placing lead anchors over plastic disks and cotton bolsters on the T-fasteners, following which the lead anchors are crimped. The extra length of the T-fasteners is cut back to the lead anchors. An additional 3-0 nylon suture is placed to secure the gastrostomy tube to the skin.

Postoperative Care

The patient is taken to the recovery room for observation before return to the hospital ward. No nasogastric tube is left. Essential medications may be given via tube immediately; feedings are begun after 24 hours and are advanced as tolerated.

Results

Many case reports of laparoscopic gastrostomy and jejunostomy have been published [3,4]. In addition, reports of the first series of patients treated with these techniques are now being published. Peitgen and coworkers [5] described 42 patients who underwent laparoscopic gastrostomy. The average operating time was 38 minutes; no patients died, 4.7% had major complications, and 9.4% had minor complications [5]. Murayama and coworkers [6] have reported on 81 patients who underwent laparoscopic gastrostomy, laparoscopic jejunostomy, or both. The operative times was 39 minutes (laparoscopic gastrostomy), 63 minutes (laparoscopic jejunostomy), and 85 minutes (for both procedures). No procedure-related deaths occurred, and the incidence of complications, including gastrointestinal bleeding, wound infection, and failed placement, was 8%. Duh and coworkers [7] report a series of 36 patients undergoing laparoscopic jejunostomy with a mean operation time of 75 minutes, no major complications, and feedings routinely begun at 24 hours after surgery.

Laparoscopic Ileostomy and Colostomy

Enteric diversion procedures are performed in various circumstances, resulting in intestinal perforation, obstruction, or inflammation (Table 9-2). Standard "open" techniques for the creation of diverting ileostomies or colostomies are safe and effective and can often be done through minimal laparotomy incisions. However, some patients requiring these procedures may previously have had abdominal surgery or have metastatic disease with peritoneal or mesenteric implants. These circumstances limit the ability of minimal incisions to create diverting ileostomy or colostomy. Moreover, open procedures are usually complicated by postoperative ileus and longer hospitalization.

The application of laparoscopic techniques for temporary or permanent enteric diversion offers several distinct advantages. Creation of an ileostomy or colostomy permits thorough inspection of the abdominal cavity for secondary problems that would probably remain undetected with use of a minimal "open" laparotomy approach. In addition, laparoscopic enteric diversion provides the opportunity to perform additional procedures, including diagnostic biopsies, feeding gastrostomy, or feeding jejunostomy. A further technical advantage of laparoscopic diversion is that the proximal and distal intestinal limbs can be examined for torsion and tension after creation of the stoma. As with most laparoscopic procedures, manipulation of the bowel is minimal and intestinal function recovers rapidly, thus allowing patients to begin immediate feedings. A regular diet is well tolerated, the diverting ostomy functions normally, and the patients can be discharged 24 to 48 hours after surgery, especially if counseling and training in the care of the stoma are provided before admission.

Although many minimally invasive techniques for the creation of diverting colostomies and ileostomies exist, the laparoscopic approach is being used with increasing frequency. Diversion can be in the form of a loop, an end ostomy alone, or an endostomy with combined mucous fistula.

Surgical Technique

Preoperative considerations are often limited in cases of acute perforation, ischemia, or obstruction, but a minimum of considerations should include intravenous antibiotics at induction of anesthesia. Under elective circumstances, both mechanical and antibiotic bowel preparations should be administered on the day before surgery. In either case, after induction of anesthesia, a urinary bladder catheter and nasogastric tube are essential to decompress the stomach and bladder. In most cases, both tubes can be removed upon completion of the operation.

Figures 9-38 through 9-45 depict the surgical technique for laparoscopic enteric diversion.

Table 9-2. Indications for enteric diversion procedures

Perforation	Volvulus
Diverticulitis	Intussusception
Cancer	Ogilvie's syndrome
Crohn's disease	Inflammatory bowel disease
Ischemia	Crohn's disease
Obstruction	Ulcerative colitis
Unresectable cancer	Toxic megacolon

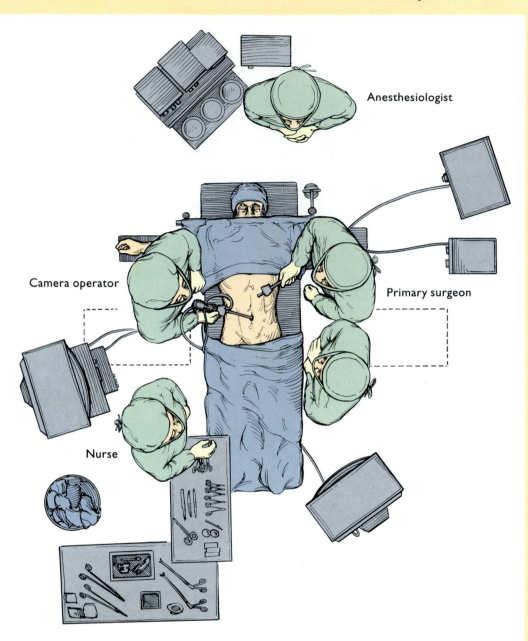

Anesthesiologist

Camera operator

Primary surgeon

Nurse

FIGURE 9-38.

Operative set-up for laparoscopic sigmoid colostomy. With the patient in the supine position, the entire abdomen is scrubbed and draped widely. The primary surgeon is positioned on the side of the patient where the ostomy is to be located. The camera operator is usually located opposite the primary surgeon. Video monitors are positioned at the foot of both sides of the operating table in direct view of the surgeons. After general anesthesia is established, a CO_2 pneumoperitoneum pressurized to 15 mm Hg is achieved at the umbilicus by using the closed (Veress needle) or open (Hasson trocar) technique. The laparoscope is then inserted through a 10-mm port and the peritoneal cavity is inspected. The presence of significant adhesions that prevent mobilization of the bowel segment to be diverted may obligate insertion of additional ports in order to provide adequate mobilization. Additional procedures (biopsies, feeding tubes, and so forth) may be performed at this time.

Procedure

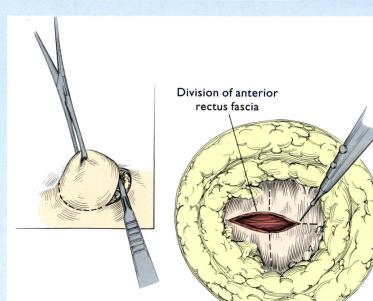

Division of anterior rectus fascia

FIGURE 9-39.

Creation of the stoma site. After mobilization of the ileum or colon, a stoma is made on the abdominal wall at a site overlying the segment for diversion, usually in a position that allows the intestine to pass through the rectus muscle. An Allis clamp is used to grasp the skin at the site of the stoma and an ellipse of skin is excised. After removal of a portion of the subcutaneous fat, a cruciate incision is made through the anterior rectus fascia with an electrocautery. The underlying rectus muscle is split by using a Kelly clamp, the posterior rectus fascia is divided, but the peritoneum is not incised.

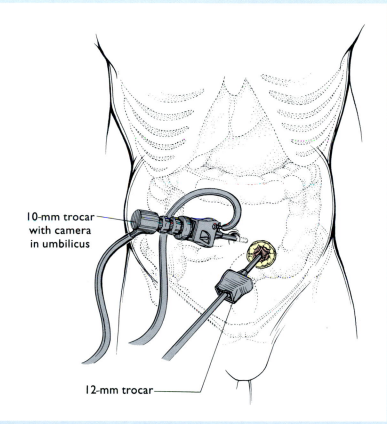

10-mm trocar with camera in umbilicus

12-mm trocar

FIGURE 9-40.

Insertion of 12-mm port through the ostomy site. A 10-mm trocar is placed in the periumbilical region, and a laparoscopic camera is placed through the trocar after insufflation of CO_2 into the abdominal cavity. A 12-mm trocar is inserted through the defect created in the skin, rectus fascia, rectus muscle, and through the peritoneum into the peritoneal cavity.

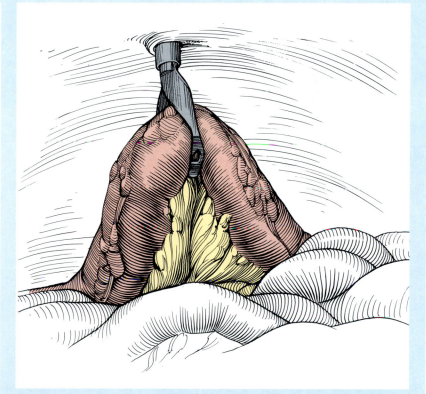

FIGURE 9-41.

A laparoscopic Babcock clamp is used to grasp the antimesenteric border of a mobile segment of the sigmoid colon. This site is selected after demonstration that it can be drawn to the anterior abdominal wall without tension while the pneumoperitoneum is maintained. At this point, the trocar has been placed through the previously created stoma. The defect in the peritoneum is opened to accommodate the bowel with temporary loss of the pneumoperitoneum. The Babcock clamp is used to withdraw the loop of sigmoid colon through the defect in the anterior abdominal wall with simultaneous removal of the trocar. The loop of sigmoid colon reseals the abdominal cavity, allowing a pneumoperitoneum to be reestablished. The abdominal cavity and the mesentery of the sigmoid colon are then visually inspected to confirm the absence of tension or torsion on the sigmoid colon.

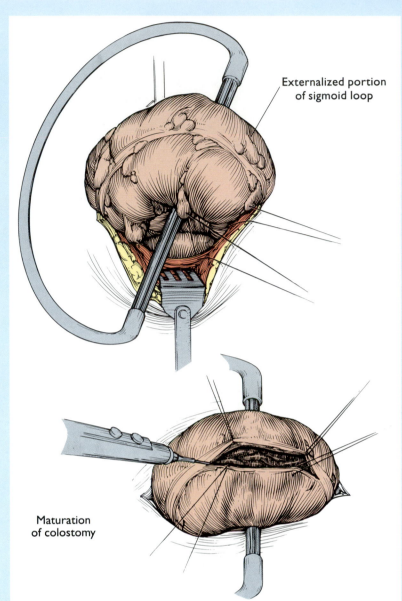

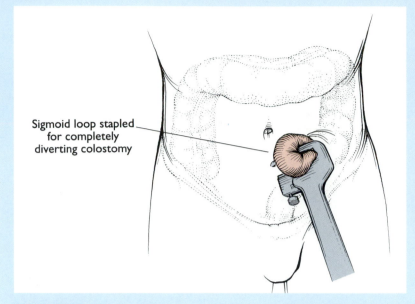

Externalized portion
of sigmoid loop

Maturation
of colostomy

FIGURE 9-42.

Maturing the stoma. Once the sigmoid loop is brought through the site of the stoma, it is matured as a double-barreled loop colostomy as shown here. A red-rubber catheter is passed through the mesentery of the colon and between the colon and the skin to ensure that the colon does not return into the peritoneal cavity. The colostomy is matured by opening the colon along a tenia and placing full-thickness interrupted 3-0 chromic sutures through the colon, approximating the mucosa and the skin.

Sigmoid loop stapled
for completely
diverting colostomy

FIGURE 9-43.

Alternatively, a loop of colon brought through the anterior abdominal wall is converted to a completely diverting colostomy by placing a TA-55 staple line across the distal limb. Maturation of the stoma is accomplished by opening the proximal limb along a tenia and placing full-thickness interrupted 3-0 chromic sutures through the colon, approximating the mucosa and the skin.

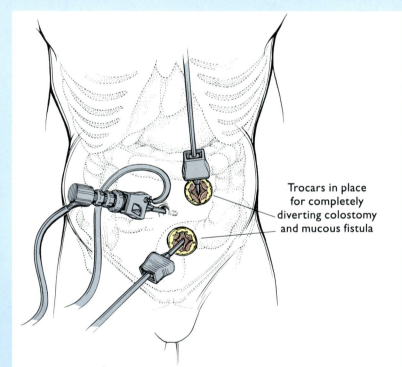

Trocars in place
for completely
diverting colostomy
and mucous fistula

FIGURE 9-44.

Creation of an end colostomy and mucous fistula. If a distal (defunctionalized) segment of intestine is longer than 10 mm above the peritoneal reflection, a completely diverting colostomy and mucous fistula can be created. In this case, two stoma sites are selected and prepared as previously described.

Procedure

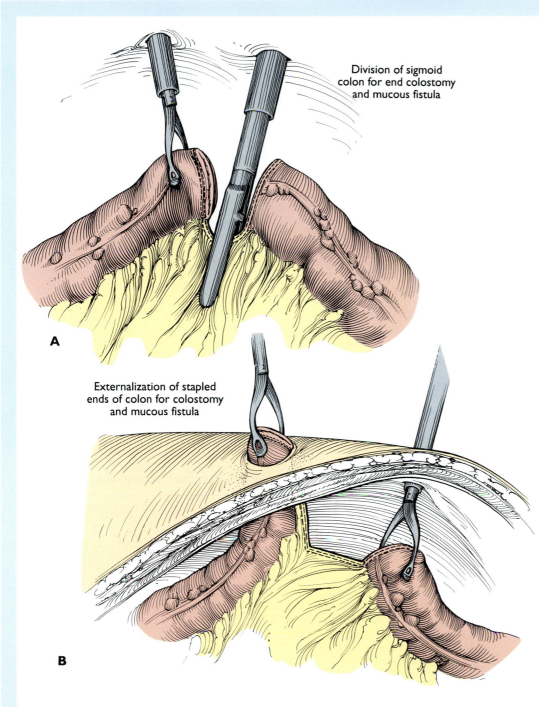

Division of sigmoid colon for end colostomy and mucous fistula

A

Externalization of stapled ends of colon for colostomy and mucous fistula

B

FIGURE 9-45.

Creation of an end-colostomy and mucous fistula continued. **A**, By using the two stomal sites shown in Figure 9-11, trocars of 10- or 12-mm diameter are passed through the sites. An appropriate segment of the sigmoid colon is selected for creation of an end colostomy and mucous fistula. The ability to mobilize the colon to the anterior abdominal wall is ensured, and a defect is created in the mesentery by sharp dissection at the site of the end colostomy with endoscopic scissors and the electrocautery. An endoscopic stapler is introduced through the 12-mm trocar and is used to divide the sigmoid colon, creating two stapled ends. After division of the sigmoid colon, vascular staples are used to divide the mesentery of the sigmoid colon. This second staple line in the mesentery allows the two ends of the colon to be separated as an end colostomy and a mucous fistula. **B**, A Babcock clamp is passed through the trocar to bring the proximal colon through the prepared stoma after the peritoneum is divided. The distal segment of colon is simultaneously withdrawn by using a second Babcock clamp through the other stoma to create the mucous fistula. Reestablishment of pneumoperitoneum after placement of the stomas as an end colostomy and mucous fistula allows inspection of the abdominal cavity to exclude tension or torsion.

Postoperative Care

Care is dictated by the patient's preoperative condition. In a patient having elective surgery, it is unnecessary to leave a nasogastric tube. Liquids may be begun on postoperative day 1 and advanced as tolerated.

Results

Several case reports have described the techniques of laparoscopic cecostomy [8], ileostomy [9], and colostomy [10]. Several groups have also reported their initial series of patients undergoing laparoscopic enteric diversion. Hollyoak and coworkers [11] retrospectively reviewed laparoscopic compared with open diverting ileostomy. They found decreased operating time, decreased time to return of bowel function, and decreased length of hospital stay in the laparoscopic group. Ludwig and coworkers [12] reviewed 24 laparoscopic diversion procedures (including both colostomy and ileostomy) performed at the Cleveland Clinic and found a median operative time of 60 minutes, median blood loss of 50 mL, and median time of return of bowel function of 1 day; one case was converted to an open procedure and one major complication occurred (pulmonary embolism in a patient with metastatic cancer). In Sweden, Almqvist and coworkers [13] performed a prospective study of laparoscopic fecal diversion in which the laparoscopic procedures took no longer to perform than traditional open procedures, no major complications were encountered, and all patients began oral intake on the first postoperative day. Oliveira and coworkers [14] presented a retrospective experience of laparoscopic enteric diversion in which patients had a mean operative time of 76 minutes, mean return of bowel function of 3.1 days, and a mean length of hospitalization of 6.2 days.

Summary

In summary, laparoscopy can be used safely to divert the fecal stream in selected patients who do not otherwise require laparotomy.

References

1. Gauderer MW, Ponsky JL, Izant RJ Jr: Gastrostomy without laparotomy: a percutaneous endoscopic technique. *J Pediatr Surg* 1980, 15:872–875.

2. Grant JP: Percutaneous endoscopic gastrostomy. Initial placement by single endoscopic technique and long-term follow-up. *Ann Surg* 1993, 217:168–174.

3. O'Regan PJ, Scarrow GD: Laparoscopic jejunostomy. *Endoscopy* 1990, 22:39–40.

4. Edelman DS, Unger SW, Russin DR: Laparoscopic gastrostomy. *Surg Laparosc Endosc* 1991, 1:251–253.

5. Peitgen K, Walz MK, Krause U, *et al.*: First results of laparoscopic gastrostomy. *Surg Endosc* 1997, 11:658–662.

6. Murayama KM, Johnson TJ, Thompson JS: Laparoscopic gastrostomy and jejunostomy are safe and effective for obtaining enteral access. *Am J Surg* 1996, 172:591–594.

7. Duh QY, Senokozlieff-Englehart AL, Siperstein AE, *et al.*: Prospective evaluation of the safety and efficacy of laparoscopic jejunostomy. *West J Med* 1995, 162:117–122.

8. Duh QY, Way LW: Diagnostic laparoscopy and laparoscopic cecostomy for colonic pseudo-obstruction. *Dis Colon Rectum* 1993, 36:65–70.

9. Weiss UL, Jehle E, Becker HD, *et al.*: Laparoscopic ileostomy. *Br J Surg* 1995, 82:1648.

10. Lyerly HK, Mault JR: Laparoscopic ileostomy and colostomy. *Ann Surg* 1994, 219:317–322.

11. Hollyoak MA, Lumley J, Stitz RW: Laparoscopic stoma formation for faecal diversion. *Br J Surg* 1998, 85:226–228.

12. Ludwig KA, Milsom JW, Garcia-Ruiz A, *et al.*:Laparoscopic techniques for fecal diversion. *Dis Colon Rectum* 1996, 39:285–288.

13. Almqvist PM, Bohe M, Montgomery A: Laparoscopic creation of loop ileostomy and sigmoid colostomy. *Eur J Surg* 1995, 161:907–909.

14. Oliveira L, Reissman P, Nogueras J, *et al.*: Laparoscopic Creation of Stomas. *Surg Endosc* 1997, 11:19–23.

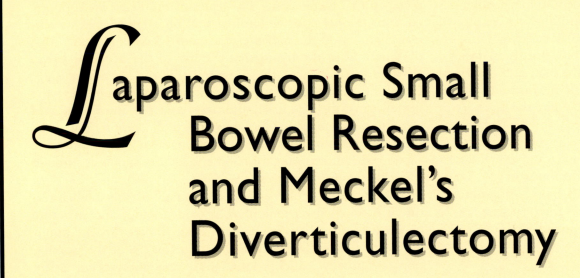

Laparoscopic Small Bowel Resection and Meckel's Diverticulectomy

Aurora D. Pryor
Steve Eubanks

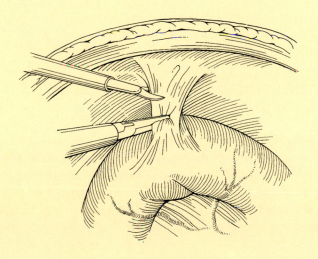

Since Bernheim's initial description of laparoscopy in the U.S. literature in 1911 [1], laparoscopy was predominantly used in the field of gynecology. Only in the past decade has laparoscopy in general surgery gained widespread acceptance. With the now prevalent use of exploratory laparoscopy and the increased availability of laparoscopic instrumentation, the number of conditions for which laparoscopic management is favored has increased. Laparoscopic handling of a variety of small bowel conditions, including obstruction [2,3,4], Meckel's diverticula [5], inflammatory bowel disease, foreign bodies, and cancer is now possible. Reports have also described successful laparoscopic management of perforated jejunal diverticulitis [6] and gallstone ileus [7]. Despite the diversity of the underlying abnormalities involved, the technique of laparoscopic bowel resection remains relatively constant. In this chapter we discuss the pathophysiology and presentation of two clinical scenarios that easily yield to laparoscopic management: Meckel's diverticula and small bowel obstruction. The technique for small bowel resection is then discussed, as it applies to these two processes and to the management of small bowel disease in general.

Anatomy

The small intestine consists of three roughly defined portions: the duodenum, the jejunum, and the ileum. The duodenum extends from the pylorus to the ligament of Treitz and is approximately 25 to 30 cm long [8]. At the ampulla of Vater in the midsection of the duodenum, the biliary and pancreatic systems join with the gut lumen to contribute their products to digestion. From this point on, the duodenum courses in a retroperitoneal location. Because of this anatomy, the duodenum is more

difficult to access from a surgical standpoint than the remainder of the small bowel and is not generally considered for "generic" small bowel resection.

The small bowel proper begins beyond the ligament of Treitz; the small bowel consists of the jejunum and ileum. From the ligament of Treitz to the ileocecal valve, the small bowel is approximately 6 to 7 meters long. The jejunum and ileum are supported from the posterior abdominal wall on a fan shaped mesentery. The root of the mesentery is about 15 cm long, extending obliquely from the ligament of Treitz to the ileocecal valve. Between the layers of the mesentery lie the vascular supply (derived from the superior mesenteric artery and draining to the portal vein), the lymphatic drainage, and the autonomic and somatic nerve supply. The parasympathetic supply is derived from the posterior vagus, and the sympathetic supply from the superior mesenteric ganglion. Somatic sensory supply is through the lesser splanchnic nerves (T9–T10).

The most common congenital anomaly of the small intestine is Meckel's diverticulum. The epidemiology and structure of Meckel's diverticula can easily be remembered by the popular "rule of twos." They typically occur in 2% of the population, are usually 2 inches long, most commonly occur 2 feet from the ileocecal valve, and may commonly contain 2 types of ectopic mucosa (gastric and pancreatic). Meckel's diverticula arise when the connection between the yolk sac and the midgut, the omphalomesenteric duct (OMD), fails to completely obliterate and involute in early gestation. Approximately 90% of these cases results in a true diverticulum from the antimesenteric border of the small intestine—a Meckel's diverticulum (Figure 10-1). A paired system of arteries, the vitelline arteries, follows the OMD from the aorta to the yolk sac. The right vitelline artery eventually becomes the superior mesenteric artery and the left generally involutes by the seventh week. A large artery, which is an abnormal remnant of the distal right vitelline artery, is commonly seen on the external surface of a Meckel's diverticulum.

Pathophysiology, Presentation, and Differential Diagnosis

Small Bowel Obstruction
Normal motility of the small bowel serves both to mix the intraluminal contents with enteric secretions, thus facilitating digestion, and to effect transit from one specialized area of the bowel to the next. As a direct result, the intraluminal bacterial counts rise progressively the more distal in the bowel one samples.

Mechanical bowel obstruction disturbs the transit of luminal contents. The resultant accumulation of volume in the bowel causes distension of the bowel and waves of pain as peristalsis attempts to push liquid past the obstruction. The pain is diffusely localized in the periumbilical region. In addition, stasis of intraluminal contents results in rapid bacterial overgrowth. In the presence of a closed loop obstruction or strangulation, bacterial translocation, bowel infarction, and perforation may result.

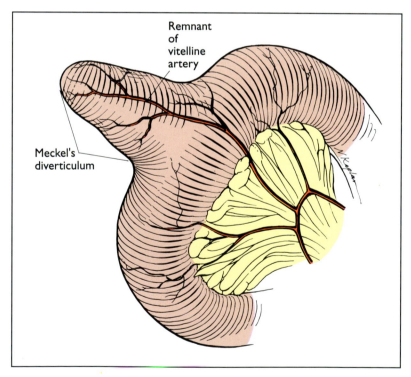

FIGURE 10-1.

Meckel's diverticulum.

The patient presents with a history of abdominal pain, distention, nausea, vomiting, and obstipation. There may be focal pain at the site of a hernia. The duration of pain prior to the onset of emesis, degree of distention, as well as the character of the emesis may serve to suggest how proximal or distal the obstruction is. The patient may report several prior similar episodes.

On examination, the patient is usually mildly to moderately distended and has no evidence of peritoneal irritation (unless perforated). Bowel sounds are present and often are described as "tinkling" or coming in "waves and rushes." Radiographic examination reveals distended loops of small bowel, air-fluid levels, and absence of distal gas. Cardinal signs and symptoms that mandate exploration include fever, tachycardia, continuous abdominal pain, leukocytosis, and peritoneal irritation, as well as a complete obstruction.

The possible etiologies of small bowel obstruction are many (Table 10-1). The three most common causes (adhesions, hernia or tumor) can often be treated laparoscopically.

Meckel's Diverticulum

Meckel's diverticula carry an approximately 4% risk of complications throughout life [9]. Over 40% of complications occur before the age of 10 years [10]. The type of complication and the clinical presentation vary greatly with age—gastrointestinal bleeding and intussusception are more common in children whereas intestinal obstruction and inflammation predominate in adults. The incidence of reported complication rates [9–18], therefore, varies significantly with the distribution of the population being studied (Table 10-2).

The most frequent complication overall is probably intestinal obstruction. Obstruction can result from a variety of mechanisms including intussusception, volvulus around fibrous or adhesive bands, or incarceration within an inguinal or femoral hernia (Littre hernia). In children, obstruction is often caused by intussusception that typically presents with intermittent crampy abdominal pain and expulsion of dark red "current jelly" stools. In the adult population, obstruction from Meckel's diverticula is usually indistinguishable from classic small bowel obstruction, except that patients may not have undergone previous celiotomy. The diagnosis may be established by physical examination, small bowel contrast examinations, and enteroclysis.

The next most frequent complication is gastrointestinal bleeding and it is the most common mode of presentation in children [19]. Although some controversy exists, bleeding usually results from ulceration of the ileum caused by the secretion of acid from adjacent gastric mucosa within the diverticulum. The amount of blood loss varies from occult bleeding to frank bright red hemorrhage per rectum with circulatory collapse [11]. It has been stated that children are more likely to present with hematochezia where-

Table 10-1. Etiology of small bowel obstruction

Cause	Incidence, %
Adhesion	75
Hernia	8
Internal	20
External	80
Malignant tumor	8
Volvulus	3*
Inflammatory bowel disease	1
Intussusception	<1
Gallstone ileus	<1
Radiation enteritis	<1
Intra-abdominal abscess	<1
Bezoar	<1

*Varies greatly with region of the world. May represent up to 50%.

Table 10-2. Complications of Meckel's diverticula

Study	Soltero and Bill [9]	Yamaguchi and coworkers [10]	Mackey and Dineen [11]	Williams [12]	Leijonmarck and coworkers [13]
Location	Seattle	Japan	New York	Adelaide	Stockholm
Year	1976	1978	1983	1981	1986
Patients, n	202	583*	68	1806*	112
Complications					
Obstruction	31%	40%	25%	16%	32%
Intussusception	NR	14	9	11	3
Inflammation	24	13	7	25	30
Hemorrhage	25	12	23	31	11
Perforation	12	8	12	NR	19
Littre's hernia	4	5	7	11	3
Umbilical fistula	3	3	3	4	NR
Other†	1	5	4	2	2

*Combined series.
†Neoplasms [13,14,15], foreign body impaction [16], fecalith [17], diverticular calculi [18], regional enteritis [17], trauma [10], myxoglobulosis [10].
NR—not reported.

as adults usually present with melena [19]. The diagnosis may be established by radioisotope scanning with 99mTc pertechnetate, first developed in 1967 by Harden and coworkers [20], which readily identifies the presence of gastric mucosa. When at least 1.8 cm² of gastric mucosa is present in the diverticulum, a positive scan will result. It should be noted, however, that Meckel's scans have a fairly high false-negative rate (due to the frequent absence of gastric mucosa) and are much more reliable in children than in adults. Angiography may also be helpful in establishing the diagnosis if active bleeding or a patent left vitelline artery can be demonstrated. Infrequently, perforation of the ilium or diverticulum may be the first presenting sign and the diagnosis may be established by plain abdominal radiograph.

The third most common mode of presentation (second most common in adults) is diverticulitis. The clinical scenario is similar to acute appendicitis. The differential diagnosis is broad and includes cholecystitis, Crohn's disease, and peptic ulcer disease. It is thought that the fairly high mortality rate of diverticulectomy (6% in some series) may be attributed to the frequent delay in diagnosis of Meckel's diverticulitis. Radiologic examinations are usually not helpful and the diagnosis is most often confirmed by surgical exploration.

The development of complications in Meckel's diverticula (Table 10-2) has led many authors to advocate routine diverticulectomy when diverticula are discovered during abdominal exploration performed for other reasons [21]. More recent data, however, illustrate that the risks of routine diverticulectomy probably outweigh the benefits for most patients [9], and routine incidental diverticulectomy is no longer recommended. However, as diverticular complications are strongly related to the age of the patient and the morphology of the diverticulum, it seems reasonable to perform selective incidental diverticulectomy if the patient is very young, if the diverticlum is attached to the umbilicus by an omphalomesenteric band, or if the diverticulum has a narrow neck, configurations believed to carry significant risks of bowel entrapment or torsion [11–13,19,22,23].

Surgical Technique

Although the surgical approach to small bowel resection may vary depending on the underlying abnormality, several basic principles are inherent to the procedure. These are outlined in Figures 10-2 through 10-12.

Set-up

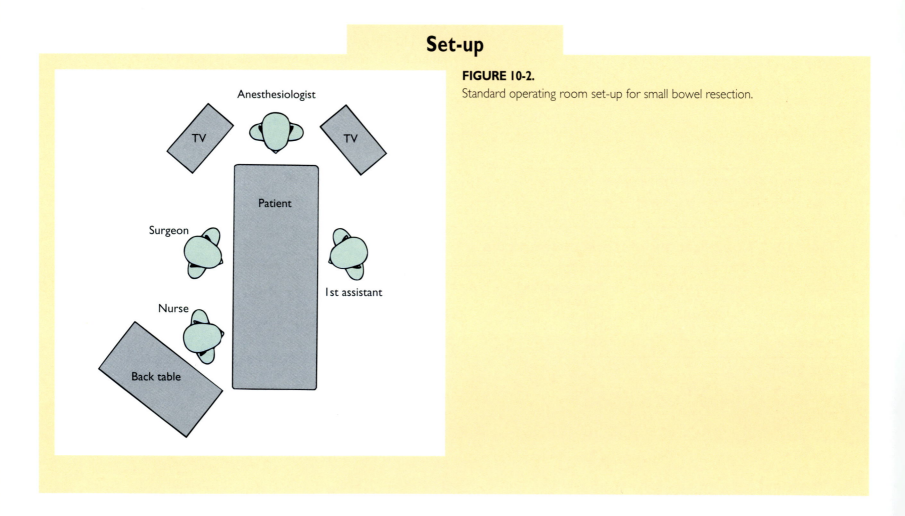

FIGURE 10-2.

Standard operating room set-up for small bowel resection.

Set-up

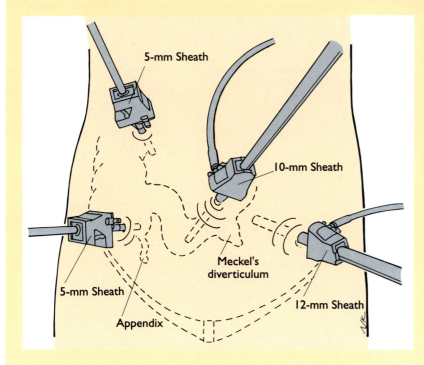

5-mm Sheath

10-mm Sheath

Meckel's diverticulum

5-mm Sheath

Appendix

12-mm Sheath

FIGURE 10-3.

Access to the peritoneal cavity is gained infraumbilically via a closed (Veress needle) or open (Hasson trocar) technique. Following CO_2 insufflation to 15 mm Hg, the laparoscope is inserted via the 10-mm sheath. Five-mm sheaths are placed in the right upper quadrant and right lower quadrant. A single 12-mm sheath is placed in a variable position to permit use of the stapling device. With the sheaths in place, abdominal exploration is performed; the gallbladder, appendix, cecum, and pelvis should be thoroughly inspected.

Procedure

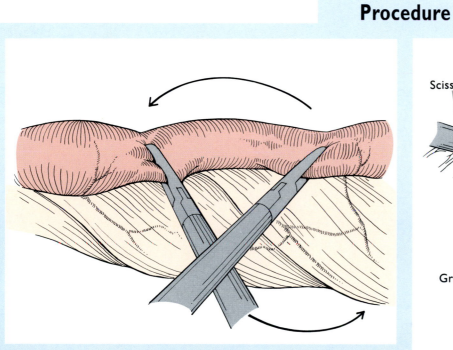

FIGURE 10-4.

The entire small bowel is "run" from the ligament of Treitz to the terminal ileum to identify the area of concern.

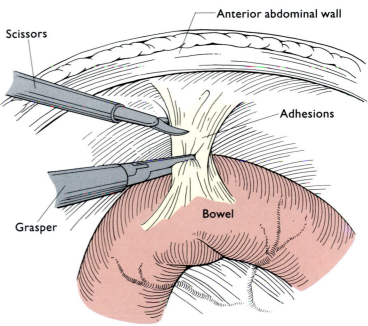

Anterior abdominal wall

Scissors

Adhesions

Grasper

Bowel

FIGURE 10-5.

Adhesions that interfere with visualization of the bowel or that may cause obstruction are lysed by using graspers and bipolar cautery scissors.

Procedure

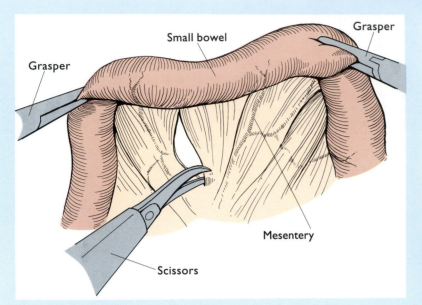

FIGURE 10-6.

A window is created in the mesentery adjacent to the segment for resection by using cautery and blunt or sharp dissection.

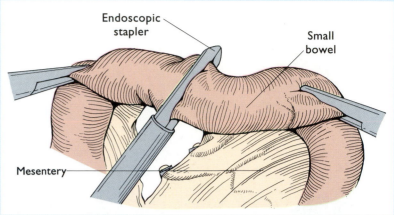

FIGURE 10-7.

The endoscopic bowel stapling device is used to divide the small bowel. A markedly dilated bowel may require more than one application of the stapler to completely divide the bowel.

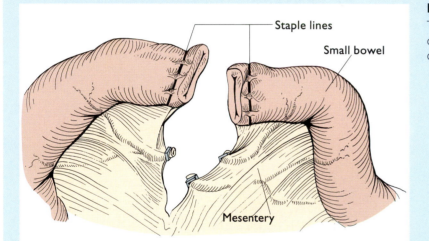

FIGURE 10-8.

The divided small bowel is demonstrated. The endoscopic stapler simultaneously divides the intestine and applies staples to prevent the spillage of bowel contents. The staple lines are also hemostatic in most situations.

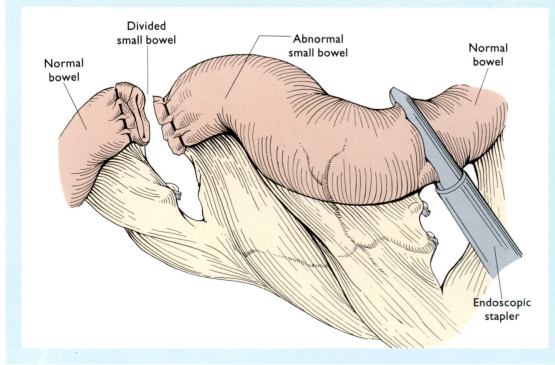

FIGURE 10-9.

A second site is selected for division of the small bowel.

Procedure

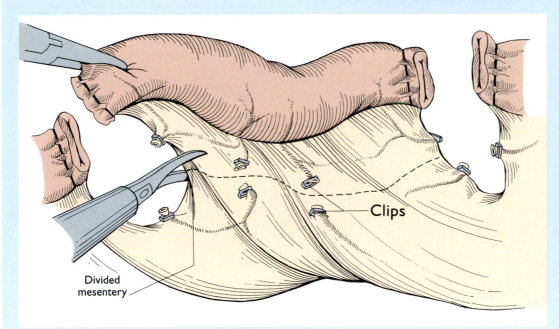

FIGURE 10-10.
The mesentery of the abnormal small bowel is divided. This can be accomplished using cautery (monopolar or bipolar), hemostatic titanium clips with sharp dissection, or with a vascular endoscopic stapler.

Clips

Divided
mesentery

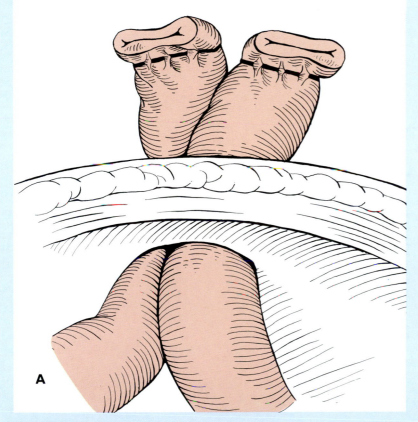

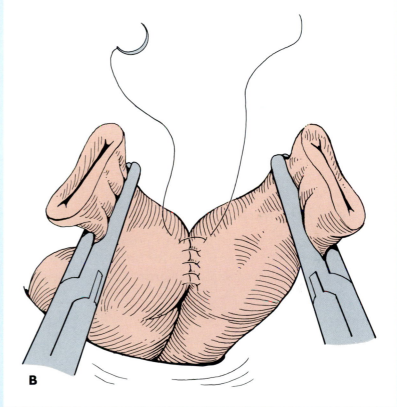

FIGURE 10-11.
A, The specimen is removed from the abdomen. **B**, The anastomosis is performed at the level of the skin using sutures or staples. (*Continued*)

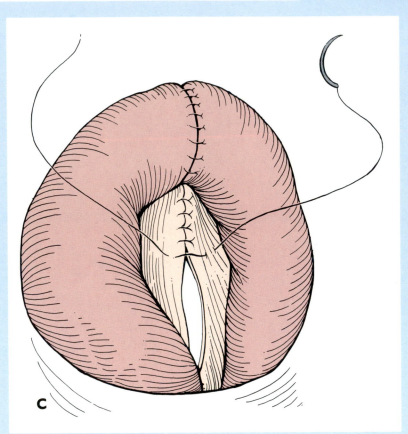

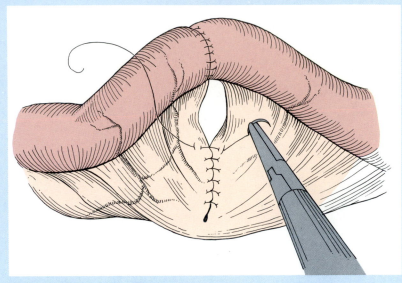

FIGURE 10-12.
Alternatively, the anastomosis and closure of the mesenteric defect may be performed intracorporeally.

FIGURE 10-11. (*Continued*)
C, The mesenteric defect is closed with sutures.

Alternative Surgical Technique for Meckel's Diverticula

Resection of a Meckel's diverticulum can proceed as in the standard small bowel resection, particularly for broad-base diverticula or those associated with bleeding. For narrow diverticula, however-er, simple staple excision is possible if the lumen is not jeopardized (*See* Figures 10-13 through 10-17). When a Meckel's diverticulum is being resected by simple excision, careful frozen section analysis must be done to avoid leaving any residual ectopic mucosa.

Alternative Procedure

FIGURE 10-13.
Resection of a Meckel's diverticulum. If its base is narrow and simple staple excision would not be expected to compromise the lumen, then the line of resection should be at the base of the diverticulum. If the diverticulum has a broad base, short segment small bowel resection will be necessary. Either procedure may be performed expeditiously using laparoscopic techniques.

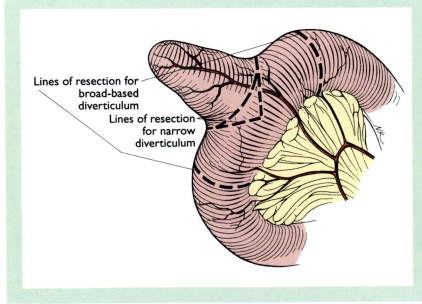

Lines of resection for broad-based diverticulum

Lines of resection for narrow diverticulum

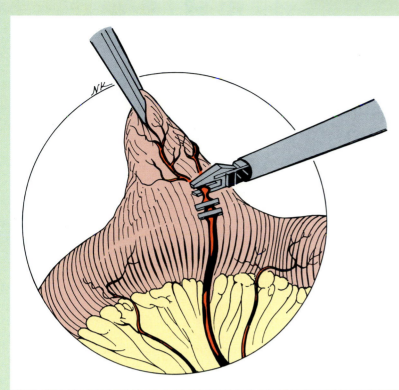

FIGURE 10-14.

If a large persistent vitelline artery is encountered, it may be doubly ligated with clips. A thorough search should be made for a persistant vitelline artery since this structure can be quite large and may not be adequately controlled with the stapling device.

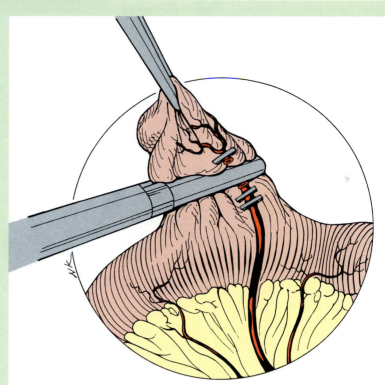

FIGURE 10-15.

Simple resection is performed with the stapling device. The tip of the diverticulum is grasped with forceps and the diverticulum positioned within the stapler delivered through a left lower quadrant sheath.

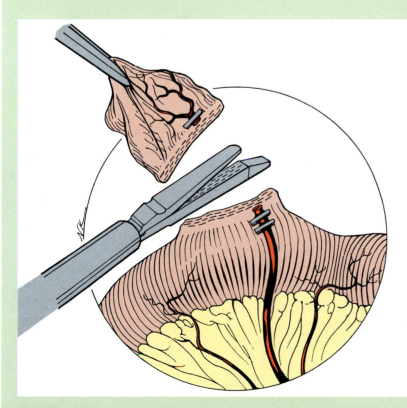

FIGURE 10-16.

The stapler is fired.

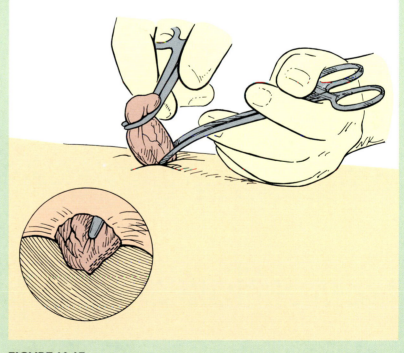

FIGURE 10-17.

The specimen can usually be delivered through the umbilical incision under direct vision.

References

1. Bernheim BM: Organoscopy: cystoscopy of the abdominal cavity. *Ann Surg* 1911, 53:764–767.

2. Adams S, Wilson T, Brown AR: Laparoscopic management of acute small bowel obstruction. *Aust N Z J Surg* 1993, 63:39–41.

3. Keating J, Hill A, Schroeder D, Whittle D: Laparoscopy in the diagnosis and treatment of acute small bowel obstruction. *J Laparoendosc Surg* 1992, 2:239–244.

4. Franklin ME, Dorman JP, Pharand D: Laparoscopic surgery in acute small bowel obstruction. *Surg Laparosc Endosc* 1994, 4:289–296.

5. Atwood SEA, McGrath J, Hill ADK, Stephens RB: Laparoscopic approach to Meckel's diverticulectomy. *Br J Surg* 1992, 79:211.

6. Cross MJ, Snyder SK: Laparoscopic-directed small bowel resection for jejunal diverticulitis with perforation. *J Laparoendosc Surg* 1993, 3:47–49.

7. Franklin ME, Dorman JP, Schuessler WW: Laparoscopic treatment of gallstone ileus: a case report and review of the literature. *J Laparoendosc Surg* 1994, 4:265–272.

8. Dresner LS, MacArthur S, Wait RB: Small intestine. In: *Surgery: A Problem Solving Approach*, edn 2. Edited by Davis JH, Sheldon GF, Drucker WR, *et al.* Baltimore: Mosby–Year Book; 1995:1314–1360.

9. Soltero MJ, Bill AH: The natural history of Meckel's diverticulum and its relation to incidental removal: a study of 202 cases of diseased Meckel's diverticulum found in King County, Washington, over a fifteen year period. *Am J Surg* 1976, 132:168–173.

10. Yamaguchi M, Takeuchi S, Awazu S: Meckel's diverticulum: investigation of 600 patients in Japanese literature. *Am J Surg* 1978, 136:247–249.

11. Mackey WC, Dineen P: A fifty year experience with Meckel's diverticulum. *SGO* 1983, 156:56–64.

12. Williams RS: Management of Meckel's diverticulum. *Br J Surg* 1981, 68:477–480.

13. Leijonmarck C-E, Bonman-Sandelin K, Frisell J: Meckel's diverticulum in the adult. *Br J Surg* 1986, 73:146–149.

14. Kusumoto H, Yoshitake H, Mochida K, Kumashiro R, Sano C, Inutsuka S: Adenocarcinoma in Meckel's diverticulum: report of a case and review of 30 cases in the English and Japanese literature. *Am J Gastroenterol* 1992, 87:910–913.

15. Weinstein EC, Dockerty WB, Waugh JH: Neoplasms of Meckel's diverticulum. *Ant Abstr Surg* 1963, 116:103–111.

16. Velanovich V, Ledbetter D, McGahren E, Nuchtern J, Schaller R: Foreign bodies within a Meckel's diverticulum. *Arch Surg* 1992, 127:864.

17. DeBartolo HM, van Heerden JA: Meckel's diverticulum. *Ann Surg* 1976, 183:30–33.

18. Newmark H, Halls J, Silberman R *et al.*: Two cases showing the radiologic appearance of Meckel's stone. *Am J Gastroenterol* 1979, 73:193–196.

19. Turgeon DK, Barnett JL: Meckel's diverticulum. *Am J Gastroenterol* 1990, 85:777–781.

20. Harden RMG, Alexander WD, Kennedy I: Isotope uptake and scanning of the stomach in man with 99mTc-pertechnetate. *Lancet* 1967, 1:1305–1307.

21. Garretson DC, Frederich ME: Meckel's diverticulum. *AFP* 1990, 42:115–119.

22. Foglia RP: Meckel's diverticulum. In *Pediatric Surgery*, edn 2. Edited by Ashcraft KW, Holder TM. Philadelphia: W.B. Saunders Company; 1993:435–439.

23. Oldham KT, Wesley JR: The pediatric abdomen. In *Surgery: Scientific Principles and Practice*. Edited by Greenfield LJ, Mulholland MW, Oldham KT, Zelenock GB. Philadelphia: J.B. Lippincott Company; 1993:1872–1873.

Laparoscopic Appendectomy

Pierre DeMatos

Kirk A. Ludwig

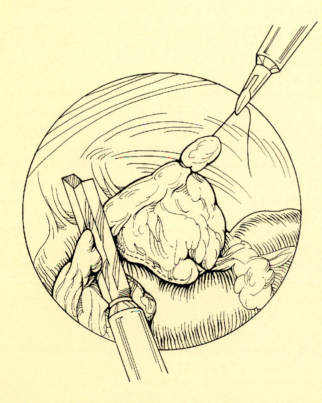

Although the first reported appendectomy was performed in 1735, it took over 150 years to recognize acute appendicitis as a clinical entity amenable to surgical therapy (Table 11-1). The standard open surgical approach via a right lower quadrant incision first suggested by McArthur [1] and McBurney [2] in 1894 has stood the test of time and has been the mainstay of treatment for acute appendicitis. Appendectomy has become one of the most frequently performed surgical procedures in the United States; approximately 12% of males and 23% of females undergo appendectomy during their lifetime [3].

Because of improvements in anesthesia, perioperative surgical care, and early diagnosis, the reported mortality of acute appendicitis is as low as 0.05% for patients with nonperforated cases and 0.27% for patients with perforation [4]. Despite these advances, significant problems still remain in the treatment of acute appendicitis. Routine appendectomy for acute appendicitis still carries a wound infection rate of approximately 5% [5,6]. Mostly because of delay in diagnosis, appendiceal perforation still occurs in 13% to 29% of cases, with its attendant increased risk for wound infection, intra-abdominal abscess formation, systemic septic complications, and death. The rate of negative appendectomies, or the percentage of those patients explored for appendicitis in which the appendix is histologically normal, remains constant at roughly 10% to 20%, depending on the institution [6,7]. These problems, coupled with the rapid evolution of laparoscopic surgical methods, have led to the development of the technique of laparoscopic appendectomy, first performed by Kurt Semm in 1982 [8]. Consideration of the laparoscopic approach is perhaps the first significant advance in the treatment of acute appendicitis for over 100 years.

Anatomy

The vermiform appendix is a narrow tubular structure arising from the posterior cecum at the confluence of the taenia coli. It is usually stated that the appendix is 1 cm wide and about 10 cm long, although variations in size and location are the rule [9]. The position of the appendiceal tip is especially inconstant. The "normal" location in the right lower quadrant overlying the sacral promontory is observed in only about 40% of cases (Figure 11-1). Other common locations include posterior to the cecum (retrocecal), in the pelvis (pelvic appendix), and posterior to the terminal ileum (retroileal). The relative frequencies of the various appendiceal positions are highly disputed.

Pathophysiology, Presentation, and Differential Diagnosis

Acute appendicitis is caused by obstruction followed by infection. Because of the presence of a fecalith, lymphoid hyperplasia, or tumor, the lumen of the appendix becomes obstructed and the resultant luminal distention leads to the sensation of poorly localized crampy pain via stimulation of the visceral afferent nerves of the appendix and small intestine. The pain is usually periumbilical in location and it is not unusual for the patient to report discomfort rather than frank pain. Also, at this stage the patient may report anorexia and nausea.

As with all epithelial-lined structures in the body, obstruction of the appendix eventually leads to stasis and infection. Intraluminal bacteria invade the appendiceal wall, and serosal inflammation results. When the inflamed serosa contacts the parietal peritoneum, the somatic nerves of the peritoneum are stimulated and the previous nonspecific pain becomes localized to the right lower quadrant. At this point, the patient may also exhibit vomiting, fever, chills, or diarrhea.

Abdominal tenderness is the sine qua non of acute appendicitis. Tenderness usually occurs in the right lower quadrant and may or may not be located at McBurney's point (two thirds the distance from umbilicus to the right anterior superior iliac spine). Many specific clinical signs may be elicited in acute appendicitis (Table 11-2) although none are as reliable as the sum of the clinical picture.

Vital signs and laboratory studies may also be helpful when acute appendicitis is suspected. Minor elevations in pulse and temperature are frequent, although body temperatures above 38.5°C are rare in uncomplicated cases. It is often stated that less than 4% of patients with acute appendicitis have entirely normal white blood cell and differential counts [10]; their presence, however, should not preclude continued observation or exploration.

Table 11-1. Milestones in the diagnosis and treatment of appendicitis

Year	Investigator	Location	Contribution
1735	Claudius Amyland	England	First report of appendectomy (via a scrotal incision for hernia and fecal fistula)
1771	Lorenz Heister	Germany	First autopsy description of abscess adjacent to a gangrenous appendix
1827	François Melier	France	Described six autopsy cases of appendiceal gangrene and first suggested surgical removal
1848	Henry Hancock	England	First reported drainage of a periappendiceal abscess
1880	Lawson Tait	England	First appendectomy for gangrenous appendix (not reported until 1890)
1883	Abraham Groves	Canada	Appendectomy for acute inflammation (not reported until 1934)
1886	Reginald Fitz	USA	First used the term "appendicitis" and described its clinical syndrome
1886	R.J. Hall	USA	Removed a perforated appendix during an exploration for incarcerated inguinal hernia
1887	Edward R. Cutler	USA	Performed appendectomy for unruptured appendicitis (reported in 1889)
1982	Kurt Semm	Germany	First report of laparoscopic appendectomy

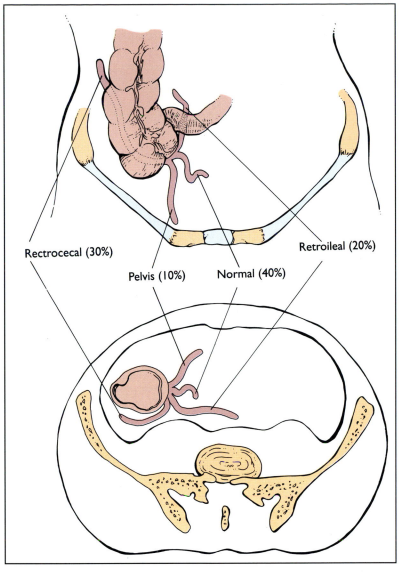

FIGURE 11-1.

The variability of the appendiceal tip. Bottom portion shows sagittal section; numbers in parentheses indicate frequencies of anatomic location.

Rectrocecal (30%)

Retroileal (20%)

Pelvis (10%)

Normal (40%)

Exhaustive lists for the differential diagnosis of acute appendicitis have been presented (Table 11-3). For practical purposes, however, the most common alternative diagnoses include gastroenteritis, pelvic inflammatory disease, urinary tract infection, tubal (ectopic) pregnancy, pyelonephritis, mittelschmerz (ovulatory pain, ruptured follicular cyst), diverticulitis, ureterolithiasis, and Crohn's disease. Because of the myriad conditions that can easily mimic acute appendicitis, it is not uncommon for a normal appendix to be found at the time of operation [6,7]. The most frequent final diagnoses are depicted in Figure 11-2.

Appendectomy may be performed via an open or laparoscopic approach. The traditional open procedure has the advantage of proven success and should probably continue to be used for cases of acute appendicitis in which the diagnosis is fairly cer-

Table 11-2. Clinical signs of acute appendicitis

Sign	Indication
Pain on gentle percussion	Peritoneal inflammation
Pain on coughing	Peritoneal inflammation
Rebound tenderness	Peritoneal inflammation
Rovsing's sign (pain in the right lower quadrant on palpation of the left lower quadrant)	Peritoneal inflammation
Voluntary muscle guarding	Peritoneal inflammation
Cutaneous hyperesthesia (increased tactile sensation of the skin of the right lower quadrant)	Peritoneal inflammation
Psoas sign (increased pain on flexion of the hip)	Irritation of the psoas muscle
Obturator sign (increased pain on internal rotation of the flexed thigh)	Irritation of the obturator internus muscle
Pain on rectal examination	Possible pelvic appendix

Table 11-3. Differential diagnosis of acute appendicitis

Gastroenteritis	Perinephric abscess
Pelvic inflammatory disease	Hydronephrosis
Urinary tract infection	Omental torsion
Tubal (ectopic) pregnancy	*Yersinia* enterocolitis
Pyelonephritis	Psoas abscess
Mittelschmerz (ovulatory pain; ruptured follicular cyst)	Rectus sheath hematoma
Diverticulitis	Cecal ulcer
Ureterolithiasis	Intestinal obstruction
Crohn's disease	Ovarian torsion
Acute cholecystitis	Ruptured corpus luteum cyst
Carcinoma of the cecum or ascending colon	Endometriosis
Meckel's diverticulitis	Congenital ureteropelvic junction obstruction
Perforated duodenal ulcer	Amebiasis
Pneumonia	Liver abscess
Osteomyelitis	Malaria
Typhoid fever	Mesenteric thrombosis
Acute porphyria	Pancreatitis
Hepatitis	Spontaneous bacterial peritonitis
Diabetes mellitus	

tain. Proponents of laparoscopic appendectomy, however, generally feel that the visual abdominal survey is superior to the exploratory capabilities of a McBurney incision and that it is most useful in cases in which the diagnosis is uncertain [11–13]. Other purported advantages of the laparoscopic approach are listed in Table 11-4. Although laparoscopic appendectomy has been safely performed in cases of acute appendicitis [14–19], perforation [15,17,18], and appendicitis during pregnancy [20] and childhood [19], the alleged advantages have never been confirmed through large randomized clinical trials.

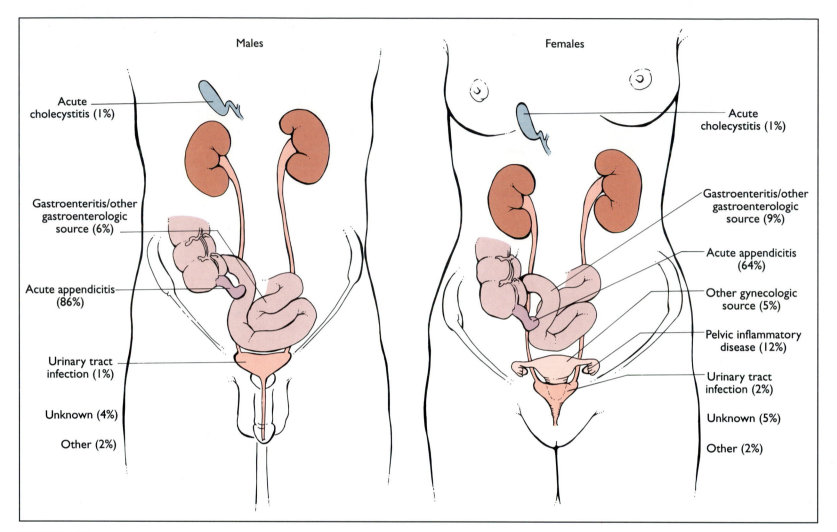

FIGURE 11-2.

Left, Final diagnoses in 636 male patients explored for acute appendicitis. **Right**, Final diagnoses in 364 female patients explored for acute appendicitis. (*From* Lewis and coworkers [7]; with permission.)

Table 11-4. Possible advantages of laparoscopic appendectomy

Increased diagnostic accuracy
Reduction in the negative appendectomy rate
Superior abdominal visualization
Decreased need for ancillary radiologic studies
Limitation of diagnostic delay
Decreased wound infection rate
Decreased postoperative pain
Decreased major complication rate
Decreased hospital stay
Earlier return to full activity
Technically easier to perform incidental appendectomy during cholecystectomy
Decreased intra-abdominal adhesion formation
Decreased cost

Surgical Technique

Figures 11–3 through 11–15 depict the surgical technique for laparoscopic appendectomy.

Set-up

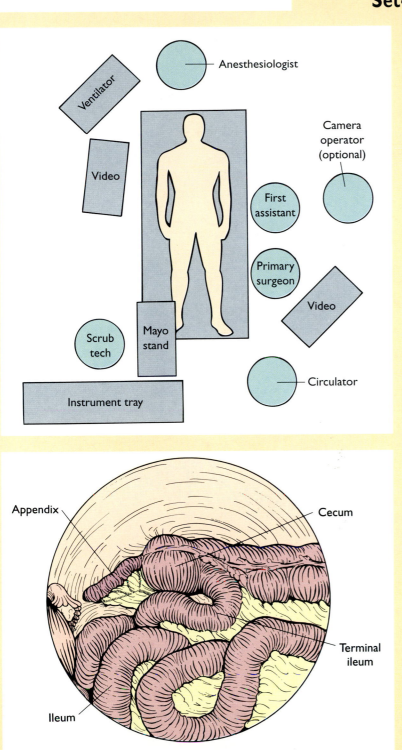

FIGURE 11-3.
Operative set-up for laparoscopic appendectomy. A preoperative dose of antibiotics is administered when the decision for operative intervention is made. Foley and nasogastric catheters are placed after induction of general anesthesia. Unlike in laparoscopic cholecystectomy, it is most helpful to position the video monitors as shown rather than at the head of the table.

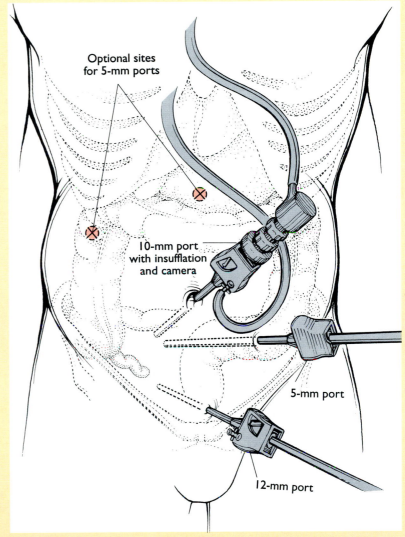

FIGURE 11-4.
The patient is placed in the 30° Trendelenburg position with the arms tucked at the sides. Access to the peritoneal cavity is gained infraumbilically by using a 10-mm sheath via a closed (Veress needle) or open (Hasson trocar) technique. After CO₂ insufflation to 15 mm Hg, the laparoscope is inserted via the 10-mm sheath and the peritoneal cavity is inspected. The liver, gallbladder, small intestine, portions of the large intestine, bladder, uterus, and ovaries can usually be visualized. At this time, the cecum and appendix are identified in the right lower quadrant.

FIGURE 11-5.
Two additional sheaths are placed under laparoscopic guidance, with abdominal transillumination and avoidance of the epigastric vessels. A 5-mm sheath is placed in the left lower quadrant at the mid-clavicular line, and a 12-mm sheath is introduced in the suprapubic midline. Slight alterations in sheath placement may be desired according to the observed location of the appendix within the abdomen. As with all cannula placement strategies, sheaths should be at least 5 fingerbreadths from each other to minimize instrument crossing during the dissection. If the exposure is difficult, an additional 5-mm sheath may be placed in the epigastrium or right upper quadrant.

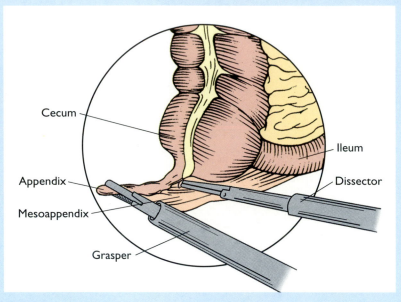

FIGURE 11-6.

The dissection is performed with the patient in 30° Trendelenburg position and tilted slightly to the left. By using a grasper inserted through the suprapubic port, the appendix and mesoappendix are retracted anterolaterally.

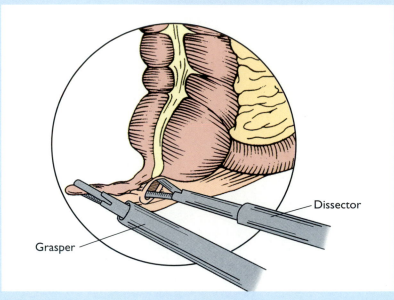

FIGURE 11-7.

The dissection of the mesoappendix is begun by using pointed-tipped forceps. A window is developed through the mesoappendix near the base of the appendix.

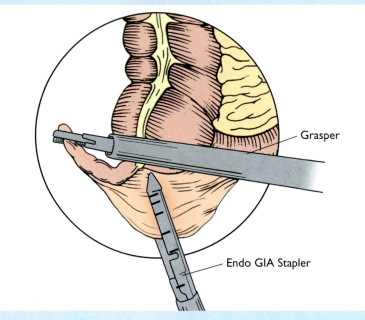

FIGURE 11-8.

A grasper introduced through the left lower quadrant port puts the mesoappendix on stretch toward the anterior abdominal wall, while an Endo-GIA (US Surgical Corp., Norwalk, CT) stapler is used to ligate and divide.

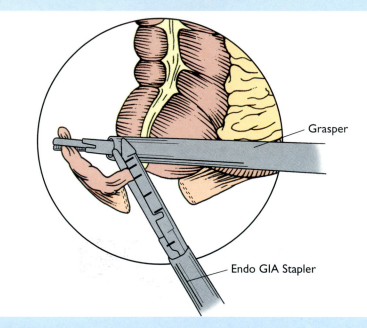

FIGURE 11-9.

The Endo-GIA stapler (US Surgical Corp., Norwalk, CT) is then used to divide the appendix at its base.

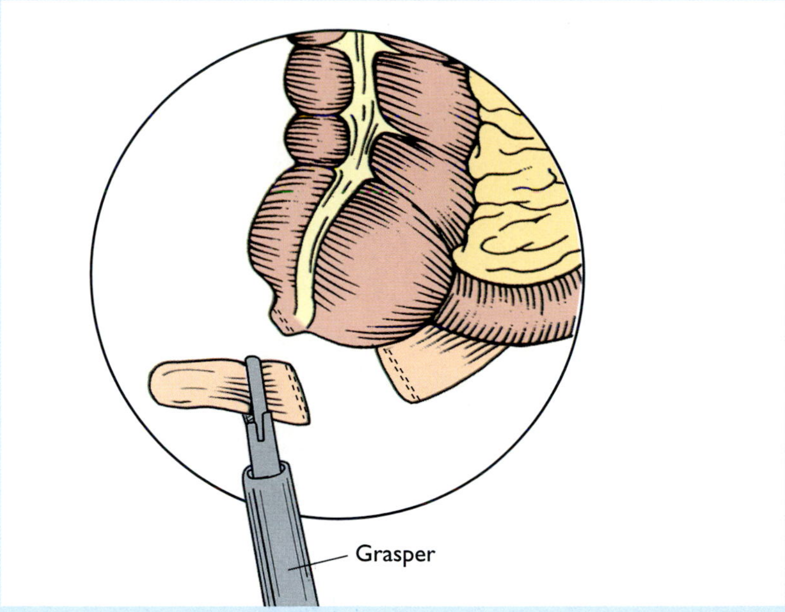

Procedure

FIGURE 11-10.
One advantage of laparoscopic appendectomy is the ability to remove the appendix without contacting the wound edges; this theoretically lessens the risk for wound infection. After division of the appendix, the tip is grasped with a forceps via the 12-mm sheath and withdrawn entirely into the sheath.

Grasper

FIGURE 11-11.
The sheath and forceps are removed as a unit, with the appendix protected inside the sheath.

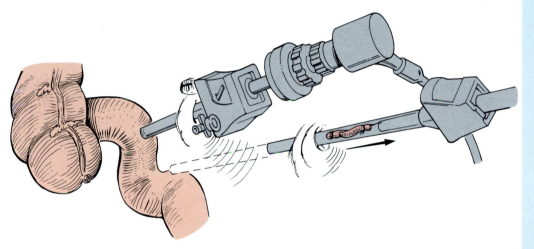

FIGURE 11-12.
If the appendix is large and friable, it may be inserted into a specially designed sterile sac (Endo-catch; US Surgical Corp., Norwalk, CT) for retrieval. As the sac is partially withdrawn into the 12-mm sheath, it closes around the appendix. The sheath and sac are then removed as a unit.

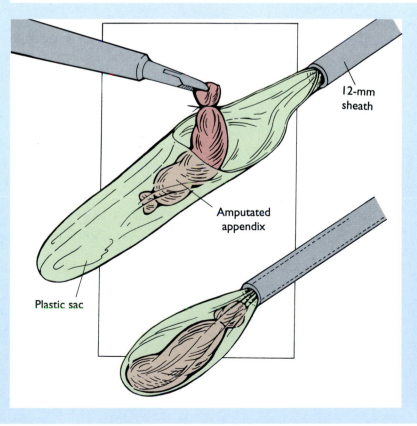

12-mm sheath

Amputated appendix

Plastic sac

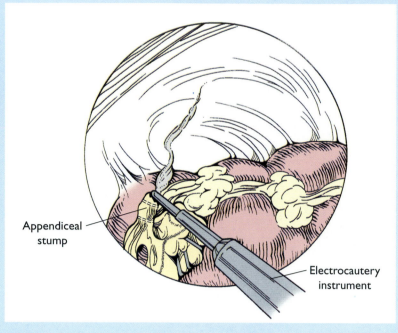

FIGURE 11-13.

The residual mucosa of the appendiceal stump is cauterized completely. Some authors recommend inversion of the appendiceal stump [30,31] although, as in open appendectomy, this is probably not necessary [32].

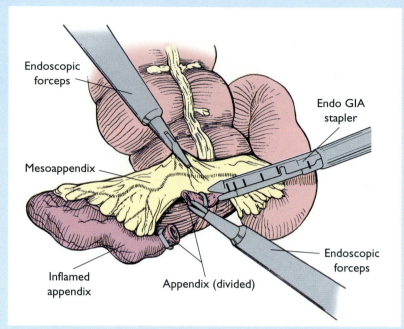

FIGURE 11-14.

Retrograde appendectomy. If the appendiceal tip or body is gangrenous and the base is relatively uninvolved, it may be advantageous to divide the base before dissection of the mesoappendix and involved segment. This procedure has been termed "retrograde appendectomy" and may limit soilage of the abdominal cavity and facilitate the dissection. This approach can be performed successfully with a laparoscope [12,13]. The base is ligated and divided using the Endo-GIA (US Surgical Corp., Norwalk, CT) stapler, or it may be ligated using an endoscopic loop suture and divided sharply. The mesoappendix is divided in a similar fashion, and the appendix is removed.

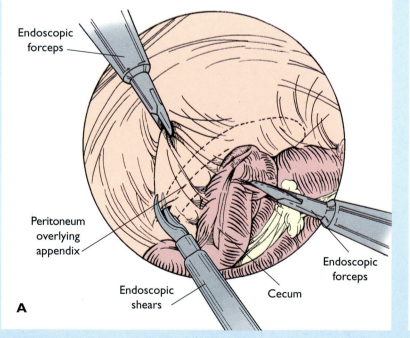

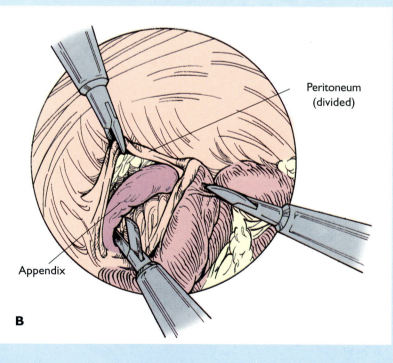

FIGURE 11-15.

Laparoscopic removal of a retrocecal appendix is challenging, but successful cases have been reported [14]. **A**, First, the peritoneum overlying the appendix is divided by using the endoscopic shears. Care must be taken to avoid injury to the right colon. **B**, After the appendiceal base is fully exposed, appendectomy is performed in a retrograde fashion as previously described.

Results

Excluding case reports and series with fewer than 40 cases, nearly 7000 laparoscopic appendectomies have been reported to date (Table 11-5). In general, the results have been excellent. For all patients studied, conversion to open appendectomy was required only 6% of the time. Major complications and wound infections occurred in 3% and 1.4% of cases, respectively. The most common major complication is pelvic abscess, which has become more prevalent with surgeons' increasing willingness to undertake more difficult appendectomies (*eg*, gangrenous and perforated) using the laparoscopic approach.

Published reports have taken the form of retrospective reviews [12,14–50], retrospective comparisons [51–72], prospective nonrandomized trials [73–81], and prospective randomized trials [30,82–96]. The safety and efficacy of this procedure have been clearly demonstrated by retrospective comparisons and nonrandomized trials. Its superiority over the conventional open technique, however, remains unproven. Some prospective trials have reported decreased rates of complications [84] and wound infections [73,75,82–85], improvements in pain and pain control [82–85,89,95–97], shortened hospital stay [73,74,76,82, 84,87,96–98], and decreased time to return to full activity [73,74,

11-5. Reported results of laparoscopic appendectomy between 1987 and 1998 (Series reporting ≥ 40 cases)

Study	Cases, n	Perforated appendices, n	Open conversion, n	Wound infection, n	Major complications, n
Nowrazadan and coworkers [52]	87	NR	6	1	3 (SBO)
Champault and coworkers [63]	50	6	6	0	3 (abscess)
Sosa and coworkers [62]	41	8	4	3	3 (abscess in 2, significant atelectasis in 1)
Naffis and coworkers [47]	51	8	0	0	
Neal and coworkers [51]	53	1	14	0	9 (ileus in 5, abscess in 2, SBO in 1, acute renal failure in 1)
Varlet and coworkers [64]	200	0	10	1	8 (abscess in 2, pulmonary complications in 3, hemorrhage in 2, intraoperative intestinal perforation in 1)
Bouillot and coworkers [79]	234	10	29	1	3 (intraoperative bladder perforation, abscess, peritonitis)
Jain and coworkers [48]	75	14	9	1	2 (abscess)
Martin and coworkers [87]	81	10	13	3	4 (abscess in 3, abdominal wall hematoma in 1)
Ortega and coworkers [88]	167	28	11	4	6 (abscess)
DesGroseilliers and coworkers [65]	100	19	12	2	2 (abscess)
Heinzelman and coworkers [66]	102	NR	18	NR	13
Chao and coworkers [80]	100	12	0	2	2 (abscess)
Karim and O'Regan [49]	69	8	8	0	4 (ileus in 2, diarrhia in 2)
Hansen and coworkers [89]	79	11	7	2	3 (SBO in 2, chest infection in 1)
Mutter and coworkers [90]	50	NR	6	1	2 (fever)
Tang and coworkers [67]	108	28	NR	NR	4 (abscess)
Henle and coworkers [91]	87	5	NR	6	1 (abscess)
Kluiber and Hartsman [68]	234	NR	NR	2	13 (abscess)
Hart and coworkers [92]	44	4	4	3	3 (abscess)
Richards and coworkers [69]	189	31	NR	1	4 (abscess in 4, ileus in 4)
Panton and coworkers [70]	101		31	2	3 (abscess in 2, trocar site hemorrhage in 1)
Moberg and Montgomery [71]	43	NR	11	2	3 (fever and diarrhea in 2, ileus in 1)
Chiarugi and coworkers [93]	77	5	6	3	14 (ileus in 5, abscess in 4, fever in 2, enteritis in 1, trocar site hemorrhage in 1, appendiceal artery hemorrhage in 1)
Reiertsen and coworkers [94]	42	6	0	1	2 (abscess)
Kazemier and coworkers [95]	96	16	12	0	7 (ileus in 5, ileal perforation in 1, pneumonia in 1)
Macarulla and coworkers [96]	106	5	9	1	2 (abscess, hemoperitoneum)
Hale and coworkers [50]	174	NR	13	2	NR
Greason and coworkers [81]	44	0	0	0	1 (postlaparoscopy pain)
Fallahzadeh and coworkers [72]	60	0	NR	NR	1 (bowel perforation)
Totals	6977	347	385	86	
Weighted percentages		7.3%	6.2	1.4%	

NR—not reported; SBO"small bowel obstruction.

76,84–86,88,89,92,94,98,99]. Other studies, however, have not shown a benefit in terms of patient outcome [30,72,76]. Furthermore, any cost savings realized by the decreased length of stay and convalescence are probably offset by increased expenditures in the operating room [57,69,73,76–78,87,96,97,100].

In conclusion, laparoscopic appendectomy can be performed safely and reliably and represents an important technique in the armamentarium of the general surgeon. The notion that it has become the procedure of choice in all cases of suspected appendicitis is not supported by the currently available data. It seems most beneficial in patients in whom the diagnosis is in question, patients for whom full visualization of the abdominal cavity is critical, or patients with compelling need or preference for early return to physical activity. As with most laparoscopic procedures, laparoscopic appendectomy should be applied selectively on the basis of the clinical setting, hospital environment, and surgeon's experience.

References

1. Strohl EL, Diffenbaugh WG: The historical background of the gridiron or muscle-splitting incision for appendectomy. *Ill Med J* 1969, 135:287–288.

2. McBurney C: The incision made in the abdominal wall in cases of appendicitis, with a description of a new method of operating. *Ann Surg* 1894, 20:38–43.

3. Addiss DG, Shaffer N, Fowler BS, Tauxe RV: The epidemiology of appendicitis and appendectomy in the United States. *Am J Epidemiol* 1990, 132:910–925.

4. Luckman R: Incidence and case fatality notes for acute appendicitis in California: a population-based study of the effects of age. *Am J Epidemiol* 1989, 129(suppl):905–918.

5. Berry J, Malt RA: Appendicitis near its centenary. *Ann Surg* 1984, 200:567–575.

6. Pappas TN, Gale F, Ross RP: Appendicitis can be treated safely with a negative appendectomy rate of 10%. *Digestive Surgery* 1989, 6:74–77.

7. Lewis FR, Holcroft JW, Boey J, Dunphy JE: Appendicitis: a critical review of diagnosis and treatment in 1,000 cases. *Arch Surg* 1975, 110:677–684.

8. Semm KI: Advances in pelviscopic surgery. *Curr Probl Obstet Gynecol* 1982, 5:32–34.

9. Kelley HA, Hurdon E: *The Vermiform Appendix and Its Disease.* Philadelphia: Saunders; 1905.

10. Sasso RD, Hanna EA, Moore DL: Leukocytic and neutrophilic counts in acute appendicitis. *Am J Surg* 1970, 120:563–566.

11. Engström L, Fenyö G: Appendectomy: assessment of stump invagination versus simple ligation. *Br J Surg* 1985, 72:971–972.

12. Nowzaradan Y, Westmoreland J, McCarver CT, Harris RJ: Laparoscopic appendectomy for acute appendicitis: indications and current use. *J Laparoendosc Surg* 1991, 1:247–257.

13. Schultz LS, Pietrafitta JJ, Graber JN, Hickok DF: Retrograde laparoscopic appendectomy: report of a case. *J Laparoendosc Surg* 1991, 1:111–114.

14. Geis WP, Miller CE, Kokoszka JS, et al.: Laparoscopic appendectomy for acute appendicitis: rationale and technical aspects. *Contemp Surg* 1992, 40:13–19.

15. Klaiber C, Wagner M, Metzger A: Various stapling techniques in laparoscopic appendectomy: 40 consecutive cases. *Surg Laparosc Endosc* 1994, 4:205–209.

16. Cox MR, McCall JL, Padbury RT, et al.: Laparoscopic surgery in women with a clinical diagnosis of acute appendicitis. *Med J Aust* 1995, 162:130–132.

17. Valla JS, Limonne B, Valla V, et al.: Laparoscopic appendectomy in children: report of 465 cases. *Surg Laparosc Endosc* 1991, 1:166–172.

18. el Ghoneimi A, Valla JS, Limonne B, et al.: Laparoscopic appendectomy in children: report of 1,379 cases. *J Pediatr Surg* 1994, 29:786–789.

19. Schreiber JH: Results of outpatient laparoscopic appendectomy in women. *Endoscopy* 1994, 26:292–298.

20. Meinke AK, Kossuth T: What is the learning curve for laparoscopic appendectomy? *Surg Endosc* 1994, 8:371–375.

21. Mohsen AA: Endocoagulator control of the mesoappendix for laparoscopic appendectomy. *J Laparoendosc Surg* 1994, 4:435–440.

22. Corso FA: Laparoscopic appendectomy. *Int Surg* 1994, 79:247–250.

23. Vargas HI, Tolmos J, Klein SR, et al.: Laparoscopic appendectomy in the 1990's. *Int Surg* 1994, 79:242–246.

24. Charoonratana V, Chansawang S, Maipang T, Totemchokchyakarn P: Laparoscopic appendicectomy. *Eur J Surg* 1993, 159:235–237.

25. Cox MR, McCall JL, Wilson TG, et al.: Laparoscopic appendicectomy: a prospective analysis. *Aust N Z J Surg* 1993, 63:840–847.

26. Schiffino L, Mouro J, Karayel M, et al.: Laparoscopic appendectomy: a study of 154 consecutive cases. *Int Surg* 1993, 78:280–283.

27. Pier A, Götz F, Backer C: Laparoscopic appendectomy in 625 cases: from innovation to routine. *Surg Laparosc Endosc* 1991, 1:8–13.

28. Götz F, Pier A, Bacher C: Modified laparoscopic appendectomy in surgery. *Surg Endosc* 1990, 4:6–9.

29. Pier A, Götz F, Bacher C, Ibald R: Laparoscopic appendectomy. *World J Surg* 1993, 17:29–33.

30. Laparoscopic versus open appendicectomy: prospective randomised trial. *Lancet* 1993, 342:633–637.

31. Ludwig KA, Cattey RP, Henry LG: Initial experience with laparoscopic appendectomy. *Dis Colon Rectum* 1993, 36:463–467.

32. Paul MG, Kim D, Tylka BL, et al.: Laparoscopic surgery in a mobile army surgical hospital deployed to the former Yugoslavia. *Surg Laparosc Endosc* 1994, 4:441–447.

33. Miller JP: Laparoscopic appendectomy. *Pediatr Ann* 1993, 22:663–667.

34. Scott-Conner CE, Hall TJ, Anglin BL, Muakkassa F: Laparoscopic appendectomy: initial experience in a teaching program. *Ann Surg* 1992, 215:660–668.

35. Goh P, Tekant Y, Kum CK, et al.: Technical modification to laparoscopic appendectomy. *Dis Colon Rectum* 1992, 35:999–1000.

36. Pelosi MA, Pelosi MA 3d: Laparoscopic appendectomy using a single umbilical puncture (minilaparoscopy). *J Reprod Med* 1992, 37:588–594.

37. Byrne DS, Bell G, Morrice JJ, Orr G: Technique for laparoscopic appendicectomy. *Br J Surg* 1992, 79:574–575.

38. Richards W, Watson D, Lynch G, et al.: A review of the results of laparoscopic versus open appendectomy. *Surg Gynecol Obstet* 1993, 177:473–480.

39. Daniell JF, Gurley LD, Kurtz BR, Chambers JF: The use of an automatic stapling device for laparoscopic appendectomy. *Obstet Gynecol* 1991, 78:721–723.

40. Cristalli B, Chiche R, Izard V, Levardon M: Douleurs pelviennes de la femme Èvaluation d'une technique d'appendicectomie intra-péritonéale per-clioscopique. *Ann Chir* 1991, 45:529–533.

41. O'Regan PJ: Laparoscopic appendectomy. *Can J Surg* 1991, 34:256–258.

42. Bonanni F, Reed J 3rd, Hartzell G, et al.: Laparoscopic versus conventional appendectomy. *J Am Coll Surg* 1994, 179:273–278.

43. Saye WB, Rives DA, Cochran EB: Laparoscopic appendectomy: three years' experience. *Surg Laparosc Endosc* 1991, 1:109–115.

44. McKernan JB, Saye WB: Laparoscopic techniques in appendectomy with argon laser. *South Med J* 1990, 83:1019–1020.

45. Schreiber JH: Early experience with laparoscopic appendectomy in women. *Surg Endosc* 1987, 1:211–216.

46. Gangal HT, Gangal MH: Laparoscopic appendicectomy. *Endoscopy* 1987, 19:127–129.

47. Naffis D: Laparoscopic appendectomy in children. *Semin Pediatr Surg* 1993, 2:174–177.

48. Jain A, Mercado PD, Grafton KP, et al.: Outpatient laparoscopic appendectomy. *Surg Endosc* 1995, 9:424–425.

49. Karim SS, O'Regan, PJ: Laparoscopic appendectomy: a review of 95 consecutive cases of appendicitis. *Can J Surg* 1995, 38:449–453.

50. Hale DA, Molloy M, Pearl RH, *et al.*: Appendectomy. A contemporary appraisal. *Ann Surg* 1997, 225:252–261.

51. Neal GE, McClintic EC, Williams JS: Experience with laparoscopic and open appendectomies in a surgical residency program. *Surg Laparosc Endosc* 1994, 4:272–276.

52. Nowzaradan Y, Barnes JP Jr, Westmoreland J, Hojabri M: Laparoscopic appendectomy: treatment of choice for suspected appendicitis. *Surg Laparosc Endosc* 1993, 3:411–416.

53. Cohen MM, Dangleis K: The cost-effectiveness of laparoscopic appendectomy. *J Laparoendosc Surg* 1993, 3:93–97.

54. Schirmer BD, Schmieg RE Jr, Dix J, *et al.*: Laparoscopic versus traditional appendectomy for suspected appendicitis. *Am J Surg* 1993, 165:670–675.

55. Lansdown M, Kraly Z, Milkins R, Royston C: Conventional versus laparoscopic surgery for acute appendicitis. *Br J Surg* 1993, 80:1349–1350.

56. Tate JJ, Chung SC, Dawson J, *et al.*: Conventional versus laparoscopic surgery for acute appendicitis. *Br J Surg* 1993, 80:761–764.

57. Schroder DM, Lathrop JC, Lloyd LR, *et al.*: Laparoscopic appendectomy for acute appendicitis: is there really any benefit? *Am Surg* 1993, 59:541–548.

58. Fritts LL, Orlando R 3d: Laparoscopic appendectomy: a safety and cost analysis. *Arch Surg* 1993, 128:521–525.

59. Naver LP, Kock JP, Bokmand S: Primary experiences with laparoscopic appendectomy. *Ugeskr Laeger* 1994, 156:3775–3777.

60. Buckley RC, Hall TJ, Muakkassa FF, *et al.*: Laparoscopic appendectomy: is it worth it? *Am Surg* 1994, 60:30–34.

61. Pruett B, Pruett J: Laparoscopic appendectomy: have we found a better way? *J Miss State Med Assoc* 1994, 35:347–351.

62. Sosa JL, Sleeman D, McKenney MG, *et al.*: A comparison of laparoscopic and traditional appendectomy. *J Laparoendosc Surg* 1993, 3:129–131.

63. Champault G, Belhassen A, Rizk N, *et al.*: Appendicectomie. McBurney or laparoscopie? *J Chir* 1993, 130:5–8.

64. Varlet F, Tardieu D, Limonne B, *et al.*: Laparoscopic versus open appendectomy in children: comparative study of 403 cases. *Eur J Pediatr Surg* 1994, 4:333–337.

65. Desgroseilliers S, Fortin M, Lokanathan R, *et al.*: Laparoscopic appendectomy versus open appendectomy: retrospective assessment of 200 patients. *Can J Surg* 1995, 38:178–182.

66. Heinzelmann M, Simmen HP, Cummins AS, *et al.*: Is laparoscopic appendectomy the new gold standard? *Arch Surg* 1995, 130:782–785.

67. Tang E, Ortega AE, Anthone GJ, *et al.*: Intraabdominal abscesses following laparoscopic and open appendectomies. *Surg Endosc* 1996, 10:327–328.

68. Kluiber RM, Hartsman B: Laparoscopic appendectomy. *Dis Col Rectum* 1996, 39:1008–1011.

69. Richards KF, Fisher KS, Flores JH, *et al.*: Laparoscopic appendectomy: comparison with open appendectomy in 720 patients. *Surg Laparosc Endosc* 1996, 6:205–209.

70. Panton ON, Samson C, Segal J, *et al.*: A four-year experience with laparoscopy in the management of appendicitis. *Am J Surg* 1996, 171:538–541.

71. Moberg AC, Montgomery A: Appendicitis: laparoscopic versus conventional operation. *Surg Laparosc Endosc* 1997, 7:459–463.

72. Fallahzadeh H: Should a laparoscopic appendectomy be done? *Am Surg* 1998, 64:231–233.

73. Gilchrist BF, Lobe TE, Schropp KP, *et al.* Is there a role for laparoscopic appendectomy in pediatric surgery? *J Pediatr Surg* 1992, 27:209–214.

74. Kollias J, Harries RH, Otto G, Hamilton DW, Cox JS, Gallery RM: Laparoscopic versus open appendicectomy for suspected appendicitis: a prospective study. *Aust N Z J Surg* 1994, 64:830–835.

75. Lujan Mompean JA, Robles Campos R, Parrilla Paricio P, Soria Aledo V, Garcia Ayllon J: Laparoscopic versus open appendicectomy: a prospective assessment. *Br J Surg* 1994, 81:133–135.

76. Reiertsen O, Trondsen E, Bakka A, Andersen OK, Larsen S, Rosseland AR: Prospective nonrandomized study of conventional versus laparoscopic appendectomy. *World J Surg* 1994, 18:411–416.

77. Apelgren KN, Molnar RG, Kisala JM: Laparoscopic is not better than open appendectomy. *Am Surg* 1995, 61:240–243.

78. Apelgren KN, Molnar RG, Kisala JM: Is laparoscopic better than open appendectomy? *Surg Endosc* 1992, 6:298–301.

79. Bouillot JL, Salah S, Fernandez F, *et al.*: Laparoscopic procedure for suspected appendicitis. A prospective study in 283 consecutive patients. *Surg Endosc* 1995, 9:957–960.

80. Chao C, Tsai CT, Wu WC: Complete two-handed laparoscopic appendectomy: report of 100 cases. *J Formos Med Assoc* 1995, 94:679–682.

81. Greason KL, Rappold JF, Liberman MA: Incidental laparoscopic appendectomy for acute right lower quadrant abdominal pain. *Surg Endosc* 1998, 12:233–235.

82. McAnena OJ, Auston O, Hederman WP, Gorey TF, Fitzpatrick J, O'Connell PR: Laparoscopic versus open appendicectomy. *Lancet* 1991, 338:693.

83. McAnena OJ, Austin O, O'Connell PR, Hederman WP, Gorey TF, Fitzpatrick J: Laparoscopic versus open appendicectomy: a prospective evaluation. *Br J Surg* 1992, 79:818–820.

84. Attwood SE, Hill AD, Murphy PG, Thornton J, Stephens RB: A prospective randomized trial of laparoscopic versus open appendectomy. *Surgery* 1992, 112:497–501.

85. Kum CK, Ngoi SS, Goh PM, Tekant Y, Isaac JR: Randomized controlled trial comparing laparoscopic and open appendicectomy. *Br J Surg* 1993, 80:1599–1600.

86. Frazee RC, Roberts JW, Symmonds RE, *et al.*: A prospective randomized trial comparing open versus laparoscopic appendectomy. *Ann Surg* 1994, 219:725–731.

87. Martin LC, Puente I, Sosa JL, *et al.*: Open versus laparoscopic appendectomy. A retrospective randomized comparison. *Ann Surg* 1995, 222:256–262.

88. Ortega AE, Hunter JG, Peters JH, *et al.*: A prospective, randomized comparison of laparoscopic appendectomy with open appendectomy. Laparoscopic Appendectomy Study Group. *Am J Surg* 1995, 169:208–212.

89. Hansen JB, Smithers BM, Schache D, *et al.*: Laparoscopic versus open appendectomy: prospective randomized trial. *World J Surg* 1996, 20:17–21.

90. Mutter D, Vix M, Bui A, *et al.*: Laparoscopy not recommended for routine appendectomy in men: results of a prospective randomized study. *Surgery* 1996, 120:71–74.

91. Henle KP, Beller S, Rechner J, *et al.*: Laparoskopische vs konventionelle Appendektomie: eine prospektive, randomisierte Studie. *Chirurg* 1996, 67:526–530.

92. Hart R, Rajgopal C, Piewes A, *et al.*: Laparoscopic versus open appendectomy: a prospective randomized trial of 81 patients. *Can J Surg* 1996, 39:457–462.

93. Chiarugi M, Buccianti P, Celona G, *et al.*: Laparoscopic compared with open appendicectomy for acute appendicitis: a prospective study. *Eur J Surg* 1996, 162:385–390.

94. Reiertsen O, Larsen S, Trondsen E, *et al.*: Randomized controlled trial with sequential design of laparoscopic versus open appendicectomy. *Br J Surg* 1997, 84:842–847.

95. Kazemier G, de Zeeuw GR, Lange JF, *et al.*: Laparoscopic vs open appendectomy: a randomized clinical trial. *Surg Endosc* 1997, 11:336–340.

96. Macarulla E, Vallet J, Abad JM, *et al.*: Laparoscopic versus open appendectomy: a prospective randomized trial. *Surg Laparosc Endosc* 1997, 7:335–339.

97. Vallina VL, Velasco JM, McCulloch CS: Laparoscopic versus conventional appendectomy. *Ann Surg* 1993, 218:685–692.

98. Cox MR, McCall JL, Toouli J, *et al.*: Prospective randomized comparison of open versus laparoscopic appendectomy in men. *World J Surg* 1996, 20:263–266.

99. Laine S, Rantala A, Gullichsen R, *et al.*: Laparoscopic appendectomy: is it worthwile? *Surg Endosc* 1997, 11:95–97.

100. Minné L, Varner D, Burnell A, *et al.*: Laparoscopic vs open appendectomy: prospective randomized study of outcomes. *Arch Surg* 1997, 132:708–712.

*L*aparoscopic Colectomy and Abdominoperineal Resection

Alan P. Kypson
Kirk A. Ludwig

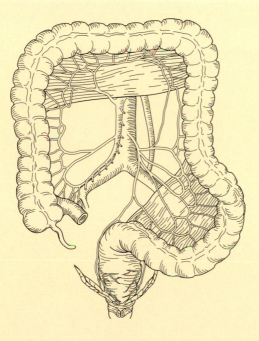

The introduction and rapid acceptance of laparoscopic chole-cystectomy in the late 1980s created a new era in abdominal surgery and inspired surgeons to apply laparoscopic techniques to colorectal surgery. Early success in the laboratory led to the application of laparoscopic colectomy for benign human diseases such as Crohn's disease and diverticulitis. As experience was gained, the technique was applied not only to all portions of the colon and rectum but to malignant disease as well. Whereas the field of laparoscopic biliary surgery developed quickly, laparo-scopic colorectal surgery has been slow to develop and evolve, in large part because of the degree of difficulty, oncologic concerns, and the difficulty in demonstrating dramatic advantages for the laparoscopic approach. New techniques and instruments are being developed to make these operations more applicable. Ongoing studies are addressing concerns about the actual bene-fits of this approach, and thorough follow-up of the long-term benefits of laparoscopic colectomy for cancer is ongoing to ensure locoregional clearance of tumor, recurrence rates, and long-term survival that are comparable to those of the conven-tional standard of open surgery. Clearly, laparoscopic colorectal surgery is still evolving.

Anatomy

Many aspects of the anatomy of the colon are important when a laparoscopic resection is being considered (Fig. 12-1). The colon has both intraperitoneal and retroperitoneal segments. As the ileum enters the cecum, there are critical associations with iliac and gonadal vessels and with the right ureter. Most of the right colon is retroperitoneal, and as the ascending colon approaches the liver, there are associations with the gallbladder, duodenum, pancreas, and potentially the common bile duct. The transverse colon overlies the body of the pancreas and is attached to the stomach by the omentum. The descending colon begins at the left colic flexure (splenic flexure) and courses retroperitoneally until it becomes the sigmoid colon, which is intraperitoneal. Special attention must be paid to the left ureter, gonadal vessels, and iliac vessels, all of which lie in the left iliac fossa. The sym-pathetic nerves travel down the aorta and lie just behind the inferior mesenteric artery. The sympathetic nerve trunk branch-es just over the sacral promontory, giving rise to right and left hypogastric nerves. These nerves should be avoided and protect-ed during dissections of the left colon and rectum.

The major blood supply of the right colon is the ileocolic artery. The right colic artery is typically a branch of the ileocolic artery and supplies the right colon to the hepatic flexure [1]. The middle colic artery supplies the hepatic flexure to the splenic flexure. Its course varies, and its structure branches. The inferior mesenteric artery supplies the descending and sigmoid colon and proximal rectum. Each of the major colonic arteries communicates peripherally in the mesentery to form a rich anas-tomotic network.

The venous drainage follows the arterial supply; the proximal and transverse colon drain into the superior mesenteric vein, and the descending and sigmoid colon drain predominantly into the inferior mesenteric vein. Similarly, the lymphatic drainage of the colon follows the major arterial channels, first through the epicolic lymph nodes near the colonic wall. The second level of nodal structures consists of pericolic lymph nodes in the mesentery along the branches of the supplying arteries. The third level of lymph nodes is at the base of the colonic mesentery near the inferior or superior mesenteric arter-ies. Finally, terminal nodes at the base of the colic vessels anasto-mose with periaortic lymph channels.

FIGURE 12-1.

Anatomy of the colon.

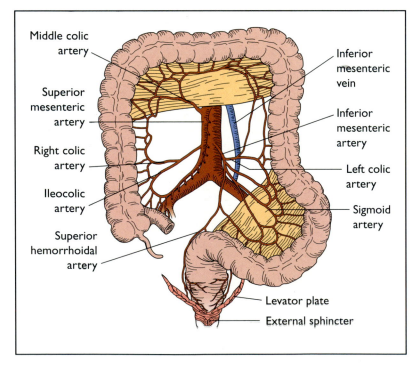

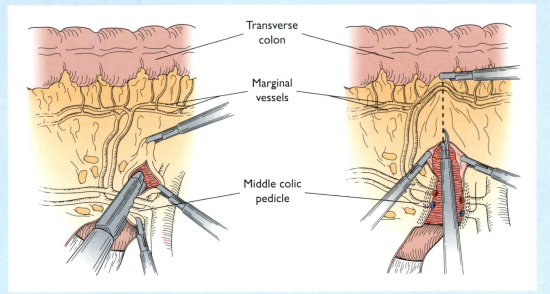

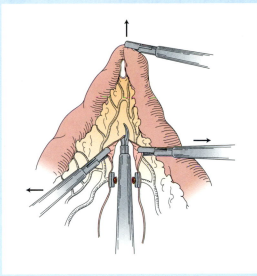

FIGURE 12-7.

Dissection continues up the colic gutter from the ventral aspect of the right colonic mesenteric root, continuing medially until the peritoneal reflection of the middle colic vessels is seen. The reflection is sharply divided, and underlying tissue is dissected to isolate the middle colic vessels. The vascular pedicle is divided in a manner similar to that used for the ileocolic vessels. Subsequently, just to the left of the vessels, the peritoneum is incised and the mesocolon is transected up to the edge of the transverse colon. Marginal vessels are divided with clips as needed. Greater omental attachments to the transverse colon are transected at the distal resection line up to the edge of the transverse colon. (*Adapted from* Milsom and Bohm [2]; with permission.)

FIGURE 12-8.

Next, the proximal resection line is identified and the ileal mesentery is dissected, starting from the ileocolic pedicle. The marginal vessels are clipped and divided up to the edge of the ileum. (*Adapted from* Milsom and Bohm [2]; with permission.)

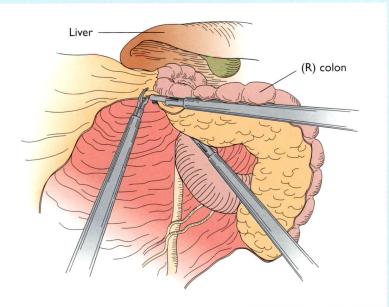

FIGURE 12-9.

At this point, the right colon is completely detached from retroperitoneal structures by using medial traction on the colon, starting at the cecum. Only the lateral peritoneal attachments still need to be divided. As the hepatic flexure is approached, the scissor electrocautery is adequate for most hemostasis, but some clipping of small vessels may be judicious. Ultrasonic shears can be used as well. This dissection is continued until the colon is freed up to the distal resection line. If the resection is being performed for malignant disease, the transverse colon and ileum are divided with the laparoscopic stapler. The umbilical cannula is changed to a 15-mm port, and a laparoscopic retrieval bag is inserted. The specimen is collected and removed as the umbilical port site is enlarged appropriately. The distal and proximal resection margins are exteriorized, and a conventional ileocolic anastomosis is completed. For benign disease, it is usually preferable to simply mobilize the bowel completely, as illustrated, and then simply exteriorize through an enlarged umbilical site. The mesentery and anastomosis can be managed conventionally. Resection of the right colon is usually unnecessary for ileocecal Crohn's disease. The right colon is mobilized only to allow sufficient length for exteriorization. For Crohn's disease, extraction sites and port sites should not be placed at potential ileostomy sites. (*Adapted from* Milsom and Bohm [2]; with permission.)

Laparoscopic Left Colectomy

Figures 12-10 through 12-21 depict the surgical technique for left colectomy.

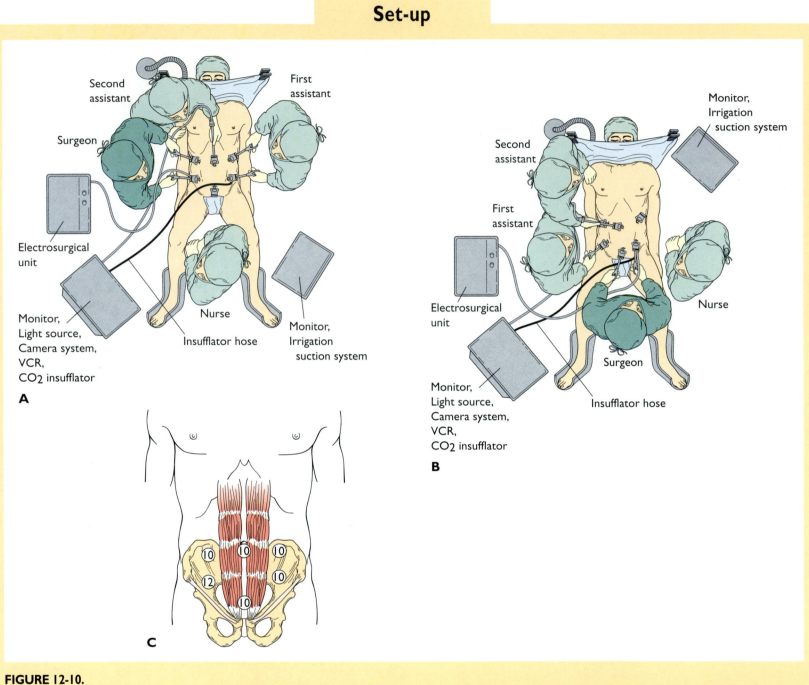

Set-up

FIGURE 12-10.

For operations on the left or sigmoid colon, the patient is placed in the modified lithotomy position by using Dan Allen stirrups (Dan Allen Co., Bedford Heights, OH). The hips and knees are slightly flexed so that the thighs are almost parallel to the floor. The patient is rolled to the right and placed in the Trendelenburg position. For splenic flexure mobilization, reverse Trendelenburg position is used. Initially, the surgeon and second assistant (cameraperson) are on the patient's right side, and the first assistant stands on the patient's left side (A). During mobilization of the splenic flexure, the surgeon stands between the patient's legs and both assistants stand on the right (B). The trocar sites are as depicted: a 10-mm umbilical trocar, a 10- and 12-mm trocar in the right lateral abdominal wall, two 10-mm trocars in the left lateral abdominal wall, and a 10-mm suprapubic port for use in splenic flexure mobilization (C). (*Adapted from* Milsom and Bohm [2]; with permission.)

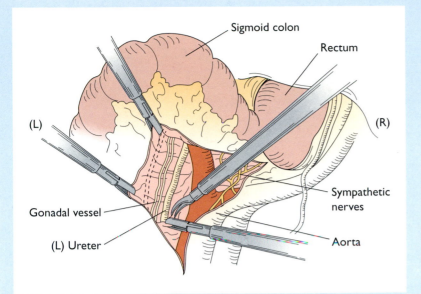

FIGURE 12-11.

Dissection is begun with cephalad and lateral retraction of the mesosigmoid by the assistant using a laparoscopic Babcock clamp and a grasper. The peritoneum immediately to the right of the inferior mesenteric artery at the level of the sacral promontory is incised. This incision is carried cephalad toward the origin of the inferior mesenteric artery. Blunt and sharp dissection is then used to sweep the inferior mesenteric vessels ventrally and to identify the left ureter and gonadal vessels, which are swept posteriorly. Dissection proceeds medial to lateral in a plane between the mesocolon and retroperitoneum. (*Adapted from* Milsom and Bohm [2]; with permission.)

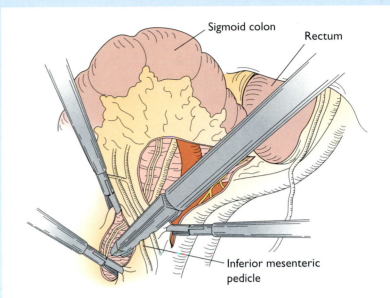

FIGURE 12-12.

Once the origin of the inferior mesenteric artery is identified, the peritoneum is incised over and to the left of the pedicle, toward the inferior mesenteric vein (which typically travels with the ascending branch of the left colic artery). A peritoneal window is created lateral to the inferior mesenteric artery. With careful attention paid to the ureter, the inferior mesenteric artery is ligated by using the endoscopic 30-mm vascular stapler. The vascular pedicle is left with a length of approximately 1.0 to 1.5 cm so that additional ligature can be applied if needed. (*Adapted from* Milsom and Bohm [2]; with permission.)

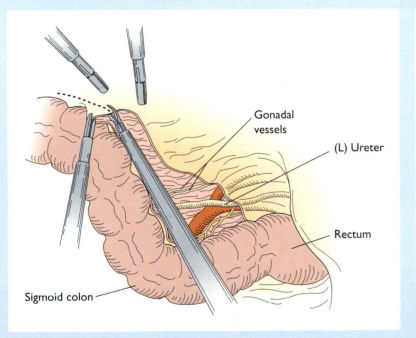

FIGURE 12-13.

Gentle caudal and medial retraction using a Babcock clamp and grasper is applied and the lateral attachments of the left colon are now dissected free. Sharp as well as blunt dissection is used to mobilize the left colon. (*Adapted from* Milsom and Bohm [2]; with permission.)

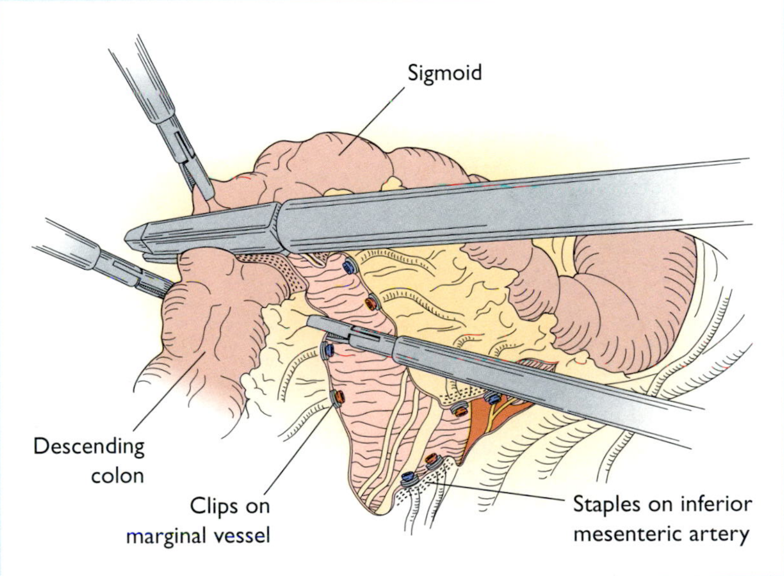

FIGURE 12-14.

Attention is then turned to the mesosigmoid of the proximal resection line. By using the technique of tissue triangulation, the mesocolon is transected up to the colonic edge. Small vessels are managed with the electrocautery scissors, whereas the marginal vessel typically requires clip placement. Ultrasonic shears may be useful for this dissection. The colon is divided with the 30-mm endoscopic stapler; two applications are generally required. (*Adapted from* Milsom and Bohm [2]; with permission.)

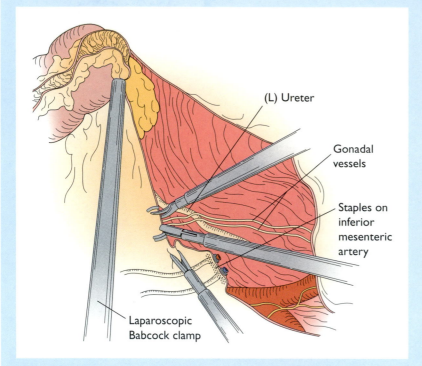

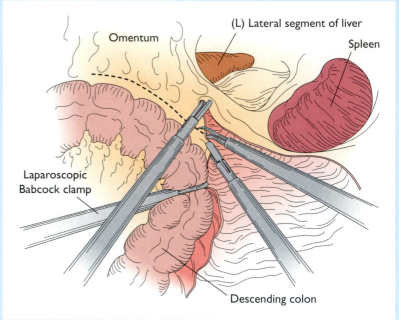

FIGURE 12-15.

The splenic flexure is then mobilized. The assistant provides medial and caudal traction by working from the right side of the patient through the right sided ports. The surgeon moves to a position between the legs and works in a cephalad direction through the suprapubic and left lower quadrant ports. The laparoscopic scissors or ultrasonic shears are used to lift the descending colon off of Gerota's fascia. The plane of dissection is close to the colon: the surgeon should keep the dissection medial. (*Adapted from* Milsom and Bohm [2]; with permission.)

FIGURE 12-16.

Continuing the caudal and medial retraction of the colon, the lateral attachments of the colon are divided. In the area of the splenic flexure, the greater omentum is visualized and must be carefully separated from the colon to ensure adequate mobilization of the flexure. As the splenic flexure and transverse colon come into view, the surgeon may prefer working through the left upper and lower quadrant ports. The dissection should proceed to the right as far as deemed necessary to allow the descending colon to reach the pelvis. Additional length on the descending and distal transverse colon can be obtained by dividing the inferior mesenteric vein alongside the duodenum just at the inferior edge of the pancreas. Clips or the endoscopic stapler can be used. (*Adapted from* Milsom and Bohm [2]; with permission.)

FIGURE 12-17.

Next, the rectum is mobilized as far distally as required toward the pelvic floor, starting with posterior mobilization just behind the fascia propria of the mesorectum. Sympathetic nerve trunks are thus protected. If the proper plane is entered, there should essentially be no bleeding. Anterior dissection is taken to a level below the anterior peritoneal reflection, as far as necessary. (*Adapted from* Milsom and Bohm [2]; with permission.)

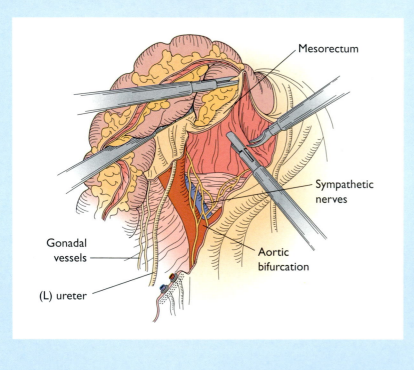

Procedure

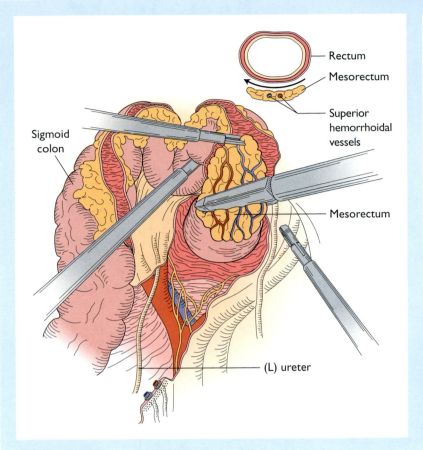

FIGURE 12-18.

The mesorectum is then separated from the rectum by use of sharp and blunt dissection. The mesorectum contains only two major vessels (the superior hemorrhoidals) that require particular attention. These vessels run posterior and medial through the mesorectum and can be managed with one application of the endoscopic stapler after the mesorectum has been thinned down using electrocautery scissors or ultrasonic shears. (*Adapted from* Milsom and Bohm [2]; with permission.)

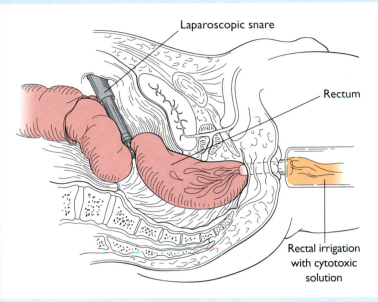

FIGURE 12-19.

Once the distal resection line is freed of its mesorectum, an endoscopic snare is used to occlude the rectum below the tumor and above the resection line. At this point, a distal rectal washout with Betadine solution (Purdue Frederick, Norwalk, CT) or sterile water is performed transanally; this may reduce the risk for implantation of exfoliated tumor cells. (*Adapted from* Milsom and Bohm [2]; with permission.)

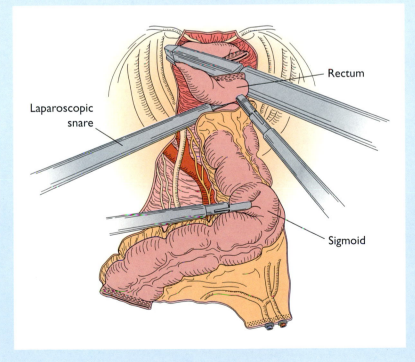

FIGURE 12-20.

The rectum is divided with two or three applications of the 30-mm endoscopic stapler just below the snare. The specimen is immediately placed in a bowel bag, which is then closed shut. The left-lower-quadrant incision is lengthened with a 3- to 5-cm muscle-splitting incision, and the specimen is removed from the peritoneal cavity. Next, the mobilized descending colon is delivered through the same incision, and a purse-string suture is placed around the cut edge of the colon after the previously placed staples are excised. The anvil of a circular 31- or 28-mm stapler is then inserted and secured. This end of the bowel is then returned to the abdomen, and the abdominal incision is closed in an air- and water-tight fashion. The abdomen is reinsufflated, and the circular stapler with a suture around the plastic spike is introduced via the anus. The device is opened, and the spike is driven through the top of the rectal stump, directly through or immediately adjacent to the transverse staple line. A grasper is then used to pull on the suture to remove the spike from the center post. (*Adapted from* Milsom and Bohm [2]; with permission.)

Procedure

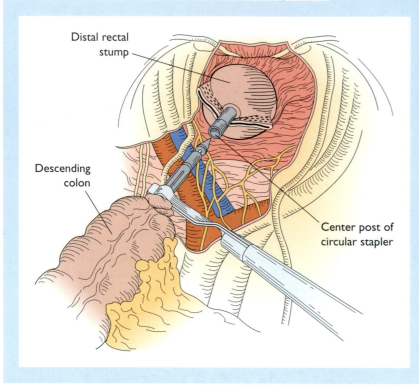

FIGURE 12-21.

A standard double-stapling technique is used to form the colorectal anastomosis. A Babcock instrument is used to place the center rod of the anvil into the center post of the transanally placed stapler. The stapler is then closed and fired in the usual fashion. The anastomotic donuts are checked for completeness. The pelvis is filled with saline, and air is insufflated via the rectum with a proctoscope to assure an airtight anastomosis.

The techniques described are used to manage malignant disease. For benign disease, typically diverticulitis, the sequence differs slightly. The operation still begins with division of the inferior mesenteric artery, distal to the left colic artery. The sigmoid is then mobilized laterally. At this point, however, the dissection is immediately taken distally as the proximal rectum is mobilized. The mesorectum and rectum are divided as illustrated (Fig. 12-18 and 12-20). With benign disease, of course, distal irrigation is unnecessary. Now the descending colon and splenic flexure are mobilized as needed, and the bowel is extracted through the enlarged site of the left-lower-quadrant port. After extraction, a soft and pliable proximal resection line is chosen. A pursestring suture is placed to secure the anvil and center rod of the staple gun. The proximal bowel is returned to the abdomen and the anastomosis is fashioned as described. (*Adapted from* Milsom and Bohm [2]; with permission.)

Laparoscopic Abdominoperineal Resection

Set-up

Initial positioning of the patient, position of the surgical team, and position of cannulas are similar to those used for laparoscopic left colectomy described earlier (Fig. 12-10). The left-lower-quadrant cannula must be placed at the premarked stoma site. Video monitors are moved to the patient's knees as dissection of the rectum commences.

Procedure

Initial dissection is similar to the initial steps of the laparoscopic left colectomy (Fig. 12-11 though 12-14). The inferior mesenteric artery is taken with the stapler, the sigmoid mesentery is mobilized from medial to lateral, the mesentery is divided and the left colon is divided with the linear stapler. Dissection of the rectum proceeds down into the pelvis in the avascular plane just outside of the fascia propria of the mesorectum.

Procedure

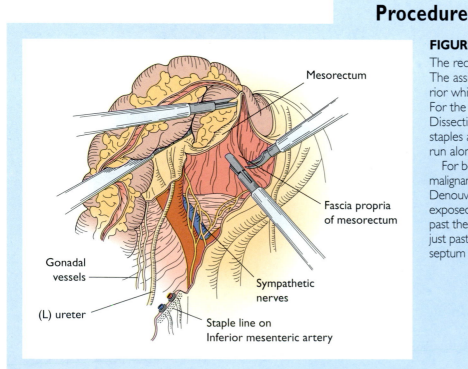

FIGURE 12-22.

The rectum is completely mobilized to the pelvic floor, starting posteriorly. The assistant, on the patient's left, provides strong traction right, left, and anterior while the rectum is pulled up out of the pelvis. Good retraction is the key. For the anterior mobilization, the assistant pushes the rectum down forcefully. Dissection in the proper plane is nearly bloodless. In most patients, no clips or staples are needed laterally because the middle hemorrhoidal vessels actually run along the pelvic floor muscles, not in the "lateral ligament."

For benign disease, the anterior dissection is kept close to the rectal wall. For malignant disease, however, the dissection should proceed anterior to Denouvier's fascia. In this case, the prostate and seminal vesicles are clearly exposed. Dissection from above concludes when the rectum has been mobilized past the tip of the coccyx posteriorly and laterally. The anterior dissection is taken just past the level of the seminal vesicles in men and well into the rectovaginal septum in women. (*Adapted from* Milsom and Bohm [2]; with permission.)

Procedure

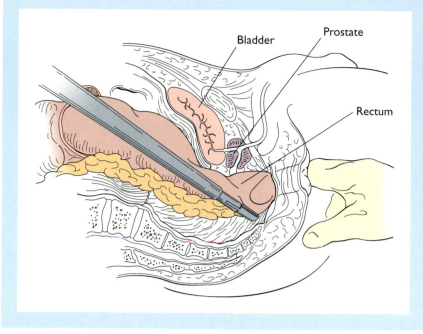

Bladder

Prostate

Rectum

FIGURE 12-23.

To check progress from above, the surgeon can place a gloved finger into the anus or, in women, the vagina. After complete mobilization of the rectum, the perineal portion of the operation begins. Pneumoperitoneum is now released, and perineal excision of the anus and the rectum is performed in a standard manner. An endoscopic grasper is next passed through the cannula located at the selected colostomy site, and the distal end of the descending colon is grasped and pulled to the anterior wall. The colostomy is then created by withdrawing the cannula, dilating the fascia with two fingers, and then pulling the bowel end up to the skin level. Visualization via the laparoscope is necessary to ensure that the descending colon has not twisted. The pelvis is then copiously irrigated by placing the patient in a head-up position. A silicon drain is placed into the pelvis. The perineum is closed and the colostomy is matured in the usual fashion. (*Adapted from* Milsom and Bohm [2]; with permission.)

Conclusions

Laparoscopic colon resection has proven to be feasible and safe when performed by well-trained surgeons [3–9]. Most groups initiated their experience with laparoscopic colectomy on benign processes of the right colon. After initial experience, laparoscopic applications of colorectal surgery were expanded to include malignant and inflammatory disease throughout the colon. In general, indications for laparoscopic surgery of the colon do not differ from those for conventional surgery. These indications include but are not limited to diverticular disease, Crohn's disease, and cancer. Many concerns have been raised about the use of these techniques for malignant diseases: the intraoperative identification of the site of abnormality, the adequacy of nodal clearance, and the possibility of port-site recurrence. Theoretical advantages of laparoscopic colorectal surgery include less pain, quicker recovery of intestinal motility, shorter hospital stay, and a quicker return to normal lifestyle.

Laparoscopic surgery is possible in inflammatory diseases of the intestinal tract if the patient is medically stable. In most cases, vital structures can be properly isolated, but the sequelae of inflammatory disease, such as abscess, fistulae, and severe distortion of anatomy, may require conversion to open surgery. Acutely ill patients with hemodynamic instability from bowel abnormalities are, in most cases, not candidates for laparoscopic colon surgery. However, minimally invasive surgery for stable patients with inflammatory disease offers theoretical advantages. In a recent review by Ludwig and coworkers [10], 14 of 31 patients with Crohn's disease underwent laparoscopic ileocecectomy with favorable results and median time to discharge of 6 days. Similar results have been reported by others [11,12].

Elective resection for chronic diverticular disease may lend itself nicely to a laparoscopic resection. Thorough knowledge of anatomy and identification and protection of vital pelvic structures are required if laparoscopic surgery is being contemplated for diverticular disease, because the inflammation associated with this abnormality can make dissection difficult. Contraindications would include

large intra-abdominal abscess or diverticular phlegmon, complex fistulization, and perforation with peritonitis. Nevertheless, when laparoscopic surgery is performed at the appropriate time, recent studies have shown promising results. In a retrospective study, Liberman and coworkers [13] compared 14 patients who underwent laparoscopic colectomy with a control group of 14 matched patients who underwent open surgery. Eleven of the 14 anastomoses were created intraperitoneally. Mean operative times did not differ between the two groups, and time to ability to receive a liquid diet (2.9 vs 6.1 days) and postoperative stay were significantly less (6.3 compared with 9.2 days) in the laparoscopic group.

Many question have been raised about the appropriateness of laparoscopy for the treatment of colorectal cancer. Current standard of care dictates that a wide margin proximal and distal to the area of abnormality exist and that high ligation of the vessels and an excision of the tissues containing the lymphatic bed of the tumor be performed. Conventional surgical oncologic principles exist and are the basis of well-known long-term results. New techniques, such as laparoscopic surgery, must prove themselves not only in terms of morbidity and mortality but also in terms of recurrence and survival rates. Only after randomized trials have been completed will we be able to widely recommend laparoscopic surgery. In patients with metastatic disease, resection of the tumor for palliative purposes can often be readily done by using laparoscopic techniques. Contraindications to laparoscopic resection of colorectal cancer include infiltrating tumors, large and bulky tumors (those greater than 8 cm in diameter), or obstructing tumors.

The lack of tactile feedback during laparoscopic procedures necessitates accurate preoperative and intraoperative identification of the diseased area. Several methods may be used to achieve this goal. Fortunately, a large percentage of cancers are externally evident on the colonic surface. For small or intraluminal lesions, preoperative barium enema can be used to delineate the anatomic location. Laparoscopic dissection performed solely according to an endoscopist's report can be perilous. If a lesion has been removed before surgery, endoscopic identification and marking of the site with India ink may be necessary [14]. It is imperative, upon removal, that the specimen be opened to confirm the presence of the pathologic lesion.

The issue of adequacy of lymph node dissection in operations for cancer has been under review. In a multicenter retrospective study of 66 patients, Falk and coworkers [4] found no statistically significant difference in the number of lymph nodes removed in sigmoid and right colectomy specimens compared with conventional controls. Other studies have also found that the laparoscopic approach is similar to open surgery in providing adequate lymphadenectomy specimens [3,15,16]. A cadaveric study of laparoscopic right and left colectomies [17] reported that the anatomic extent of a laparoscopic resection does not differ from that obtained by conventional resection techniques. This serves, at least initially, as evidence that an adequate oncologic resection can be performed successfully through a laparoscopic approach.

Port site metastasis has been a concern as laparoscopic techniques have been applied for treatment of malignant disease [18–20]. Most reports of this problem are anecdotal and therefore provide little quantitative information. Direct tumor manipulation is not a prerequisite for port site tumor implantation [21]. Although the mechanism of these recurrences is unknown, it probably relates to the abdominal-wall trauma imposed during the cannula insertion, coupled with implantation of an adequate inoculum of exfoliated cells during the procedure. Therefore, certain operative principles should be adhered to: 1) minimal manipulation of the diseased segment; 2) occlusion of the proximal and distal ends of the intestinal segment; 3) placement of the specimen in an endoscopic bag as soon as possible; and 4) intraoperative protection of the extraction wound with a wound protector. Irrigation of cannula sites with a cytotoxic agent is also advisable. Early reports raised many questions about the incidence of port site recurrence; more recent studies suggest that port site recurrence does not occur more frequently than does wound implantation after conventional surgery [22]. A retrospective multicenter analysis of 372 patients conducted by the Clinical Outcomes of Surgical Therapy (COST) study group revealed four recurrences (1.3% of resectable cases) involving port sites or the abdominal wall [5], a rate consistent with the incidence of abdominal wound implantation for open colectomy [22,23]. Only one of the four patients died of widespread cancer. The other three underwent resection of their port site recurrence and remained free of disease thereafter.

The advantages and disadvantages of laparoscopic colorectal surgery are not entirely known and will take years of intense study to determine. Recent reports indicate that the postoperative stay is significantly shorter for patients undergoing laparoscopic colectomy [24–26]. In addition, although the operative times are longer, patients become ambulatory sooner and experience earlier return of bowel function, even though the mechanism for this is unclear [15, 24,25,27]. Reports indicate that patients return to normal activity at an earlier date than those undergoing traditional colectomy. Most cost-benefit analyses, however, have not reported a benefit in hospital costs when comparing laparoscopic to traditional colon resection [4,15,28]. Furthermore, it becomes significantly more expensive, both in terms of operating room costs and hospital costs, when a laparoscopic case is converted to open. It remains to be seen whether there is an overall cost benefit from earlier mobilization and return to work. Intense scrutiny and long-term follow-up in the context of randomized studies are needed to satisfactorily answer these as well as other questions surrounding the appropriate role of laparoscopic colorectal surgery.

References

1. Garcia-Ruiz A, Milsom JW, Ludwig KA, *et al.*: Right colonic arterial anatomy. *Dis Colon Rectum* 1996, 39:906–911.

2. *Laparoscopic Colorectal Surgery.* Edited by Milsom JW, Bohm B. New York: Springer-Verlag; 1996.

3. Peters WR, Bartels TL: Minimally invasive colectomy: are the potential benefits realized? *Dis Colon Rectum* 1993, 36:751–756.

4. Falk PM, Beart RW Jr, Wexner SD, *et al.*: Laparoscopic colectomy: a critical appraisal. *Dis Colon Rectum* 1993, 36:28–34.

5. Fleshman JW, Nelson H, Peters WR, *et al.*: Early results of laparoscopic surgery for colorectal cancer. Retrospective analysis of 372 patients treated by Clinical Outcomes of Surgical Therapy (COST) Study Group. *Dis Colon Rectum* 1996, 39:S53–S58.

6. Fielding GA, Lumley J, Nathanson L, *et al.*: Laparoscopic colectomy. *Surg Endosc* 1997, 11:745–749.

7. Fowler DL, White SA, Anderson CA: Laparoscopic colon resection: 60 cases. *Surg Laparosc Endosc* 1995, 5:468–471.

8. Lumley JW, Fielding GA, Rhodes M, *et al.*: Laparoscopic-assisted colorectal surgery: lessons learned from 240 consecutive patients. *Dis Colon Rectum* 1996, 39:155–159.

9. Wexner SD, Reissman P, Pfeifer J, *et al.*: Laparoscopic colorectal surgery: analysis of 140 cases. *Surg Endosc* 1996, 10:133–136.

10. Ludwig KA, Milsom JW, Church JM, *et al.*: Preliminary experience with laparoscopic intestinal surgery for Crohn's disease. *Am Surg* 1996, 171:52–56.

11. Reissman P, Salky BA, Edye M, *et al.*: Laparoscopic surgery in Crohn's disease. *Surg Endosc* 1996, 10:1201–1204.

12. Liu CD, Rolandelli R, Ashley SW, *et al.*: Laparoscopic surgery for inflammatory bowel disease. *Am Surg* 1995, 61:1054–1056.

13. Liberman MA, Phillips EH, Carroll BJ, *et al.*: Laparoscopic colectomy vs traditional colectomy for diverticulitis. *Surg Endosc* 1996, 10:15–18.

14. Kim SH, Milsom JW, Church JM, *et al.*: Perioperative tumor localization for laparoscopic colorectal surgery. *Surg Endosc* 1997, 11:1013–1016.

15. Van Ye T, Cattey R, Henery L: Laparoscopically assisted colon resections compare favorably with open technique. *Surg Laparosc Endosc* 1994, 4:25–31.

16. Moore JW, Bokey EL, Newland RC, *et al.*: Lymphovascular clearance in laparoscopically assisted right hemicolectomy is similar to open surgery. *Aust N Z J Surg* 1996, 66:605–607.

17. Milsom JW, Bohm B, Decanini C, *et al.*: Laparoscopic oncologic proctosigmoidectomy with colorectal anastomosis. *Surg Endosc* 1994, 8:1117–1123.

18. Fusco MA, Paluzzi MW: Abdominal wall recurrence after laparoscopic-assisted colectomy for adenocarcinoma of the colon: report of a case. *Dis Colon Rectum* 1993, 36:858–861.

19. Wexner SD, Cohen SM: Port site metastases after laparoscopic colorectal surgery for cure of malignancy. *Br J Surg* 1995, 82:295–298.

20. Fodera M, Pello MJ, Atabek U, *et al.*: Trocar site tumor recurrence after laparoscopic-assisted colectomy. *J Laparoendosc Surg* 1995, 5:259–262.

21. Siriwardena A, Samarji W: Cutaneous tumour seeding from a previously undiagnosed pancreatic carcinoma after laparoscopic cholecystectomy. *Ann R Coll Surg Engl* 1993, 75:119–120.

22. Reilly WT, Nelson H, Schroeder G, *et al.*: Wound recurrence following conventional treatment of colorectal cancer: a rare but perhaps underestimated problem. *Dis Colon Rectum* 1996, 39:200–207.

23. Lacy AM, Delgado S, Garcia-Valdecasas JC, *et al.*: Port site metastases and recurrence after laparoscopic colectomy. A randomized trial. *Surg Endosc* 1998, 12:1039–1042.

24. Lacy AM, Garcia-Valdecasas JC, Pique JM, *et al.*: Short-term outcome analysis of a randomized study comparing laparoscopic versus open colectomy for colon cancer. *Surg Endosc* 1995, 9:1101–1105.

25. Franklin ME Jr, Rosenthal D, Abrego-Medina D, *et al.*: Prospective comparison of open vs. laparoscopic colon surgery for carcinoma. Five-year results. *Dis Colon Rectum* 1996, 39:S35–S46.

26. Stage J, Schulze S, Moller P, *et al.*: Prospective randomised study of laparoscopic vs open colonic resection for adenocarcinoma. *Br J Surg* 1997, 84:391–396.

27. Gelpi JR, Dorsey-Tyler K, Luchtefeld MA, *et al.*: Prospective comparison of gastric emptying after laparoscopic-aided colectomy versus open colectomy. *Am Surg* 1996, 62:594–596.

28. Phillipson BM, Bokey EL, Moore JW, *et al.*: Cost of open versus laparoscopically assisted right hemicolectomy for cancer. *World J Surg* 1997, 21:214–217.

$\mathcal{L}$aparoscopic Cholecystectomy

Larkin J. Daniels
Edward G. Chekan

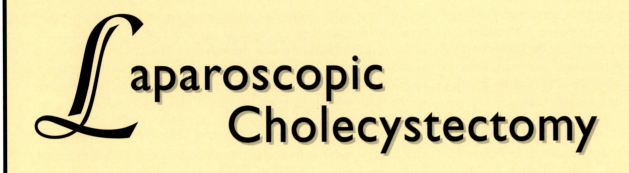

Laparoscopic Cholecystectomy

Although gallstones were first described in the fifth century by the Greek physician Alexander Trallianus, therapy for gallstone disease was delayed until 1867 when John Stough Bobbs performed the first cholecystotomy with removal of gallstones in a 32-year-old woman with hydrops of the gallbladder. This was followed in 1882 by the first cholecystectomy by Langenbuch in Berlin. His patient was discharged from the hospital 7 weeks after the new procedure. During the first half of the 20th century, the most significant advances in the field pertained primarily to improved diagnosis. The surgical treatment of gallbladder disease remained largely unchanged until the introduction of laparoscopic techniques for cholecystectomy. Although there is some debate in the literature on who deserves credit for this advancement, several investigators are listed in Table 13-1.

Anatomy

The normal anatomy of the biliary system is shown in Figure 13-1. The gallbladder is 7 to 10 cm long, with a maximal width of 2.5 to 3 cm at the fundus, and a typical volume of approximately 30 mL, although in marked distension the gallbladder can contain as much as 300 mL. It is bound to the gallbladder fossa between the right and left hepatic lobes on the undersurface of the liver. The attachment can vary from an intrahepatic location to a true mesentery. Blood supply comes via the cystic artery that arises from the right hepatic artery in 95% of cases, but it can be derived from the left hepatic, common hepatic, gastroduodenal, or superior mesenteric arteries. Double cystic arteries are found in 8% and accessory cystic arteries in 12% of patients.

The cystic duct is from 2.5 to 4 cm long. It passes very close to the free right margin of the gastrohepatic ligament, usually joining the main hepatic duct at an acute angle. Within it are many spiral folds, known as the valves of Heister, that can make catheter passage difficult in intraoperative cholangiography. Occasionally, the cystic duct can take a longer course posterior to the main hepatic duct and empty into it posteriorly.

Pathophysiology, Presentation, and Differential Diagnosis

Cholecystectomy is indicated for the treatment of symptomatic gallstone disease, acalculous cholecystitis, and, in very specific instances (*eg*, porcelain gallbladder or immunosuppression),

---

Table 13-1. Milestones in the diagnosis and treatment of gallbladder disease

Year	Investigator	Location	Procedure
1867	John Stough Bobbs	USA	First cholecystostomy
1882	Carl Langenbuch	Berlin	First cholecystectomy
1890	Ludwig Courvoisier	Basel	First choledocholithotomy
1924	Evarts Graham and Warren Cole	USA	First cholecystogram in humans
1953	Eric Yuhl	USA	First cholescintigram
1987	Phillipe Mouret	France	First laparoscopic cholecystectomy
1988	Eddie Reddick and Douglas Olsen	USA	First laparoscopic cholecystectomy in USA

Table 13-2. Differential diagnosis of cholecystitis

Acute appendicitis	Fitz-Hugh-Curtis syndrome
Duodenal ulcer	Pyelonephritis
Gastric ulcer	Gastroesophageal reflux
Acute pancreatitis	Radicular pain
Hepatitis	Coronary artery disease
Right heart failure	

Table 13-3. Advantages and disadvantages of the laparoscopic versus open approach

Advantages	Disadvantages
Smaller incisions	Equipment requirements
Less pain	More difficult to control bleeding
Rapid return to full activity	Slightly increased incidence of bile duct injury
Shorter hospital stay	Difficult to explore common bile duct
Decreased total cost	Restricted application because of to adhesions and inflammation
Fewer pulmonary effects	

asymptomatic patients. Occasionally it may be indicated with documented biliary dyskinesia or "crystal disease."

Chronic cholecystitis is characterized by recurrent bouts of right upper quadrant or epigastric pain that usually follows meals and can radiate through to the back. Frequently, the pain is accompanied by nausea, vomiting, and a feeling of abdominal fullness or bloating. Attacks typically last from 30 minutes to 24 hours. The discomfort of chronic cholecystitis is believed to represent biliary colic and not inflammation. A complex of symptoms that does not include pain is probably not due to chronic cholecystitis even if gallstones are demonstrated.

Acute cholecystitis is characterized by acute bacterial inflammation of the gallbladder, usually resulting from cystic duct obstruction secondary to calculous (95% of cases). Persistent pain and tenderness in the right upper quadrant are present in almost every case. Nausea and vomiting occur in two thirds of patients and are thought to be secondary to the rapid rise in gall-

bladder pressure. Fever is present in 80% of patients. Signs of peritoneal irritation, such as Murphy's sign, become more common as the disease progresses. The leukocyte count is elevated in 85% of cases. Common processes mimicking acute cholecystitis are summarized in Table 13-2.

Although the laparoscopic approach to cholecystectomy has significantly decreased recovery time, it should not be viewed as expanding the indications for cholecystectomy. The first decision is whether a cholecystectomy is indicated and the second decision is whether a laparoscopic or open approach is more appropriate. Although the laparoscopic approach has many advantages (Table 13-3), there are still patients in whom an open cholecystectomy is indicated.

Surgical Technique

Figures 13-2 through 13-13 depict the surgical technique for laparoscopic cholecystectomy.

FIGURE 13-1.

Normal anatomy of the biliary system.

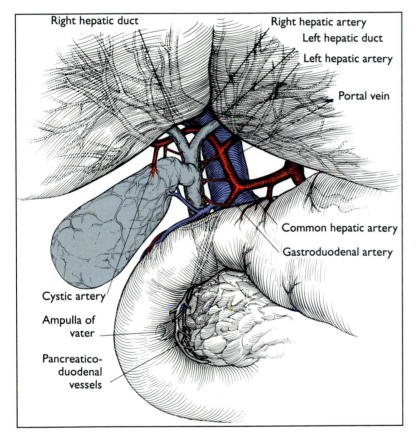

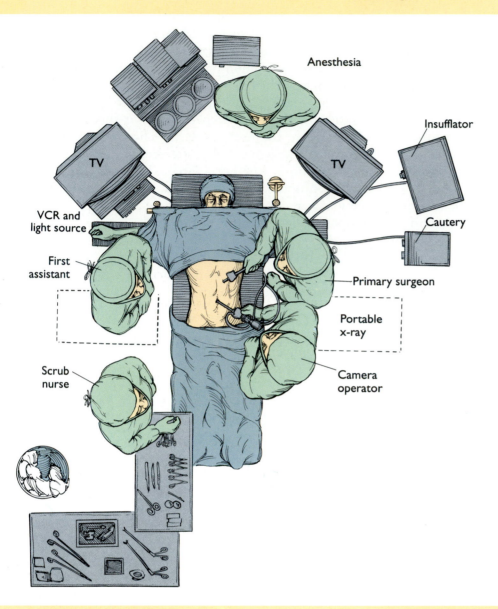

FIGURE 13-2.

Operative set-up for laparoscopic cholecystectomy. The use of a separate camera operator is optional because many surgeons prefer to operate the camera with the left hand and use the right hand for instrument manipulation. A preoperative dose of antibiotic, usually a first-generation cephalosporin, is administered before induction. A nasogastric catheter is placed after induction of general anesthesia.

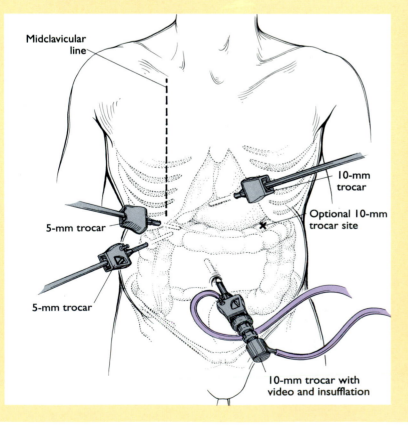

FIGURE 13-3.

The patient is placed in a 30° Trendelenburg position with arms extended. Access to the peritoneal cavity is gained infraumbilically by using a 10-mm sheath via a closed (Veress needle) or open (Hasson trocar) technique. After insufflation with carbon dioxide to 15 mm Hg, the laparoscope is inserted and the peritoneal cavity inspected. The patient is then shifted to a reverse Trendelenburg position and rolled toward the left to allow better visualization of the gallbladder and surrounding structures. Two right subcostal 5-mm trocars and an epigastric 10-mm trocar are then placed under laparoscopic direction. Occasionally, a fifth trocar is placed in the left subcostal position for retraction, allowing better visualization of hilar structures.

Procedure

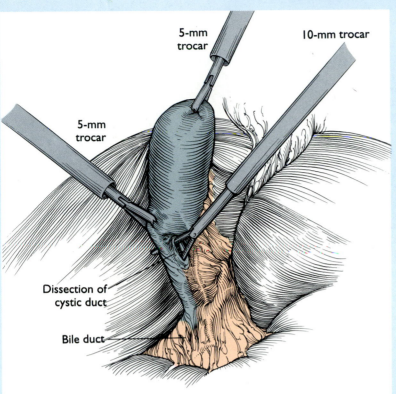

FIGURE 13-4.

With traction on the fundus of the gallbladder in a cephalad direction and on the infundibulum inferolaterally to the right, the cystic duct is placed on tension at a right angle to the common bile duct, minimizing the chance of confusing the two structures. The dissection is then begun in a right to left direction and the cystic duct identified and dissected thoroughly enough to be positive about its identity.

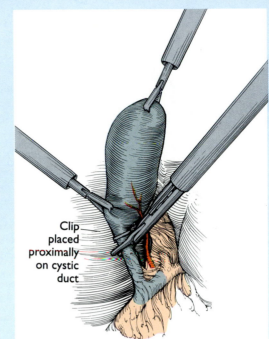

FIGURE 13-5.

At this point in the operation, the anatomical landmarks should be carefully considered. If anatomy of the infundibulum-cystic duct junction remains unclear after 30 minutes of dissection, the surgeon should strongly consider conversion to open procedure. If landmarks of the cystic duct are clear at this time, endoscopic clips should be placed at the infundibulum–cystic duct junction.

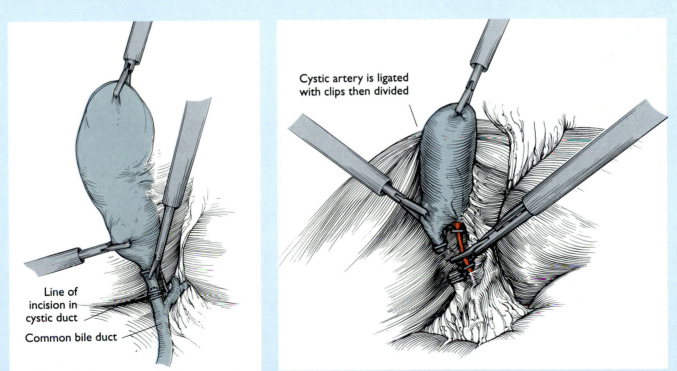

FIGURE 13-6.

At this point, cholangiography is performed if indicated. Two clips are then placed on the common duct end of the cystic duct and it is divided with scissors.

FIGURE 13-7.

Once the cystic duct has been divided, the dissection is continued toward the left, and the cystic artery is identified. The cystic artery is divided among three clips in similar fashion.

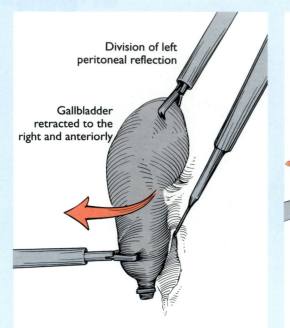

FIGURE 13-8.

The neck of the gallbladder is then rolled to the right to place the peritoneal reflection along the left margin of the gallbladder on tension. Anterior tension also greatly assists in this portion of the dissection. The peritoneal reflection is then divided by using a hook cautery instrument.

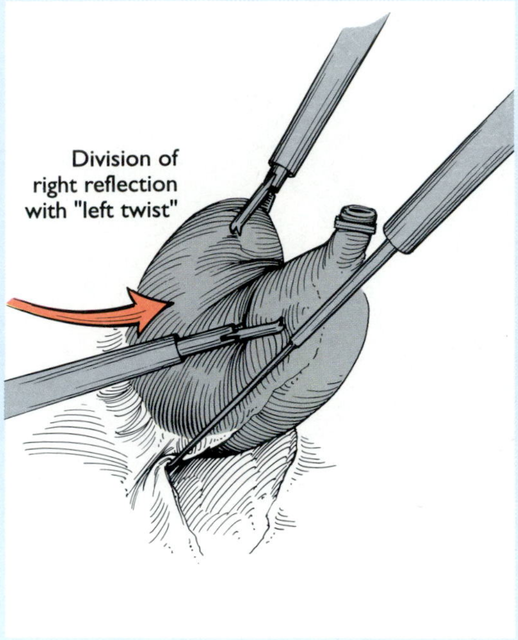

FIGURE 13-9.

In similar fashion, the right peritoneal reflection is divided by using the "left twist" maneuver to place it under adequate tension. Great care must be exercised during this dissection to identify the posterior branch of the cystic artery which occasionally branches off the cystic artery below the site of division. Should this be encountered it is doubly clipped and divided.

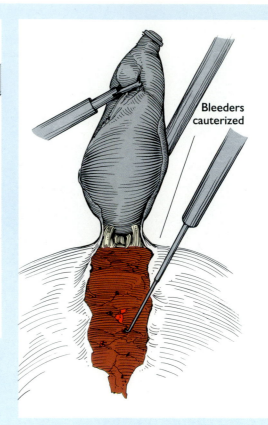

FIGURE 13-10.

With the peritoneal reflections incised, the gallbladder is separated from the liver bed by using the cautery, being careful to note any accessory bile ducts entering the gallbladder directly from the liver bed. Minor bleeding sites are controlled with electrocautery. Larger bleeding sites from hepatic sinuses can be controlled at this point with application of Gelfoam (Pharmacia & Upjohn Co.; Kalamazoo, MI) or Surgicel (Johnson & Johnson Medical; Arlington, TX) and pressure with a blunt clamp.

Procedure

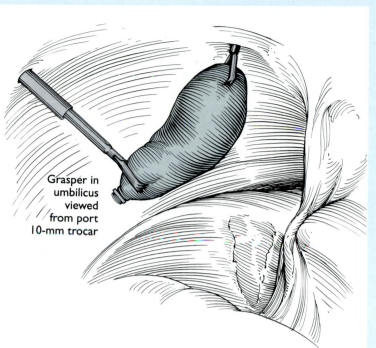

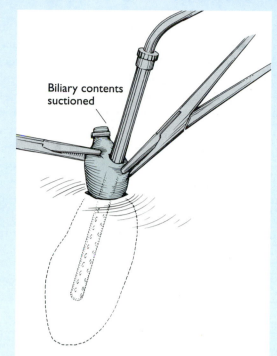

FIGURE 13-11.

After thorough irrigation of the subhepatic and periheptic spaces, the gallbladder is suspended by the fundus and the patient is returned to a flat position. The laparoscope is shifted to the subxiphoid port, and the neck of the gallbladder is grasped with the extractor inserted via the umbilical port.

FIGURE 13-12.

The neck of the gallbladder is then retracted through the abdominal wall, and the umbilical port is simultaneously removed. The laparoscope is directed to the umbilical site to ensure that no intraperitoneal spillage occurs during the extraction procedure. The gallbladder neck is then incised and bilious contents are suctioned.

Alternative Procedure

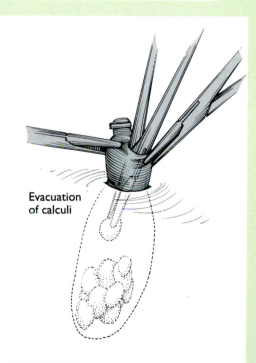

FIGURE 13-13.

Should the gallbladder prove too bulky to extract via the umbilical incision, calculi are evacuated. If the thickened gallbladder is still too large, the fascial defect is enlarged to allow for its removal.

Results

Table 13-4 highlights selected large multicenter and single-center series of laparoscopic cholecystectomy performed to date. Data clearly demonstrate that laparoscopic cholecystectomy has become a procedure implemented throughout the world with a rapidity never before seen in surgery and is now performed on a broad scale with remarkably few complications [1–22]. The conversion rates range from 1% to 8% and have been demonstrated to decline with increased operator experience. Major complications are also very rare and appear to relate to the experience of the operating surgeon.

Many recent studies have also confirmed the role of laparoscopic cholecystectomy in acute cholecystitis [23–26]. Although conversion rates are higher and operating time is frequently extended, patients who have successful laparoscopic cholecystectomy enjoy the benefits of decreased pain and recovery time, without any increase in complications.

The studies highlighted here and numerous others have shown that laparoscopic cholecystectomy has become the treatment of choice for most patients with symptomatic cholelithiasis and acute cholecystitis, providing the advantages of decreased pain and disability and, potentially, substantially decreased cost. These findings, as well as the improved desirability of the procedure, have contributed to the increased number of cholecystectomies performed in the United States each year (600,000) [27–29]. Several studies have documented an increase in cholecystectomies in the early 1990s from 22% to as high as 58% compared with rates in the late 1980s [28,29].

Table 13-4. Multicenter and single-center series for laparoscopic cholecystectomy

Multicenter series	Patients, n	Conversion, %	Mortality, %	Bile duct injury, %
Z'graggen and coworkers [1]	10,174	8.2	0.2	0.31
Adamsen and coworkers [2]	7654	6.8	0.01	0.74
MacFadyen and coworkers [3]	114,005	2.2	0.06	0.5
Regoly-Merei and coworkers [4]	26,440	5.9	0.02	0.6
Deziel and coworkers [5]	77,604	1.2	0.04	0.6
Richardson and coworkers [6]	5913	13.9	0	0.6
The Southern Surgeons Club [7]	1518	4.7	0.07	0.5
Orlando and coworkers [8]	4640	6.9	0.13	0.3
Deveney [9]	9597	NR	0.04	0.28
Go and coworkers [10]	6076	6.8	0.12	0.86
Cocks and coworkers [11]	5927	NR	NR	0.2
Single-center series				
Dubois and coworkers [12]	2006	2.1	0.05	0.7
Barkun and coworkers [13]	1300	6.2	0.08	0.38
Raute and coworkers [14]	1022	NR	0	0
Korman and coworkers [15]	343	8	0	0
Lorimer and coworkers [16]	525	4.8	0.19	0
Soper and coworkers [17]	618	2.9	0	0.2
Baird and coworkers [18]	800	2.3	0.13	0
Graffis [19]	900	2.2	0	0.11
Davis and coworkers [20]	622	4.2	0	0.16
Perissat and coworkers [21]	700	5.8	0.13	0.4

NR—not recorded.

Laparoscopic Common Bile Duct Evaluation

Choledocholithiasis is present in 8% to 15% of patients with cholelithiasis. Approximately 90% of common bile duct stones are less than 4 mm in diameter and pass into the duodenum without any intervention. Before the development of laparoscopic cholecystectomy, the question of when to perform intraoperative cholangiography was controversial. Now, with the advent of laparoscopic cholecystectomy, this subject has become an even greater point of contention among surgeons. Indications for intraoperative cholangiogram are listed in Table 13-5. Those in favor of routine cholangiography argue that this procedure should be performed because of 1) the need to evaluate for retained common bile duct stones in order to avoid another invasive procedure, 2) the need to delineate the anatomy to avoid missed common bile duct injuries, and 3) the loss of tactile perception in assessing the ducts. Arguments against routine cholangiography include 1) studies demonstrating a low incidence of clinically significant retained stones, 2) increased operative time, and 3) risk for injury to the common bile duct.

We and others [30–34] prefer a selective approach toward laparoscopic cholangiography. Many large studies have shown that laparoscopic cholecystectomy can be done safely without routine cholangiography. The available literature does not support the argument that routine cholangiography leads to a reduction in the incidence of retained common duct stones. Several large studies have demonstrated the presence of retained stones in less than 1.5% of patients who did not have cholangiography but who were well screened for risk factors for cholelithiasis. Previous studies have not shown that the use of routine cholangiography avoids bile duct injuries. Large reviews suggest that the main factor leading to bile duct injuries is inexperience of the operating surgeon [4,7,20,21]. In studies addressing the role of cholangiography, the incidence of bile duct injuries in patients undergoing laparoscopic cholecystecto-

my using a selective approach toward cholangiography ranges from 0% to 0.5% [35–42]. Thus, it is apparent that selective cholangiography can be performed with no clear increase in retained stones or bile duct injuries. The methods most commonly used for laparoscopic cholangiography are described in detail under "Surgical Technique."

Surgical Technique

Figures 13-14 through 13-20 depict the surgical technique for laparoscopic cholangiography. After adequate identification of the infundibulum–cystic duct junction, a single endoscopic clip is placed across the proximal cystic duct to prevent spillage of gallbladder contents (Figure 13-14). If the anatomy is unclear at this point, the surgeon may omit placement of this clip. Endoscopic scissors are then used to make an anterior incision along the proximal cystic duct just distal to the clip (Figure 13-15). A cholangiocatheter is passed through the superior right-sided port or through a new percutaneous puncture site overlying the cystic duct.

A variety of cholangiocatheters have been developed in recent years. Several of the more commonly used catheters are shown in Figures 13-16 to 13-18, and 13-21. By their design, the Taut (Taut, Geneva, IL) and balloon-tipped catheters prevent backflow of contrast. Other catheters are fed through a clamp and are held in place; backflow is prevented by applying the clamp when the catheter is appropriately positioned. A simple cholangiocatheter can be advanced into the cystic duct and then secured into place with a single clip at the entrance site.

The cholangiocatheter should be advanced no more than 4 to 5 mm into the cystic duct (Figure 13-19). After the catheter is secured into place and all instruments that may interfere with the cholangiogram are removed, cholangiography is performed by injecting 10 mL of half-strength Renografin (Sanofi-Winthrop; New York, NY) under fluoroscopic guidance (Figure 13-20).

Table 13-5. Indications for cholangiography	
Routine	Radiographic evidence of common duct stones
Uncertain anatomy	Dilated cystic duct
Abnormal liver function test results	Pancreatitis
Dilated common bile duct	Cholangitis
Jaundice	Single-faceted stones (during open cholecystectomy)
Multiple small stones in gallbladder	Maintenance of surgical skills

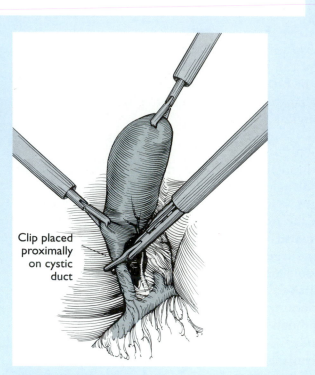

FIGURE 13-14.

The endoscopic clip applier is passed through the 10-mm epigastric sheath and a single clip is placed across the proximal cystic duct to prevent spillage of gall-bladder contents into the abdomen. If the anatomy is unclear at this point, the surgeon may omit the placement of this clip.

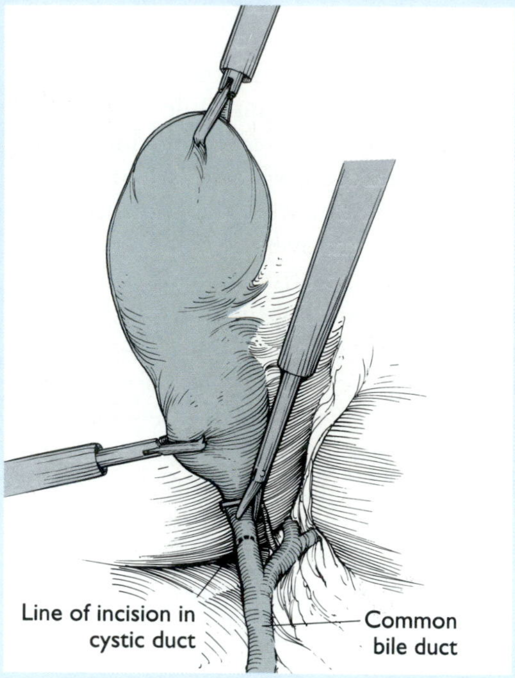

FIGURE 13-15.

Endoscopic scissors are then passed through the epigastric sheath, and the cystic duct is incised along half its circumference just distal to the previously placed titanium clip.

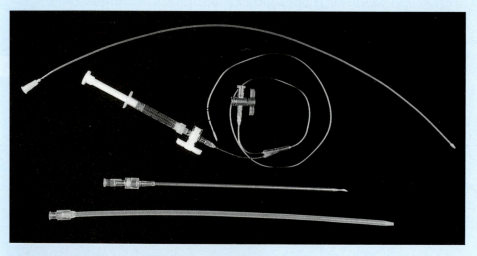

FIGURE 13-16.

Photograph of the Taut (Taut; Geneva, IL) (*top*) and balloon-tip cholangiocatheters and access cannulas. The authors use a 4-French balloon-tip cholangiocatheter (*second from the top*) passed through an Olsen cholangiogram fixation clamp (Karl Storz Endoscopy-America) in performing transcystic cholangiography. Several alternatives exist including the Taut catheter depicted (*top*) as well as standard central venous access catheters and ureteric catheters. Access into the peritoneal cavity can be obtained through one of the existing ports assisted by either a specially designed hollow-core clamp or adapter sheath (*bottom*) designed to minimize the loss of CO_2 or through a separate percutaneous puncture using a 14- or 15-gauge angiocatheter or similar catheter (*second from the bottom*). In the latter case, the puncture site is chosen to afford the optimal angle for catheter guidance into the cystic duct.

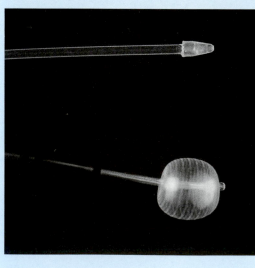

FIGURE 13-17.

The Taut and balloon-tip cholangio-catheter tips.

Procedure

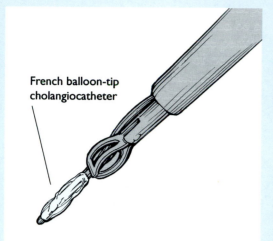

French balloon-tip cholangiocatheter

FIGURE 13-18.
The balloon-tip cholangio-catheter is placed through the hollow core of the cholangiography clamp and passed through the epigastric or mid-clavicular port into the peritoneal cavity. In situations where the retraction provided by forceps in these ports is necessary for adequate exposure, a fifth cannula may be inserted or the cholangio-catheter passed through a percutaneously placed angio-catheter obviating the need for another port.

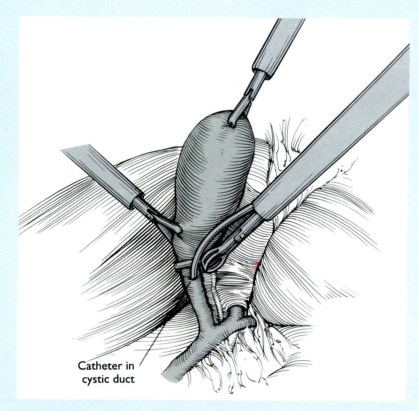

Catheter in cystic duct

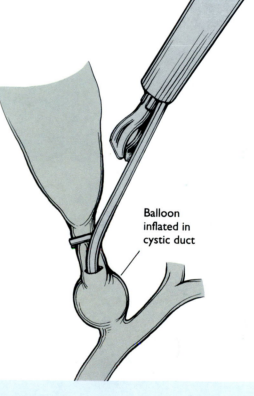

Balloon inflated in cystic duct

FIGURE 13-19.
The catheter is guided into the partially transected proximal cystic duct. When not using the cholangiogram clamp, the endoscopic grasper may be used in maneuvering the catheter. If difficulty is encountered in passing the catheter into the duct, a guidewire passed through the cholangiocatheter into the duct may facilitate this step. The catheter is inserted 4 to 5 mm.

FIGURE 13-20.
The ballloon is then inflated to secure the positioning of the catheter and prevent extravasation of contrast when injected. Before infusion of contrast, the laparoscope is removed from the abdomen and care taken to ensure that all radioopaque objects are removed from the radiographic field. Ten mL of half-strength Renografin (Sanofi-Winthrop; New York, NY) is then infused via the catheter and the radiograph obtained during infusion. Care must be taken to ensure that the tip does not migrate into the common bile duct, which will produce a cholangiogram with no retrograde flow. In the case of a cystic duct that is tightly adheres to the common bile duct, inflation of the balloon within the cystic duct may cause an indentation in the wall of the common duct, giving the false impression of a stone. Many institutions advocate the use of digital fluoroscopy in place of standard radiography.

Alternative Technique

Figures 13-21 through 13-26 depict the alternative technique of cholecystocholangiography.

Alternative Procedure

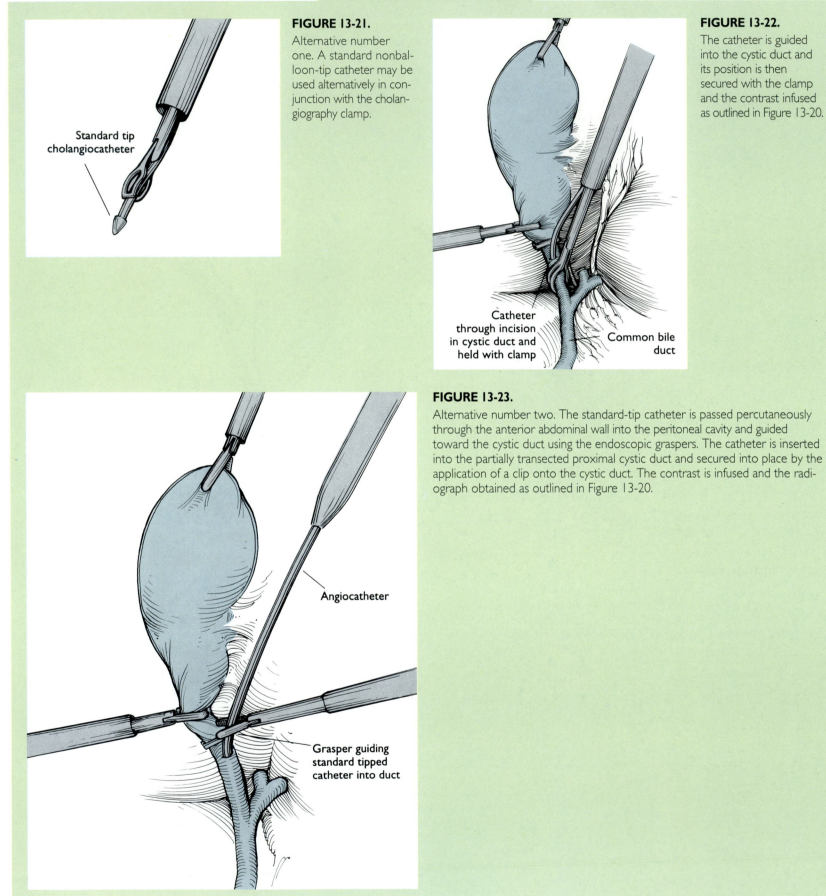

FIGURE 13-21.
Alternative number one. A standard nonballoon-tip catheter may be used alternatively in conjunction with the cholangiography clamp.

Standard tip cholangiocatheter

FIGURE 13-22.
The catheter is guided into the cystic duct and its position is then secured with the clamp and the contrast infused as outlined in Figure 13-20.

Catheter through incision in cystic duct and held with clamp

Common bile duct

FIGURE 13-23.
Alternative number two. The standard-tip catheter is passed percutaneously through the anterior abdominal wall into the peritoneal cavity and guided toward the cystic duct using the endoscopic graspers. The catheter is inserted into the partially transected proximal cystic duct and secured into place by the application of a clip onto the cystic duct. The contrast is infused and the radiograph obtained as outlined in Figure 13-20.

Angiocatheter

Grasper guiding standard tipped catheter into duct

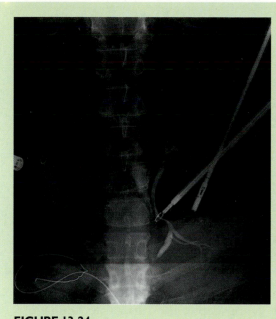

FIGURE 13-24.

Photograph of properly performed cystic duct cholangiogram.

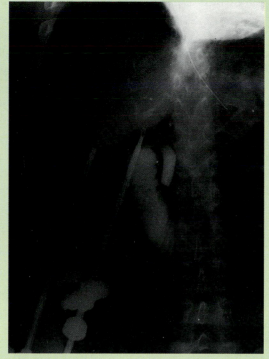

FIGURE 13-25.

Photograph of inadequate cystic duct cholangiogram.

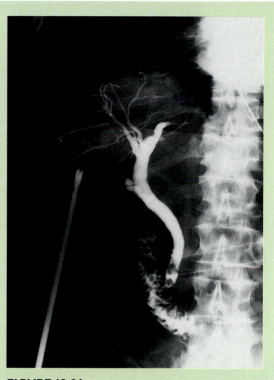

FIGURE 13-26.

Photograph of cystic duct cholangiogram with stones.

Ultrasonography of the Biliary Tree

Ultrasonography of the biliary tree has been increasingly reported over the past 4 years as an alternative to intraoperative cholangiography to evaluate anatomy and rule out choledocholithiasis. Although this test has not yet applied on a large scale, small series have reported sensitivities and specificities for choledocholithiasis similar to those seen with cholangiography [43–48]. Potential advantages of ultrasonography include simplicity, lack of adverse effects, shorter examination times, lower costs, and possibility of unlimited repetition. The application of this technology to laparoscopy will be an area to watch in the coming years.

Results

Laparoscopic cholangiography remains an integral part of the procedure of laparoscopic cholecystectomy. Although debate continues in the literature as to whether cholangiography should be performed routinely or selectively, the skill needed to perform cholangiography is imperative for any surgeon practicing cholecystectomy. Technical success, described as the ability to obtain a cholangiogram of sufficient quality to allow interpretation, has been demonstrated in large trials to be 90% to 98% in the hands of experienced operators. Complications of the procedure are few and can be readily avoided with adherence to the guidelines reviewed in this chapter.

Laparoscopic Management of Choledocholithiasis

Choledocholithiasis is defined as the presence of stones in any portion of the common bile duct, although the most frequent location is at the most narrow portion of the duct at the papilla. Stones in the common hepatic duct make up only 5% of all stones in the biliary system. To diagnose choledocholithiasis, a high index of suspicion must be maintained for all patients with gallstones. Many clinical criteria have been established in an attempt to predict which patients with choledocholithiasis are at risk for common bile duct stones (Table 13-6) [49,50]. In general, preoperative clinical, laboratory, and radiologic data are reliable in predicting the absence of choledocholithiasis in more than 95% of cases. Because of the large number of patients with gallstones, however, this still leaves a substantial number of cases in which common bile duct stones found at the time of surgery were entirely unsuspected.

Management of Choledocholithiasis

In the present era of minimally invasive surgery, endoscopic retrograde cholangiopancreatography (ERCP), and sophisticated interventional radiology, many patients with choledocholithiasis can be safely and successfully managed without the need for a right upper quadrant incision and open common bile duct exploration. Notable exceptions include patients with cholangitis, gallbladder perforation, pancreatitis, suspicion of carcinoma, or large impacted stones in which time-consuming minimally invasive techniques must often be relinquished for standard and proven medical and surgical therapy.

Patients with uncomplicated choledocholithiasis, however, are excellent candidates for minimally invasive techniques. For the purposes of the laparoscopic surgeon, these patients generally fall into two categories: 1) patients with cholelithiasis who are suspected of having choledocholithiasis as a result of their preoperative evaluation; and 2) patients who are undergoing laparoscopic cholecystectomy and are found to have choledocholithiasis intraoperatively. The management strategies for these two groups of patients are slightly different.

For patients suspected of having choledocholithiasis before surgery, the decision must be made whether to perform preoperative ERCP to retrieve the stones from the common duct. This has been termed clearing the duct. The reported success rate of ERCP for the removal of common bile duct stones before surgery approaches 95%, although this level of success may not be achieved in centers with limited ERCP experience. Also, since the positive predictive value of clinical parameters for choledocholithiasis is at best about 50%, use of routine preoperative ERCP will subject many patients to unnecessary examination. The relative indications for clearing the duct preoperatively are given in Table 13-7 and suggest a strategy for selective preoperative ERCP.

A particularly noteworthy indication for preoperative ERCP is the presence of choledocholithiasis in an elderly patient. This has the advantage of making the subsequent laparoscopic cholecystectomy more expeditious because cholangiogram or duct exploration will not be required. Furthermore, some investigators have questioned whether these patients even need a subsequent cholecystectomy, because the risk for recurrent biliary tract problems after endoscopic stone removal in elderly patients (roughly 10% in 5 years) compares favorably with the risk of cholecystectomy. Thus, not all patients with choledocholithiasis must have a cholecystectomy.

If both the laparoscopic surgeon and the endoscopist are experienced in stone removal and the patient is a good operative candidate, preoperative ERCP is not necessary; patients may be taken directly to laparoscopic cholecystectomy with plans for retrieval of stones via a laparoscopic approach or postoperatively via an endoscopic approach. Also, regardless of the extensiveness of the preoperative evaluation, some cases of choledocholithiasis will be discovered intraoperatively after cholangiography. It is in these two scenarios that there is a role for laparoscopic treatment of common bile duct stones.

Surgical Technique

Figures 13-27 through 13-36 depict the surgical technique for laparoscopic transcystic common bile duct exploration.

Table 13-6. Clinical, laboratory, radiologic, and intraoperative criteria for possible choledocholithiasis

Clinical presentation

Jaundice (present, recent, or recurrent)
Light colored feces (stools devoid of bile pigment or "acholic" stools)
Dark urine (containing bilirubin)
Fever (present or recent)

Laboratory values

Serum bilirubin > 1.2 mg/dL
Serum alkaline phosphatase > 250 U/L

Radiologic studies

Multiple small gallstones
Common bile duct diameter > 6 mm
Common bile duct calculi

Intraoperative findings

Multiple small gallstones
Common bile duct diameter > 10 mm
Cystic duct diameter > 5 mm

Table 13-7. Indications for preoperative ERCP in patients suspected of choledocholithiasis

Clinical suspicion of choledocholithiasis and:

Presence of multiple stones

Small cystic duct and/or common bile duct (may preclude safe transcystic exploration)

Elderly patient

High operative risk

Endoscopist with limited experience in stone retrieval (if eventually required postoperatively)

Surgeon with limited experience in laparoscopic treatment of choledocholithiasis

Wishes of the patient (strong desire to avoid open procedure)

ERCP—endoscopic retrograde cholangiopancreatography.

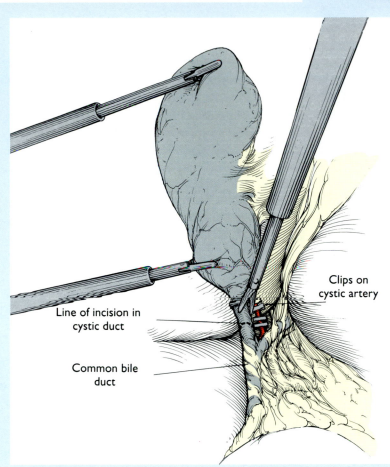

FIGURE 13-27.

The procedure is performed at the time of laparoscopic cholecystectomy after intraoperative cholangiography. The cystic artery is identified and doubly clipped. The cystic duct is identified and clipped on the gallbladder side to prevent bile and stone spillage. The cholangiocatheter is removed. If the cholangiogram has been obtained via the cystic duct, then the cystic duct incision is used for transcystic cholangioscopy. If no cystic duct incision has been made (as in the figure), then the gallbladder is retracted superomedially with traction on the cystic duct, and the duct is incised half its full diameter, approximately 1.5 to 2.0 cm proximal to its junction with the common hepatic duct.

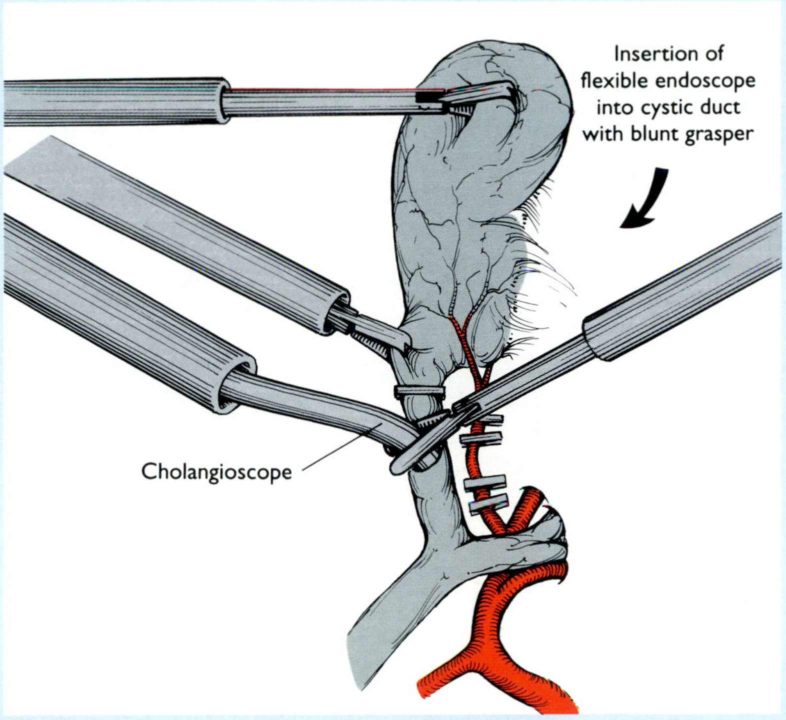

FIGURE 13-28.

A 2.7- to 3.3-mm outer diameter flexible endoscope is passed through the right upper quadrant trocar and advanced into the cystic duct. Obviously, the smaller the diameter of the endoscope, the easier passage will be. Many small scopes are available (ACMI-Circon, Olympus, Intramed Laboratories, Karl Storz Endoscopy), although they may have been originally designed as ureteroscopes or choledochoscopes. Care should be taken to grasp the scope with noncrushing forceps only. Some authors advocate the use of a hydrophilic guidewire to facilitate ductal access.

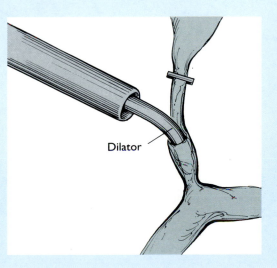

FIGURE 13-29.

If the smallest available scope cannot be advanced through the cystic duct, the cystic duct may be gently dilated with either mechanical tapered dilators or an angioplasty balloon system. Cystic duct dilatation can be safely performed up to 4 mm; dilatation beyond 8 mm is not recommended. Obviously, rigorous dilatation of a tight cystic duct should be avoided and the procedure abandoned if the cholangioscope does not pass entirely. If the cystic duct–common duct junction is disrupted by forcible dilatation, open exploration may be required for repair. The intravenous administration of glucagon, 2 mg, may also be of benefit by providing smooth muscle relaxation of the cystic duct.

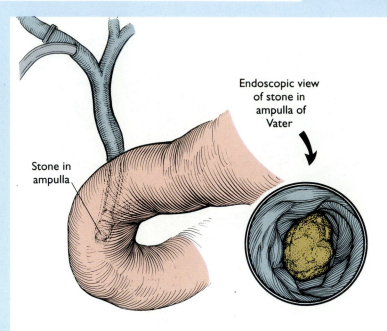

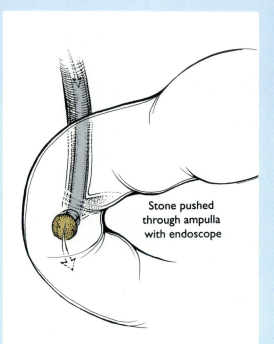

Endoscopic view of stone in ampulla of Vater

Stone in ampulla

Stone pushed through ampulla with endoscope

FIGURE 13-31.
When stones are encountered, they may often be made to pass through to the duodenum just by gently pushing with the cholangioscope.

FIGURE 13-30.
Once the cholangioscope is in the common bile duct, the video camera should be removed from the laparoscope and placed on the cholangioscope for maximum resolution. The cholangioscope is gently advanced distally in the common duct until stones are visualized (*inset*). The common hepatic duct can sometimes be visualized by gently twisting the cholangioscope superiorly to negotiate the acute angle of the junction of cystic and common hepatic ducts. Excessive effort, however, may cause tearing of the ductal system and should be avoided.

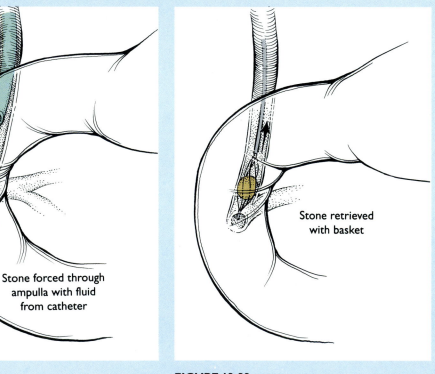

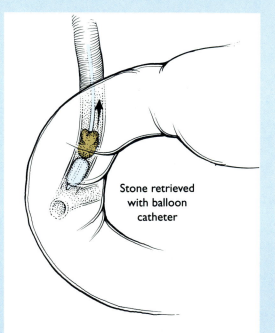

Stone forced through ampulla with fluid from catheter

Stone retrieved with basket

Stone retrieved with balloon catheter

FIGURE 13-34.
Lastly, a 3-French Fogarty embolectomy catheter may be used to retrieve the stone. This may be difficult because the stone may be withdrawn into the common hepatic duct and be rendered irretrievable.

FIGURE 13-32.
If the stones do not pass with gentle scope manipulation, several of maneuvers may be attempted. A red rubber catheter or similar device may be passed into the cystic duct for flushing of the common duct.

FIGURE 13-33.
If the cholangioscope has a sufficiently large operating channel (1–1.5 mm), then a stone basket may be used for retrieval.

Procedure

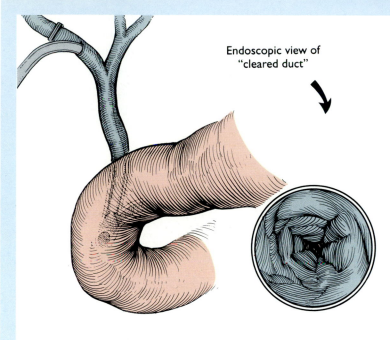

Endoscopic view of "cleared duct"

FIGURE 13-35.

When the stones have been removed, the cholangioscope is again inserted and the ampulla visualized.

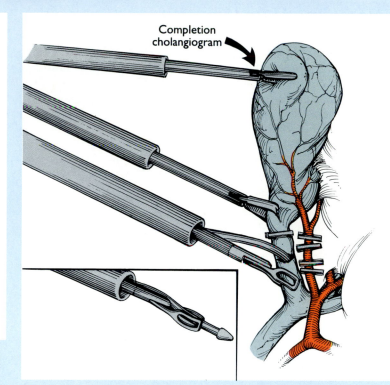

Completion cholangiogram

FIGURE 13-36.

Completion cholangiography is then performed to confirm ductal clearance. Cystic duct control after extensive dilatation and manipulation is critical. Although simple endoscopic clips may be routinely used after cholecystectomy alone, single or double endoscopic loop sutures are preferable after transcystic exploration. A subhepatic Jackson-Pratt closed-system drain is placed before closure.

Results

The reported experience in the literature for laparoscopic treatment of choledocholithiasis shows successful clearance of the duct in up to 93% to 100% of cases in some series [51–54]. However, these results come from authors with extensive experience in advanced laparoscopic techniques. Other reports in the literature also cite success rates in the range of 58% to 75% [37,39,40,55,56]; these rates are more in keeping with the experience of average general surgeons in the United States.

Although this chapter describes the most popular method of transcystic bile duct exploration, a variety of other methods for stone identification and extraction have been suggested, including the use of pulsed dye laser or electrohydraulic lithotripsy, transcystic placement of a T-tube for laser use, placement of common bile duct introducer sheaths for multiple stones, bile duct exploration under fluoroscopic control, balloon catheter–assisted antegrade stone advancement, intraoperative ultrasonography or ERCP, laparoscopic sphincter dilatation, and supraduodenal laparoscopic common bile duct exploration [57–60].

Regardless of the method used, traditional surgical principles and the useful adage of "first, do no harm" must be adhered to. As with open bile duct exploration, there are potential risks for common duct complications, especially common duct ischemia, stricture formation, and biliary sepsis. Whether endoscopic sphincterotomy is preferable to open common bile duct exploration continues to be debated, and comparison of the endoscopic technique with laparoscopic exploration has not been definitively studied to the satisfaction of most authors. However, because the reported success of endoscopic duct clearance after laparoscopic cholecystectomy is excellent (>95% in many series), and in view of the well-documented evidence that most stones less than 3.0 mm in diameter will pass spontaneously without symptoms, persisting with the laparoscopic approach in a difficult common bile duct is probably not warranted.

Summary

Over the past decade, laparoscopic cholecystectomy has largely replaced open cholecystectomy as the procedure of choice for cholelithiasis. Since the evolution of this procedure, we have seen dramatic developments of instrumentation and evolution in techniques used to remove the gallbladder and, more recently, to evaluate and manage choledocholithiasis. The tremendous growth in interest in laparoscopic cholecystectomy is exemplified by the MEDLINE database; fewer than 10 articles on the subject published before 1991 are contained in the database compared with 3256 articles published over the subsequent 7 years.

The numerous studies, which have included tens of thousands of patients, have shown the safety and efficacy of laparoscopic cholecystectomy. When the management of choledocholithiasis is being considered, it is clear that undertaking laparoscopic management of this condition should be more selective and based on the size and location of the stones, as well as the expertise of the operator. It is hoped that surgical training programs in the future will incorporate development of advanced laparoscopic training to allow safe and practical laparoscopic management of choledocholithiasis outside specialized centers. This advancement would benefit patients with gallstones in limiting the need for more than one invasive procedure.

References

1. Z'graggen K, Wehrli H, Metzger A, *et al.*: Complications of laparoscopic cholecystectomy in Switzerland: a prospective 3-year study of 10,174 patients. *Surg Endos* 1998, 12:1303–1310.

2. Adamsen S, Hansen OH, Funch-Jensen P, *et al.*: Bile duct injury during laparoscopic cholecystectomy: a prospective nationwide series. *J Am Coll Surg* 1997, 184:571–578.

3. MacFadyen BV, Vecchio R, Ricardo AE, *et al.*: Bile duct injury after laparoscopic cholecystectomy: The United States experience. *Surg Endosc* 1998, 12:315–321.

4. Regoly-Merei J, Ihasz M, Szeberin Z, *et al.*: Biliary tract complications in laparoscopic cholecystectomy: a multicenter study of 148 biliary tract injuries in 26,440 operations. *Surg Endosc* 1998, 12:294–300.

5. Deziel DJ, Millikan KW, Economou SG, *et al.*: Complications of laparoscopic cholecystectomy: a national survey of 4,292 hospitals and an analysis of 77,604 cases. *Am J Surg* 1993, 165:9–14.

6. Richardson MC, Bell G, Fullarton GM, *et al.*: Incidence and nature of bile duct injuries following laparoscopic cholecystectomy: an audit of 5913 cases. *Br J Surg* 1996, 83:1356–1360.

7. The Southern Surgeon's Club: A prospective analysis of 1518 laparoscopic cholecystectomies. *N Engl J Med* 1991, 324:1073–1078.

8. Orlando R, Russell JC, Lynch J, *et al.*: Laparoscopic cholecystectomy: a statewide experience. *Arch Surg* 1993, 128:494–498.

9. Deveney KE.: The early experience with laparoscopic cholecystectomy in Oregon. *Arch Surg* 1993, 128:627–632.

10. Go PMNYH, Schol F, Gouma DJ.: Laparoscopic cholecystectomy in the Netherlands. *Br J Surg* 1993, 80:1180–1183.

11. Cocks J, Johnson W, Cade R, *et al.*: Bile duct injury during laparoscopic cholecystectomy: a report of the Standards Sub-committee of the Victorian State Committee of the Royal Australian College of Surgeons. *Aust N Z J Surg* 1993, 63:682–683.

12. Dubois F, Berthelot G, Levard H.: Coelioscopic cholecystectomy: experience with 2006 cases. *World J Surg* 1995, 19:748–752.

13. Barkun JS, Fried GM, Barkun AN, *et al.*: Cholecystectomy without operative cholangiography: implications for common bile duct injury and retained common bile duct stones. *Ann Surg* 1993, 218:371–379.

14. Raute M, Podlech P, Jaschke W, *et al.*: Management of bile duct injuries and strictures following cholecystectomy. *World J Surg* 1993, 17:553–562.

15. Korman J, Cosgrove J, Furman M, *et al.*: The role of endoscopic retrograde cholangiopancreatography and cholangiography in the laparoscopic era. *Ann Surg* 1996, 223:212–216.

16. Lorimer JW, Fairfull-Smith RJ.: Intraoperative cholangiography is not essential to avoid duct injures during laparoscopic choelcystectomy. *Am J Surg* 1995, 169:344–347.

17. Soper NJ, Stockmann PT, Dunnegan DL, *et al.*: Laparoscopic cholecystectomy: the new 'gold standard'? *Arch Surg* 1992, 127:917–921.

18. Baird DR, Wilson JP, Mason EM, *et al.*: An early review of 800 laparoscopic cholecystectomies at a university-affiliated community teaching hospital. *Am Surg* 1992, 58:206–210.

19. Graffis R.: Laparoscopic cholecystectomy: the Methodist Hospital experience. *Surg Laparosc Endosc* 1992, 1:69–73.

20. Davis CJ, Arregui ME, Nagan RF, *et al.*: Laparoscopic cholecystectomy: the St. Vincent experience. *Surg Laparosc Endosc* 1992, 2:64–68.

21. Perissat J, Collet D, Belliard R, *et al.*: Laparoscopic cholecystectomy: the state of the art. A report on 700 consecutive cases. *World J Surg* 1992, 16:1074–1082.

22. McMahon AJ, Fullarton G, Baxter JN, *et al.*: Bile duct injury and bile leakage in laparoscopic cholecystectomy. *Br J Surg* 1995, 82:307–313.

23. Lo CM, Lui CL, Fan ST, *et al.*: Prospective randomized study of early versus delayed laparoscopic cholecystectomy for acute cholecystitis. *Ann Surg* 1998, 227:461–467.

24. Lai PBS, Kwong KH, Leung KL, *et al.*: Randomized trial of early versus delayed laparoscopic cholecystectomy for acute cholecystitis. *Br J Surg* 1998, 85:764–767.

25. Kiviluoto T, Siren J, Luukkonen P, *et al.*: Randomised trial of laparoscopic versus open cholecystectomy for acute and gangrenous cholecystitis. *Lancet* 1998, 351:321–325.

26. Lujan JA, Parilla P, Robles R, *et al.*: Laparoscopic cholecystectomy vs open cholecystectomy in the treatment of acute cholecystitis: a prospective study. *Arch Surg* 1998, 133:173–175.

27. Chen AY, Daley J, Pappas TN, *et al.*: Growing use of laparoscopic cholecystectomy in the national veterans affairs surgical risk study: effects on volume, patient selection, and selected outcomes. *Ann Surg* 1998, 27:12–24.

28. Diehl AK: Laparoscopic cholecystectomy: too much of a good thing? *JAMA* 1993, 270:1469–1470.

29. Escarce JJ, Chen W, Schwartz JS: Falling cholecystectomy thresholds since the introduction of laparoscopic cholecystectomy. *JAMA* 1995, 273:1581–1585.

30. Clair D, Carr-Locke D, Becker J, *et al.*: Routine cholangiography is not warranted during laparoscopic cholecystectomy. *Arch Surg* 1993, 128:551–555.

31. Soper N, Dunnegan D.: Routine versus selective intra-operative cholangiography during laparoscopic cholecystectomy. *World J Surg* 1992, 16:1133–1140.

32. Lillemoe K, Yeo C, Talamini M, *et al.*: Selective cholangiography: current role during laparoscopic cholecystectomy. *Ann Surg* 1992, 215:669–676.

33. Cantwell D: Routine cholangiography during laparoscopic cholecystectomy. *Arch Surg* 1992, 127:483–484.

34. Scott-Combes D: Bile duct stones and laparoscopic cholecystectomy. *BMJ* 1991, 303:1281–1282.

35. Kullman E, Borch K, Lindstrom E, *et al*: Value of routine intraoperative cholangiography in detecting aberrant bile ducts and bile duct injuries during laparoscopic cholecystectomy. *Br J Surg* 1996, 83:171–175.

36. Willekes C, Edoga J, Castronovo J, *et al.*: Technical elements of successful laparoscopic cholangiography as defined by radiographic criteria. *Arch Surg* 1995, 130:398–400.

37. Kondylis P, Simmons D, Agarwal S, *et al.*: Abnormal intraoperative cholangiography. *Arch Surg* 1997, 132:347–350.

38. Sabharwal A, Minford E, Marson L, *et al.*: Laparoscopic cholangiography: a prospective study. *Br J Surg* 1998, 85:624–626.

39. Roush T, Traverso L: Management and long-term follow-up of patients with positive cholangiograms during laparoscopic cholecystectomy. *Am J Surg* 1995, 169:484–487.

40. Fiore N, Ledniczky G, Wiebe E, *et al.*: An analysis of perioperative cholangiography in one thousand laparoscopic cholecystectomies. *Surgery* 1997, 122:817–823.

41. Yoshida J, Chijiiwa K, Yamaguchi K, *et al.*: Practical classification of the branching types of the biliary tree: an analysis of 1,094 consecutive direct cholangiograms. *J Am Coll Surg* 1995, 182:37–40.

42. Hammarstrom L, Holmin T, Stridbeck H, *et al.*: Routine preoperative infusion cholangiography versus intraoperative cholangiography at elective cholecystectomy: a prospective study in 995 patients. *J Am Coll Surg* 1996, 182:408–416.

43. Birth M, Ehlers KU, Delinikolas K, *et al.*: Prospective randomized comparison of laparoscopic ultrasonography using a flexible-tip ultrasound probe and intraoperative dynamic cholangiography during laparoscopic cholecystectomy. *Surg Endosc* 1998, 12:30–36.

44. Kelly SB, Remedios D, Lau WY, *et al.*: Laparoscopic ultrasonography during laparoscopic cholecystectomy. *Surg Endosc* 1997, 11:67–70.

45. Kubota K, Bandai Y, Sano K, *et al.*: Appraisal of intraoperative ultrasonography during laparoscopic cholecystectomy. *Surgery* 1995, 118:555–561.

46. Barteau JA, Castro D, Arregui ME, *et al.*: A comparison of intraoperative ultrasound versus cholangiography in the evaluation of the common bile duct during laparoscopic cholecystectomy. *Surg Endosc* 1995, 9:490–496.

47. Rothlin MA, Schob O, Schlumpf R, *et al.*: Laparoscopic ultrasonography during cholecystectomy. *Br J Surg* 1996, 83:1512–1516.

48. Thompson DM, Arregui ME, Tetik C, *et al.*: A comparison of laparoscopic ultrasound with digital fluorocholangiography for detecting choledocholithiasis during laparoscopic cholecystectomy. *Surg Endosc* 1998, 12:929–932.

49. Barkun A, Barkun J, Fried G, *et al.*: Useful predictors of bile duct stones in patients undergoing laparoscopic cholecystectomy. *Ann Surg* 1994, 220:32–39.

50. Koo K, Traverson W: Do preoperative indicators predict the presence of common bile duct stones during laparoscopic cholecystectomy? *Am J Surg* 1996, 171:495–499.

51. Hunter JG: Laparoscopic transcystic common bile duct exploration. *Am J Surg* 1992, 163:53–58.

52. Rhodes M, Nathanson L, O'Rourke N, *et al.*: Laparoscopic exploration of the common bile duct: lessons learned from 129 consecutive cases. *Br J Surg* 1994, 82:666–668.

53. Stoker M: Common bile duct exploration in the era of laparoscopic surgery. *Arch Surg* 1995, 130:265–269.

54. Huang S, Wu C, Chau G, *et al.*: An alternative approach of choledocholithotomy via laparoscopic choledochotomy. *Arch Surg* 1996, 131:407–411.

55. Ferguson C: Laparoscopic common bile duct exploration. *Arch Surg* 1998, 133:448–451.

56. Rhodes M, Sussman L, Cohen L, *et al.*: Randomised trial of laparoscopic exploration of common bile duct versus postoperative endoscopic retrograde cholangiography for common bile duct stones. *Lancet* 1998, 351:159–161.

57. Fitzgibbons R, Ryberg A, Ulualp K, *et al.*: An alternative technique for treatment of choledocholithiasis found in at laparoscopic cholecystectomy. *Arch Surg* 1995, 130:638–642.

58. Duensing R, Williams R, Collins J, *et al.*: Managing choledocholithiasis in the laparoscopic era. *Am J Surg* 1995, 170:619–623.

59. Berthou J, Brambs H, Dominguez J, *et al.*: Diagnosis and treatment of common bile duct stones. *Surg Endosc* 1998, 12:856–864.

60. Phillips L, Liberman M, Carroll B, *et al.*: Bile duct stones in the laparoscopic era. *Arch Surg* 1995, 130:880–886.

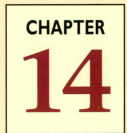

Complications of Laparoscopic Cholecystectomy

Mark W. Onaitis
Edward G. Chekan

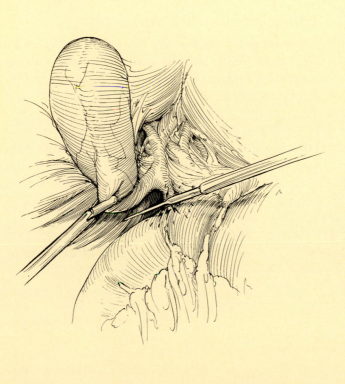

Laparoscopic cholecystectomy has been documented to be a safe and effective procedure in the treatment of symptomatic gallbladder disease. Widespread satisfaction among patients and surgeons has led to its position as the current treatment of choice for symptomatic gallstones. As the popularity of laparoscopic cholecystectomy grew, it became clear that a learning curve was associated with the procedure, during which there was a higher than expected rate of complications, especially major biliary ductal complications. This was related largely to unfamiliarity with new instruments and technology and the conversion from a three-dimensional, hands-on technique to a two-dimensional, video-assisted technique.

The early prospective study by the Southern Surgeons Club documented a low overall complication rate of less than 5% and a bile duct complication rate of 0.5% [1]. Series were reported, however, with bile duct complication rates as high as 3%, a six-fold increase from the expected rate of open cholecystectomy [2]. The follow-up study of over 9000 cholecystectomies revealed that the risk for bile duct injury in any one surgeon's experience was increased during a learning curve that primarily lasted the first 15 cases and reached nadir at 50 cases [3].

The complication rate documented by the Southern Surgeons Club has been borne out by two larger recent studies. In a prospective 3-year study in Switzerland, Z'graggen and coworkers [4] noted a bile duct injury rate of 0.31%. A Hungarian retrospective study [5] revealed a risk for biliary tract injury of 0.56%.

A review of the intraoperative videotapes that accompany many injuries reveals that nearly all biliary complications associated with laparoscopic cholecystectomy are preventable (Table 14-1). Moreover, major complications not associated with the biliary tract are also preventable if a set of simple principles is applied. Errors in the identification of ductal or arterial anatomy lead to the most dire complications, and adequate visualization of the cystic duct entering the gallbladder is the goal in every laparoscopic cholecystectomy.

Anatomy

A detailed knowledge of normal and anomalous hepatobiliary anatomy is necessary to avoid complications. Common anomalies of the hepatic arterial and biliary ductal anatomy may increase the hazards of laparoscopic cholecystectomy (Fig. 14-1). The gallbladder usually lies to the right of the common bile duct with the cystic duct-common duct union lying just above the first portion of the unmobilized duodenum. This junction may occur anywhere in the extrahepatic biliary tract, however, from the hepatic ducts above the bifurcation to the intrapancreatic common bile duct, and may occur anywhere around its circumference. In addition, anomalous accessory ducts may join the common or cystic duct directly from the hepatic parenchyma. One interesting anatomic variation recognized in 14 patients at Duke University Medical Center, Durham, North Carolina, involves a low insertion of hepatic segmental duct VII to VIII [6]. These anomalous connections or ductal structures occur in 10% to 15% of patients. Although an anomalous insertion of the cystic duct may make the dissection more tedious and identification of the anatomy difficult, major complications should not ensue, if the gallbladder cystic duct junction is identified correctly. However, identification of accessory ducts and their avoidance are critical to safe completion of laparoscopic cholecystectomy.

Aberrant anatomy of the hepatic artery, especially the right hepatic artery, is present in 15% to 20% of cases. Commonly seen patterns of the branching of the right hepatic artery include a medial right hepatic artery that runs posterior to the common duct (60%), a medial right hepatic artery that runs anterior to the common duct (25%), and an aberrant right hepatic artery arising from the superior mesenteric artery and running posterior to the common duct in 15% to 20% of the cases. The posterior or aberrant right hepatic artery is in danger in any dissection low on the cystic duct or when the common duct is misidentified as the cystic duct and dissected free in the portahepatis. The artery may be injured by cautery, clipping, laser, or traction.

Biliary Complications

Common patterns of injury have been recognized (Table 14-2). The classic injury and its variants are the most common and devastating injuries; burn injuries, bile leaks, and retained stones are also encountered.

The Classic Injury

The classic laparoscopic biliary injury results when the common bile duct or common hepatic duct is misidentified as the cystic duct during the initial dissection phase of the cholecystectomy (Fig. 14-2).

Table 14-1. Factors contributing to intraoperative injury	
Problem	**Result**
Inexperience with equipment	Poor visualization, exposure
Inadequate training, proctoring	Overconfidence, misidentification of anatomy, failure to convert to open procedure before injury
Inability to perform cholangiography	Misidentification of anatomy
Misunderstanding of electrosurgical principles	Thermal injury

Table 14-2. Patterns of injury
Classic injury: resection of extrahepatic biliary tree
Cystic duct–common duct injury
Cystic duct–right hepatic duct injury
Right hepatic duct clip/transection
Lateral common bile duct tear/laceration
Burn-induced stricture
Cystic duct leak

Variations of the classic injury

A common variation of the classic injury occurs when appropriately placed clips are applied to the proximal cystic duct, but because of inappropriate dissection and traction with tenting of the common bile duct, the distal clips are placed on the common duct. The cystic duct is then divided near the common duct junction leading to total proximal biliary leakage and obstruction of the common bile duct. Patients with short or nonexistent cystic ducts are particularly prone to this injury. Figure 14-3 depicts a variation of the classic injury.

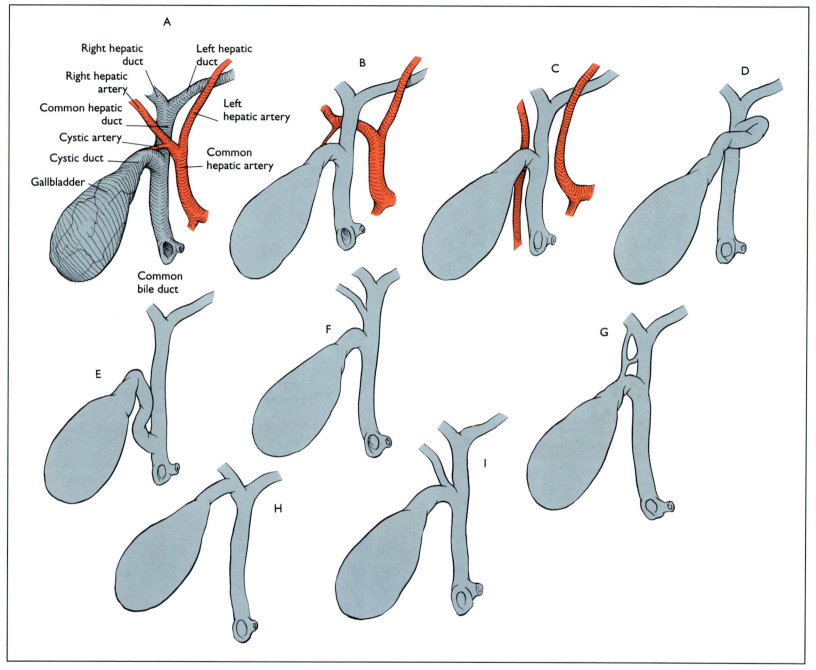

FIGURE 14-1.

Common anomalies of the hepatic arterial and biliary ductal anatomy that may increase the hazards of laparoscopic cholecystectomy. **A**, Conventional arterial and ductal anatomy. **B**, Right hepatic arterial branch posterior to the common hepatic duct. **C**, Replaced right hepatic artery arising from the superior mesenteric artery. **D** through **I**, Variants of cystic and accessory duct insertion into the extrahepatic biliary tree.

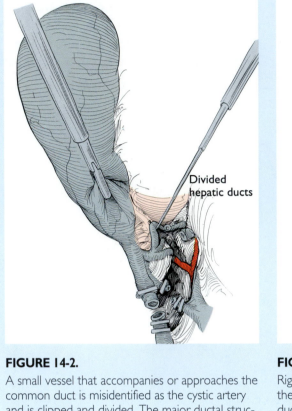

Divided hepatic ducts

Right hepatic duct clipped behind cystic duct

FIGURE 14-2.

A small vessel that accompanies or approaches the common duct is misidentified as the cystic artery and is clipped and divided. The major ductal structure is then dissected free from surrounding portal structures, clipped, divided, and removed with the gallbladder. This leads not only to common duct injury but resection of a segment of the major extrahepatic biliary tree. The injury is often associated with right hepatic arterial injury because of its proximity as the ductal structures are dissected free from what is thought to be the gallbladder bed. The proximal duct structures are transected anywhere from just below to well above the bifurcation of the hepatic duct.

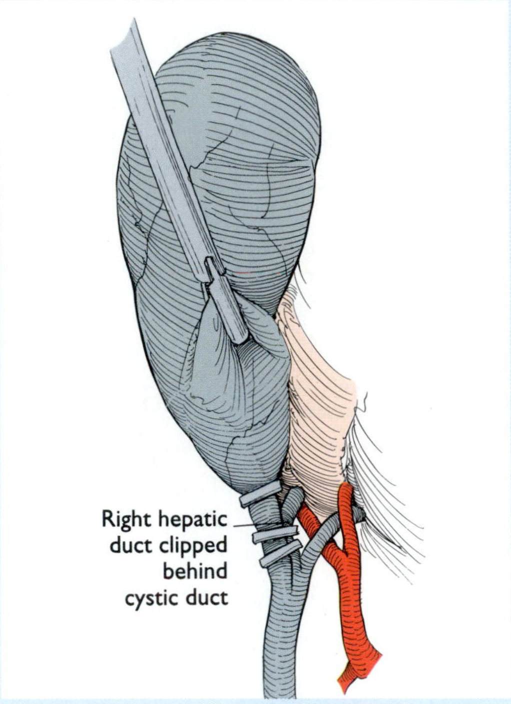

FIGURE 14-3.

Right hepatic ductal injury is prone to occur when the cystic duct has its origin from the right hepatic duct or when inappropriate cephalad retraction is applied to the infundibulum. The cystic duct is appropriately clipped in its proximal position but the distal clips are placed on the right hepatic duct, resulting in its division. Biliary leakage results, and right hepatic arterial injury is common.

Thermal Injury

The second most common type of major biliary injury occurs when excessive laser or cautery usage leads to a biliary stricture. This may occur when injudicious use of the laser or cautery is used during the initial exposure of the cystic duct (Fig. 14-4). Early instructional tapes mistakenly described division of the cystic duct with the laser or cautery instruments. Transmission of heat through the ductal structures can have disastrous results. Thermal injury leads to coagulation and disruption of the blood supply to delicate ductal structures, and normal biliary systems with their small caliber, as well as systems with anomalous blood supplies, are particularly prone to injury (Fig. 14-5). These injuries may present weeks to months after surgery and are particularly challenging to reconstruct.

Thermal Injury

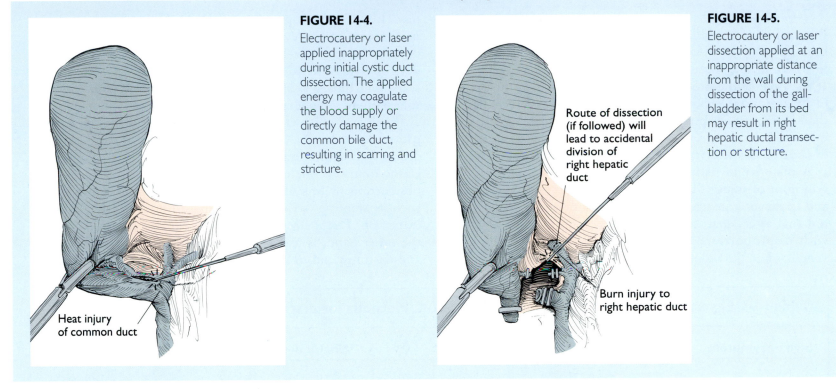

FIGURE 14-4.
Electrocautery or laser applied inappropriately during initial cystic duct dissection. The applied energy may coagulate the blood supply or directly damage the common bile duct, resulting in scarring and stricture.

Heat injury of common duct

Route of dissection (if followed) will lead to accidental division of right hepatic duct

Burn injury to right hepatic duct

FIGURE 14-5.
Electrocautery or laser dissection applied at an inappropriate distance from the wall during dissection of the gallbladder from its bed may result in right hepatic ductal transection or stricture.

Biliary Leakage

Various injuries to the biliary tree or other technical problems may lead to bile leakage after laparoscopic cholecystectomy. The classic injury and its variants, a partial tear of a ductal structure (Fig. 14-6), an injured accessory ductal structure, or the cystic duct may leak bile after surgery. Leakage from the gallbladder bed or small accessory ducts is difficult to recognize at the time of operation. Significant leakage, however, eventually results in biliary ascites or pain leading to investigation. Bile leakage in the absence of major ductal injuries usually responds to stenting, drainage of the ascites with percutaneous catheters, or a combination of the two. Leakage from the cystic duct stump may occur when clips are inappropriately placed and fall off (Fig. 14-7), or when they are placed too aggressively and cause crush necrosis of the duct. This is particularly prone to occur in cases of acute cholecystitis when the tissues are edematous and friable. Chromic gut ties may be safer than clips in the acute situation.

Biliary Leakage

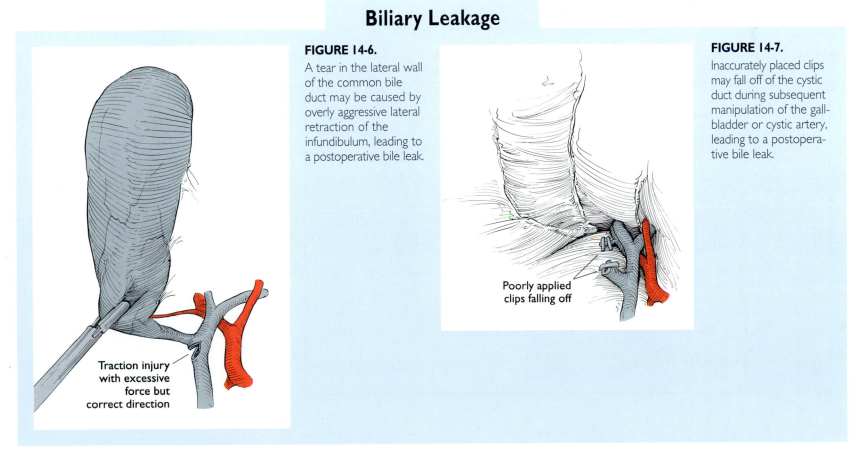

FIGURE 14-6.
A tear in the lateral wall of the common bile duct may be caused by overly aggressive lateral retraction of the infundibulum, leading to a postoperative bile leak.

Traction injury with excessive force but correct direction

Poorly applied clips falling off

FIGURE 14-7.
Inaccurately placed clips may fall off of the cystic duct during subsequent manipulation of the gallbladder or cystic artery, leading to a postoperative bile leak.

Diagnosis

Biliary injury is unlikely to be recognized at the time of the initial operation, though a review of videotapes of procedures in which injuries occur reveals that there are clues to the injury at the time of the procedure [7]. Specific clues to the presence of biliary injury include a "cystic" duct with a larger diameter than usual, presence of unexplained golden hepatic-type bile, unusual hemorrhage, hemorrhage from sites that are difficult to control, or the division of two distinct ductal structures.

A majority of patients have pain as their initial presenting symptom of injury (Table 14-3). Complete biliary obstruction and cholangitis are uncommon. Significant postoperative pain is unusual after laparoscopic cholecystectomy, and any patient with disproportional pain that persists after the procedure should undergo endoscopic retrograde cholangiopancreatogra-phy (ERCP) or computed tomography (Table 14-4). A simple noninvasive test to evaluate for a leak is radionuclide imaging done by using ^{99m}Tc-IDA. Small leaks that pool in the gallbladder fossa or Morrison's pouch may be detected with nuclear scans and biliary ascites may be present throughout the peritoneal cavity or pool in various dependent sites.

If a leak or obstruction is suspected, ERCP is the first investigational method in a treatment algorithm (Fig. 14-8). This procedure will demonstrate complete bile duct obstruction in the classic injury or one of its variants, and in cases of incomplete obstruction or leak allows for other interventional procedures such as stenting, stricture dilation, sphincterotomy, or stone extraction. Percutaneous transhepatic cholangiogram (PTC), on the other hand, is useful to delineate proximal biliary injuries and anatomy, and to identify the source of a bile leak if present.

Table 14-3. Signs and symptoms of injury

Sign or symptom	Cause
Abdominal pain	Chemical/bacterial peritonitis
Fever	Cholangitis, peritonitis
Nausea/vomiting	Peritonitis, ileus
Abdominal distension	Ileus, biloma
Jaundice	Bile duct obstruction
Anorexia	Ileus, biloma, obstruction

Table 14-4. Methods for diagnosis of injury

Method	What it demonstrates	Therapy available
Endoscopic retrograde choledochopancreat-ography	Distal ductal anatomy, leaks, sites of stricture	Papillotomy balloon, stones
Computed tomography	Bile collection, ductal dilation	Drainage of abscess/biloma
Percutaneous transhepatic cholangiography	Proximal ductal anatomy, sites of leaks, disruption, strictures	Stents for duct identification/drainage, balloon
Radionuclide methods	Bile leak/collection, obstruction	None

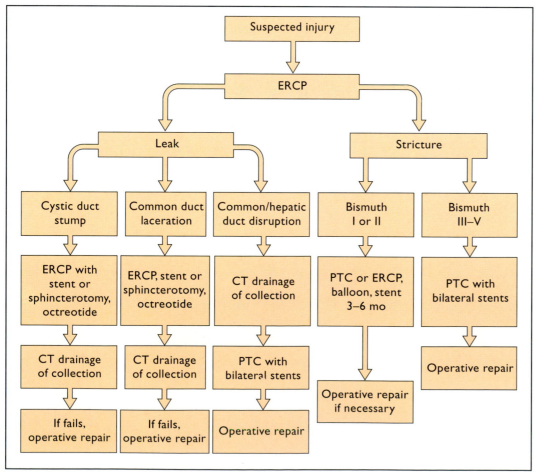

FIGURE 14-8.

Treatment algorithm for biliary injury. CT—computed tomography; ERCP—endoscopic retrograde cholangiopancreatography; PTC—percutaneous transhepatic cholangiography.

Stents placed during PTC are important for intraoperative identification of damaged ductal structures and should be placed bilaterally if exploration and repair are planned. The performance of computed tomography after the placement of percutaneous drainage tubes and injection of contrast may facilitate the drainage of bile collections and the preoperative stabilization of the patient.

Treatment

The classic injury and its variants should be treated with Roux-en-Y hepaticojejunostomy (Table 14-5). This is true whether the injury is discovered at the time of the initial operation or, as is usually the case, days to weeks after the initial procedure. Preoperative studies should adequately identify the choledochal anatomy and transhepatic stents should be placed (Fig. 14-9). Most injuries even high into the hepatic biliary radicals can be successfully treated with a Roux-en-Y hepaticojejunostomy (Fig. 14-10). It is critical that the procedure be performed by an experienced hepatobiliary surgeon, as the best chance of a long-term success is at the first attempted repair.

Thermal injury can cause stricture and scarring that is reminiscent of ductal cancer. The density and character of the damaged tissue can make intraoperative identification of the ductal anatomy and the subsequent repair very difficult. The excised scar tissue should be sent for pathologic examination. Extrahepatic duc-

Table 14-5. Treatment options for biliary injuries	
Injury	**Therapy**
Ductal disruption	Hepaticojejunostomy
Stricture	Hepaticojejunostomy, balloon/stent
Bile leak	
Disruption	Hepaticojejunostomy
Duct laceration	Repair, stent/papillotomy
Accessory duct	Hepaticojejunostomy, stent/papillotomy, ligate
Cystic duct stump	Stent/papillotomy, repair, octreotide

Treatment

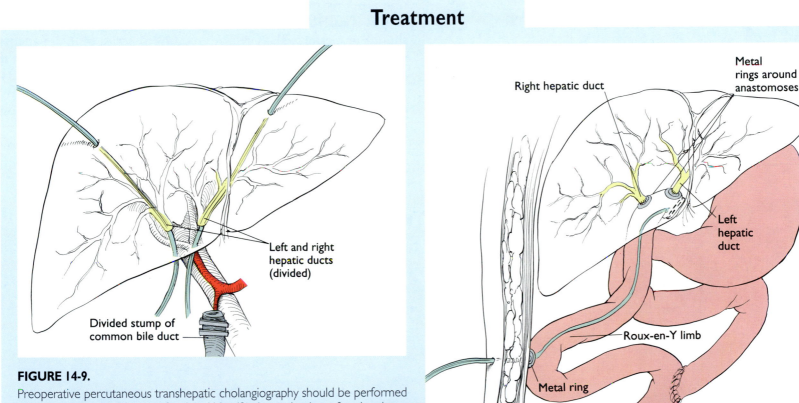

FIGURE 14-9.
Preoperative percutaneous transhepatic cholangiography should be performed and bilateral stents left in place for ductal identification at the time of exploration.

FIGURE 14-10.
Multiple anastomoses may be required, although some ducts may be filleted and anastomosed concurrently. It is critical that all scar tissue be excised and that a mucosa-to-mucosa anastomosis be performed on normal ductal tissue. The anastomoses should be marked with a radiopaque horseshoe, and the Roux-en-Y segment should be tacked to the anterior abdominal wall and marked with clips or a coronary o-ring. This allows subsequent access to the biliary tree without percutaneous transhepatic cholangiography.

tal strictures may be caused by the inappropriate placement of a biliary clip or by thermal injury. A minority of strictures are amenable to percutaneous or ERCP balloon dilatation, though most require hepaticojejunostomy. Bile leaks from the cystic duct or a minor common duct injury usually respond to percutaneous drainage alone or percutaneous drainage with endoscopic stenting. In such situations ERCP allows for diagnosis and treatment of contributory abnormalities such as retained stones. Octreotide may be useful to decrease the volume of a leak and hasten its closure.

Finally, if these measures fail, operative intervention with closure of the leak may be necessary.

Prevention of Injuries

Nearly all biliary injuries during laparoscopic cholecystectomy are preventable (Table 14-6) [1,7,8]. The fundus of the gallbladder and region of the portahepatis must be clearly in view on the operating monitor prior to beginning any dissection (Figs. 14-11 to 14-13). The operative field must not be obstructed by the stomach, duodenum, colon, or liver. Videotapes of procedures in which injuries occurred revealed that inadequate visualization, from inexperience of the surgeon or mechanical difficulties, can lead to misinterpretation of the anatomy and subsequent injury [9]. No clips should be placed and no cuts should be made in a tubular structure until the cystic duct infundibular junction has been identified with certainty.

Intraoperative cholangiography is an important adjunct to the prevention of injury [8,10]. Anomalous or accessory biliary ducts may be identified, and, in a minority of cases, the operative plan will be altered on the basis of cholangiography. Controversy concerns whether cholangiography is mandatory; however, if any question arises regarding ductal anatomy, if dissection is at all difficult, or if it is early in the experience of any surgeon, cholangiography should be performed. A recently compiled series of 171 patients with laparoscopic cholecystectomy biliary injuries indicated that if intraoperative cholangiography was performed, both the severity and Bismuth level of the injury were less severe. Moreover, in many cases, correctly interpreted cholangiograms can prevent progression from one level of severity to the next [9,11,12].

Finally, one should always maintain a conservative attitude toward conversion of laparoscopic cholecystectomy to an open

---

Table 14-6. Techniques to avoid injury

Clear, unobstructed view of the infundibulum/triangle of Calot

Firm cephalad retraction of the fundus, inferior and lateral retraction of the infundibulum

Dissection of fat/areolar tissue from infundibulum toward common duct, never vice versa

Absolute visualization of the cystic duct–gallbladder junction with no other intervening tissue

Cholangiography to confirm anatomy and rule out other abnormalities

Accessory/anomalous ducts are rare; do not over-call

A ductal structure wider than a standard clip is the common duct until proven otherwise

No cauterization or cliping blindly to control bleeding

Irrigation as often as necessary to clear the operative field and optimize visualization

Six to eight clips are the routine maximum; the need for more should lead to conversion

Asking yourself if one should convert to open surgery probably means that you should

---

Injury Prevention

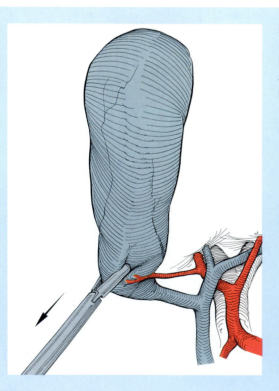

FIGURE 14-11.

Proper retraction of the gallbladder is critical to expose the cystic duct gallbladder junction. There should be maximal cephalic retraction of the fundus of the gallbladder while the infundibulum is retracted laterally and inferiorally at a 90° angle to the common bile duct. The traction should be firm but not excessive to prevent tenting of the common bile duct into the operative field.

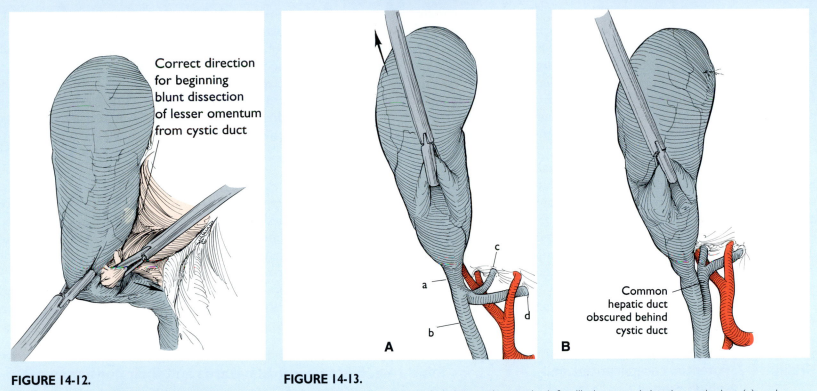

FIGURE 14-12.

The adventitial fatty tissues on the infundibulum of the gallbladder should be dissected away from the infundibulum and toward the common duct, never the opposite. This principle of dissecting away from the gallbladder holds true for the cystic artery as well.

FIGURE 14-13.

A, Inappropriate firm and cephalad retraction on the infundibulum may bring the cystic duct (*a*) and common duct (*b*) into a linear configuration. This predisposes to misidentification of the common duct as the distal cystic duct, leading to the classic injury. The right (*c*) and left (*d*) hepatic ducts are identified. **B**, Inappropriate medial and cephalad retraction of the infundibulum predisposes to common hepatic or right hepatic ductal injury, even if the cystic duct is correctly identified.

operation. Conversion to an open operation should not be viewed as a complication or as inexperience, but as an exercise in good judgment [7,10,13].

Miscellaneous Complications

Bleeding

Bleeding that is not associated with a bile duct injury may occur from the dissection bed near the porta, from the cystic artery stump, or from the gallbladder bed itself. Bleeding in the portahepatis should be considered a criterion for opening the patient, because injudicious placement of clips or imprecise cautery may injure the bile duct or worsen the bleeding. The cystic artery stump may be grasped and clips or ties reapplied as necessary. If this proves difficult because of the amount of bleeding, the patient should be opened immediately. Bleeding from the gallbladder bed may be compressed by the organ if it is still attached. Individual bleeding sites may be cauterized, and topical agents may be applied to the hepatic bed to tamponade bleeding. Ongoing bleeding that is difficult to control or is coming from the region of the porta may be associated with bile duct injury; thus, converting to open cholecystectomy is indicated.

Spilled Stones

Stones may leak from the gallbladder during the dissection of the gallbladder from its bed or upon removal of the gallbladder from the abdominal cavity (Table 14-7).

Stones that are spilled into the abdominal cavity usually cause no complications, but reports have described subhepatic and intraperitoneal abscesses caused by free-floating stones. These cases required conventional laparotomy, stone removal, and drainage of the abscess [14,15]. There have been reports of stones migrating into the hepatic substance, into the gastrointestinal tract, and through the diaphragm into the lung parenchyma, causing cholelithoptysis and cholelithorrhea [16]. If intra-abdominal stones remain, appropriate administration of antibiotics, aspiration of the bile, and irrigation of the peritoneal cavity lead to postoperative courses similar to those with unperforated gallbladders [15].

Electrosurgical Injury

The use of electrosurgery is obviously critical to the performance of laparoscopic cholecystectomy. A detailed review of the subject is beyond the scope of this chapter but has been presented elsewhere [17]. The safe use of electrosurgical techniques in laparoscopic surgery requires a basic understanding of several principles (Table 14-8).

Laparoscopic surgery is performed by using instruments that are between 30 and 50 cm long. However, the field of view on the monitor as the operation proceeds is typically 5 to 10 cm in diameter. Events related to the electric current in the proximal 20 cm of the instruments, therefore, are out of view of the surgeon. Although most instruments have adequate insulation for routine use, most of the insulated portion of the instruments is out of view. If this protective layer breaks down, electric energy to surrounding viscera can escape.

With the expansion in laparoscopic general surgery has come a vast increase in instrumentation design. One unfortunate result is the combination of metal and plastic in trocar and cannula design. Passage of a metal cannula through a plastic collar should be condemned because of its ability to set up a capacitance couple with subsequent discharge of electric energy into hollow viscera (Fig. 14-14). The use of all metal cannulas is strongly encouraged to prevent this problem.

Finally, instruments carrying monopolar current may inadvertently contact the laparoscope. If an all-metal cannula is in use, the current passes through the trocar and passes safely through the abdominal wall. However, if a plastic cannula is in use, the current may pass to adjacent organs out of view of the field of the operation, potentially causing injury. Electrocautery generates intense heat when applied to tissues. Heat conducted through the biliary tree via the cystic duct, cystic artery, or surrounding tissues during dissection can cause ischemia and stricturing of the extrahepatic or intrahepatic biliary tree. Judicious use of the cautery is advised to prevent devastating injury.

Results

Laparoscopic cholecystectomy has proven to be a very safe procedure. Ten major series, comprising 47,100 patients, were reviewed. (Table 14-9). The rate of major complications, including biliary injury and leakage, hemorrhage, infection, trocar and Veress needle injuries, and major organ system morbidity, was less than 3% [1,4–5,17–22]. Although the rate of biliary injury, clearly the most devastating complication, is extremely low, these patients present particularly challenging problems.

Table 14-7. Potential complications of spilled stones	
Abscess	Migration of stones
Subhepatic	Transdiaphragmatic
Subphrenic	Intrahepatic
Intraperitoneal	Transbronchial

Table 14-8. Electrosurgical hazards and their consequences	
Hazard	**Potential consequence**
Insulation breakdown	Spark-gap to adjacent viscera
Combination metal/plastic trocar/cannulae	Sets up capacitance couple with discharge to adjacent viscera
Narrow field of view	Electrical events occur off-screen
Loss of tactile sensation	Intense heat generated at the ends of long instruments

Electrosurgical Injury

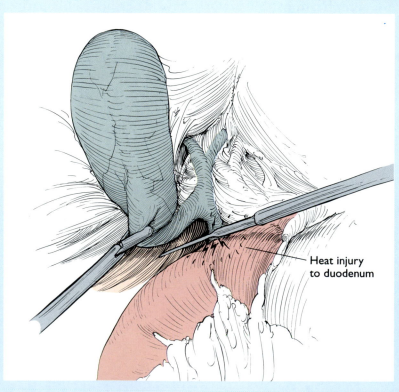

Heat injury to duodenum

FIGURE 14-14.
Discharge of energy from instruments with insulation defects or in which a capacitance couple has been established may cause a burn injury to the duodenum or colon, with subsequent perforation, or to the bile duct, with subsequent stricture.

The biliary injury encountered in open cholecystectomy consists primarily of postoperative stricture at the level of the cystic duct-common duct junction. Transected ducts are typically transected sharply and can usually be repaired primarily over a T-tube with good results, although some develop late strictures. The severity of laparoscopic cholecystectomy injuries is clearly worse, with major segments of the biliary tree removed or scarred secondary to thermal injury.

Several series detailing the management of biliary complications of laparoscopic cholecystectomy have been published. Rossi and coworkers [10] detailed the management of 11 patients who underwent biliary reconstruction after laparoscopic cholecystectomy. They emphasize several risk factors, including acute or chronic inflammation and scarring in the triangle of Calot, as well as obesity. All 11 patients underwent at least one hepaticojejunostomy for reconstruction, and two patients who had been repaired at outside hospitals underwent re-do intrahepatic hepaticojejunostomy. Patients with such injuries averaged almost 29 days in the hospital and 3 to 7 months out of work. The Mayo Clinic chronicled 22 patients with major injuries. Nineteen of these patients had injuries in the biliary tree, including 11 with Bismuth type II or higher [14]. The author emphasized the high rate of bile duct injuries and reinforced the experience of others that the injuries occurred high in the biliary tree. Soper and coworkers [13] treated 20 patients with biliary complications after laparoscopic cholecystectomy. In 15 of these patients, the injury was to the common bile duct or common hepatic duct. In 10 of these 15 patients, the common bile duct was mistaken for the cystic duct and the classic injury or one of its variants ensued. Nine of the patients had injuries at Bismuth type II or higher. Eleven of the patients required hepaticojejunostomy for treatment, with three requiring at least one reoperation for leak or stricture. At Duke University Medical Center, 50 patients, 38 with major injuries to the major bile ducts, were encountered [7]. Twenty-four patients had the classic injury or a variant. These patients underwent Roux-en-Y hepaticojejunostomy after evaluation and placement of transhepatic stents. Reoperation was necessary in five of these 38 patients. Right hepatic lobectomy was required in two patients for unreconstructible right hepatic ductal injury. Thirty-one of the 38 patients had injuries of Bismuth type II or higher, and 16 patients had injuries involving at least four individual intrahepatic ducts.

Mirza and coworkers [24] more recently described a series of 27 patients. Nine of the patients had injuries at Bismuth II or higher. Four of these patients continued to have episodes of cholangitis on follow-up, and one has developed secondary biliary cirrhosis.

Despite its overall safety, these four series document the catastrophes that may occur during laparoscopic cholecystectomy. Many of these patients are young, and continuing morbidity and a certain percentage of mortality can be expected as examination of these series continues. Careful and meticulous preparation and dissection, as well as the principles outlined earlier as specific preventive measures, must be adhered to so that these most feared complications may be avoided.

Table 14-9. Rates of injury

Study	Cases, n	Biliary injury, n(%)	Biliary leak, n(%)	Bleeding, n(%)
Litwin and coworkers [22]	2201	3(0.1)	22(1)	95(4.3)
Larson and coworkers [20]	1983	5(0.3)	7(0.4)	7(0.4)
Southern Surgeons Club [1]	1518	7(0.5)	3(0.2)	4(0.3)
Cushieri and coworkers [18]	1236	4(0.3)	0	0
Baird and coworkers [21]	800	0	3(0.4)	3(0.4)
Soper and coworkers [13]	618	1(0.2)	1(0.2)	0
Spaw and coworkers [19]	500	0	1(0.2)	1(0.2)
Z'Graggen and coworkers [4]	10174	32(.31)	39(.38)	1074(10.5)
Regoly-Merci and coworkers [5]	26440	148(.56)	476(1.8)	NR
Targarona and coworkers [23]	1630	16(.95)	NR	NR
Total	47100	216(.46)	552(1.2)	1184(2.5)

NR—Not recorded.

References

1. The Southern Surgeons Club: Prospective analysis of 1518 laparoscopic cholecystectomy. *N Engl J Med* 1991, 324:1073–1078.

2. Shanahan D, Knight M: Laparoscopic cholecystectomy. *BMJ* 1992, 304:776–777.

3. Moore MJ, Bennett CL: The learning curve for laparoscopic cholecystectomy. *Am J Surg* 1995, 170:55–59.

4. Z'graggen K, Wehrli H, Metzger A, *et al.*: Complications of laparoscopic cholecystectomy in Switzerland. *Surg Endosc* 1998, 12:1303–1310.

5. Regoly-Merei J, Ihaz M, Szeberin Z, *et al.*: Biliary tract complications in laparoscopic cholecystectomy. A muliticenter study of 148 biliary tract injuries in 26,440 operations. *Surg Endosc* 1998, 12:294–300.

6. Meyers W, Peterseim D, Pappas T, *et al.*: Low insertion of hepatic segmental duct VII-VIII is an important cause of major biliary injury or misdiagnosis. *Am J Surg* 1996, 171:187–191.

7. Branum G, Schmitt C, Baillie J, *et al.*: Management of major biliary complications after laparoscopic cholecystectomy. *Ann Surg* 1993, 217:532–541.

8. Hunter JG: Avoidance of bile duct injury during laparoscopic cholecystectomy. *Am J Surg* 1991, 162:71–75.

9. Stewart L, Hunter J, Oddsdottir M, Way LW: Prevention of bile duct injuries during laparoscopic cholecystectomy. *Surgery* 1993, in press.

10. Rossi RL, Schirmer WJ, Braasch JW, *et al.*: Laparoscopic bile duct injuries: risk factors, recognition, and repair. *Arch Surg* 1992, 127:596–602.

11. Woods MS, Traverso LW, Kozarek R, *et al.*: Characteristics of biliary tract complications during laparoscopic cholecystectomy: a multi-intitutional study. *Ann J Surg* 1994, 167:27–33.

12. Olsen D. Bile duct injuries during laparoscopic cholecystectomy. *Surg Endosc* 1997, 11:133–138.

13. Soper N, Flye MW, Brunt LM, *et al.*: Diagnosis and management of biliary complications of laparoscopic cholecystectomy. *Am J Surg* 1992, 165:663–669.

14. Ress A, Sarr M, Nagorney D, *et al.*: Spectrum and management of major complications of laparoscopic cholecystectomy. *Am J Surg* 1993, 165:655–662.

15. Lauffer J, Krahenbuhl L, Baer H, *et al.*: Clinical manifestations of lost gallstones after laparoscopic cholecystectomy: a case report with review of the literature. *Surg Laparosc Endosc* 1997, 7:103–112.

16. Assaf Y, Matter I, Sabo E, *et al.*: Laparoscopic cholecystectomy for acute cholecystitis and the consequences of gallbladder perforation, bile spillage, and "loss" of stones. *Eur J Surg* 1998, 164:425–431.

17. Odell RC: Laparoscopic electrosurgery. In *Minimally Invasive Surgery.* Edited by Hunter JG, Sackier JM. New York: McGraw-Hill Inc.; 1993:33–41.

18. Cushieri A, Dubois F, Moviel J, *et al.*: The European experience with laparoscopic cholecystectomy. *Am J Surg* 1991, 161:385–387.

19. Spaw AT, Reddick EJ, Olsen DO: Laparoscopic laser cholecystectomy: analysis of 500 procedures. *Surg Laparosc Endosc* 1991, 1:2–7.

20. Larson GM, Vitale GC, Casey J, *et al.*: Multipractice analysis of laparoscopic cholecystectomy in 1988 patients. *Am J Surg* 1992, 163:221–226.

21. Baird DR, Wilson JP, Mason EM, *et al.*: An early review of 800 laparoscopic cholecystectomies at a university-affiliated community teaching hospital. *Am Surg* 1992, 58:206–210.

22. Litwin DEM, Girotti MJ, Poulin EC, *et al.*: Laparoscopic cholecystectomy trans-Canada experience with 2,201 cases. *Can J Surg* 1992, 35:291–296.

23. Targarona E, Marco C, Balague C, *et al.*: How, when, and why bile duct injury occurs. A comparison between open and laparoscopic cholecystectomy. *Surg Endosc* 1998, 12:322–326.

24. Mirza D, Narsimhan K, Ferraz Neto B, *et al.*: Bile duct injury following laparoscopic cholecystectomy: referral pattern and management. *Br J Surg* 1997, 84:786–790.

*L*aparoscopic Liver Biopsy

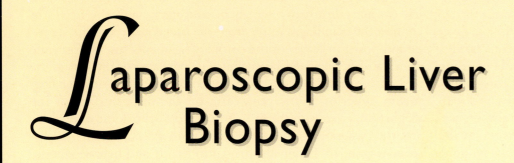

Robert B. Noone
J. E. Tuttle-Newhall

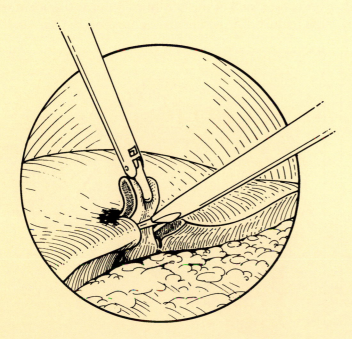

Operative management of liver disorders begins with their recognition and diagnosis. Many initiation points lead to diagnosis and treatment of specific disorders. Most often, cysts or solid lesions of the liver are found incidentally on ultrasonography or computed tomography (CT). From this point, further noninvasive or invasive tests may be performed to define the abnormality and guide therapy. Liver biopsy is one of the invasive tests the physician may choose to help in the diagnosis and management of liver disease. Indications for liver biopsy fall broadly into one of two categories: 1) diagnosis of lesions identified by an imaging study; or 2) evaluation of liver status in diseases involving the whole liver parenchyma (Table 15-1). Liver biopsy is most commonly done by using a percutaneous needle. Biopsy with this instrument is often performed blindly by using an aspiration technique (described by Menghini) or core biopsy with a Tru-cut, (Allegiance Healthcare Corp., McGraw Park, IL) needle [1,2]. Fine-needle aspiration for cytology can also be useful. Laparoscopic liver biopsy adds another dimension to the diagnostic capabilities of needle biopsy: 1) Biopsy can be done under direct vision; 2) the appearance of the liver can be assessed; 3) other abdominal abnormalities can be ascertained; and 4) surrounding structures can be visualized and biopsied to assess the possibility of metastatic disease.

Anatomy

The liver is the largest solid organ in the body, with an average mass of 1500 g in the adult. The liver resides under the rib cage (in the right upper quadrant of the abdomen) and is not palpable in the adult on physical examination. The inferior surface of the liver touches the duodenum, colon, kidney, adrenal gland, esophagus, and stomach. With the laparoscope, approximately 70% of the surface of the liver can be visualized. The anatomy of the liver, which is discussed below, describes the pertinent structures as appreciated by the laparoscope.

The reflections of the peritoneum, which attach the liver to the diaphragm, abdominal wall, and abdominal viscera are easily identified and define the topographic anatomy of the liver. There are three sets of ligaments. First is the falciform ligament, which attaches the liver to the anterior abdominal wall; the ligamentum teres hepaticus (the remnant of the umbilical vein) is incorporated in its dorsal border. Second is the anterior and posterior right and left coronary ligaments, which in continuity with the falciform connect the diaphragm of the liver; the lateral aspects of the anterior and posterior leaves of the coronary ligaments fuse to form the right and left triangular ligaments. The bare area of the liver is the area encompassed by the falciform, coronary, and triangular ligaments, superior to the vena cava, on the undersurface of the diaphragm. Even with the 30° viewing scope, the dome of the liver and the posterior ligaments are difficult to assess with the laparoscope (Figure 15-1). Finally, the gastrohepatic and hepaticoduodenal ligaments consist of the anterior layer of lesser omentum and are continuous with the left triangular ligament. The hepaticoduodenal ligament forms the anterior border of the epiploic foramen of Winslow and contains the hepatic arteries, portal vein, and extrahepatic bile ducts.

With retraction of the anterior border of the liver, the undersurface can be evaluated. The hepaticoduodenal ligament can easily be viewed, and nodes can be biopsied if necessary. The topographic right and left lobes are the portions of the liver on the respective side of the falciform ligament. The caudate (Spigelian) lobe delineated anatomically by the posterior (transverse) extension of the falciform ligament (ligamentum venosum, the remnant of the ductus venosus) on the left, and the impres-

---

Table 15-1. Indications for laparoscopic liver biopsy

Biopsy for specific lesions

Histologic diagnosis of lesion
Assessment of extent of metastatic disease

Biopsy for diffuse liver disease

Diagnosis of primary liver disease
Assessment of disease progression
Assessment of response of liver to treatment
Diagnosisis of condition of liver in metabolic disease
Defininition of involvement of liver in multisystem liver disease

---

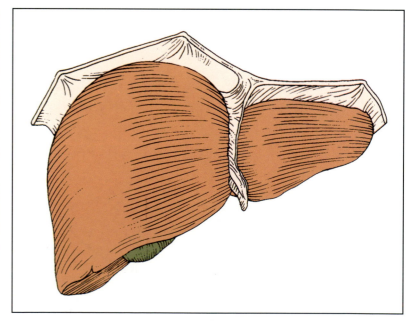

FIGURE 15-1.

A laparoscopic view of the anterior surface of the liver demonstrating the falciform and coronary ligaments. The left coronary ligament ends as the left triangular ligament.

sion of the inferior vena cava on the right, is difficult to assess because it is mostly hidden from view by the hepaticoduodenal ligament and the gastrohepatic ligament. The quadrate lobe is anterior to the caudate lobe. It is bound by the gallbladder fossa on the right, the groove of falciform ligament to the left, and by the porta hepatis posteriorly (umbilical fissure) (Figure 15-2).

The lobar anatomy, as defined by the distribution of the major branches of the portal vein, seldom conforms to the topographic right and left lobes. Cantlie first reported in 1898 that the division of the right and left lobes of the liver was not the falciform ligament, but rather a line (Cantlie's line) passing through the fossa of the gallbladder and to the left of the inferior vena cava; this plane is also called the lobar fissure. Couinaud [3] further divided each of the lobes into four segments, resulting in a total of eight subsegments: four on the right, three on the left, and one corresponding to the caudate lobe, segment I. Segments II to IV constitute the anatomical left lobe of the liver, while segments V to VIII make up the right. The caudate lobe is its own segment in the French nomenclature as described by Couinaud; anatomically, there are two branches of the portal vein in the caudate: one arising from each the right and left portal branches. Thus, the caudate is actually part of both the true left and right lobes (Figure 15-3).

Pathophysiology, Presentation, and Differential Diagnosis

The predominant application of laparoscopy in the management of liver disease is the evaluation and management of specific lesions within the parenchyma. A detailed work-up before liver biopsy allows the surgeon to determine the likelihood of success with the laparoscopic approach. Table 15-2 outlines the features of frequently observed liver lesions and the diag-

nostic imaging method of choice. Below, some of the features of the more common diseases amenable to laparoscopic evaluation are discussed.

Malignant Liver Disease

Laparoscopic evaluation is particularly useful in the assessment of malignancy, both in the liver and elsewhere. Metastatic spread can be seen on laparoscopy before it is apparent on imaging studies. Laparoscopy is most accurate when imaging suggests lesions close to the surface of the liver [2]. Most studies have demonstrated 100% specificity for laparoscopic biopsies, with sensitivity in the range of 74% to 80% [4,5]. Imaging-guided biopsy techniques also are used frequently. Prospective comparison studies between CT- or ultrasonography-guided biopsy and laparoscopic techniques have showed no difference in overall accuracy. However, because laparoscopy seems to be more sensitive for small tumors, it should be used if malignancy is suspected clinically and if findings on imaging studies are negative [5]. Table 15-3 compares the relative advantages of laparoscopy- and CT-guided liver biopsy.

Hepatocellular carcinoma must be suspected in patients with a liver mass and history of hepatitis B or C infection and in patients from an area endemic for one of these infections. Strongly positive alpha-fetoprotein level is diagnostic in these cases. If the patient is a candidate for resection, laparotomy for resection should proceed. If the patient has cirrhosis and is being considered for liver transplantation, then biopsy should not be done because of the risk for peritoneal seeding of cancer [6].

More recently, the ability of the surgeon to assess liver abnormalities intraoperatively beyond the surface has increased with the advent of laparoscopic ultrasonograph probes. These probes can be inserted through standard trocars placed in

FIGURE 15-2.

A stylized version of liver anatomy seen from the undersurface.

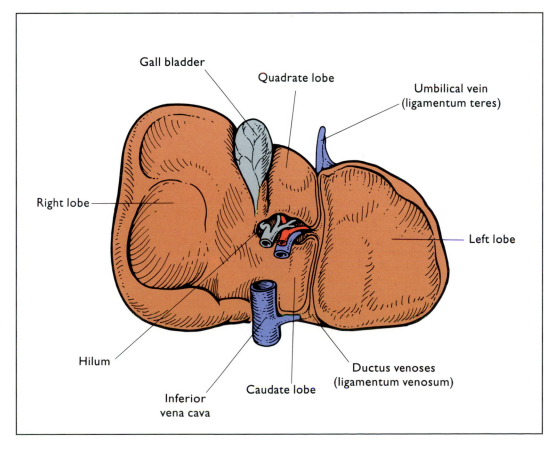

Gall bladder

Quadrate lobe

Umbilical vein (ligamentum teres)

Right lobe

Left lobe

Hilum

Ductus venoses (ligamentum venosum)

Inferior vena cava

Caudate lobe

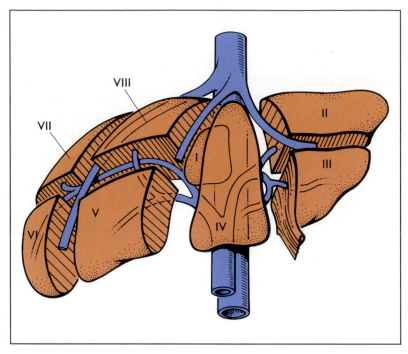

FIGURE 15-3. Segmentation of the liver according to Couinaud [3].

direct contact with the liver. With this direct contact, resolution is much greater than with surface ultrasonograph. Detailed images of the hepatic parenchyma allow for more accurate evaluation and biopsy.

Cancer Staging

The ability to visualize and biopsy multiple lesions in one procedure makes laparoscopy a powerful diagnostic tool in staging early malignant disease of the liver. It is even more impressive when one considers that lesions as small as 1 mm can be identified (compared with a 5- to 10-mm resolution of CT). More than 70% of the liver can be visualized, and, more important, surgical and autopsy studies demonstrate that in metastatic disease, about 90% of the liver metastases present on the surface [7,8]. Laparoscopy enables surgeons to detect and biopsy small lesions not only in the liver but also on the peritoneum or diaphragm; unnecessary radical surgery can be obviated when early diagnosis of metastatic disease is made. In addition, the unaffected parts of the liver can be assessed at the time of laparoscopy, and the severity of cirrhosis can be assessed. In some of these patients, transplantation may be an option.

Table 15-2. Features of frequently observed liver lesions

Disorder	Epidemiology	Signs and symptoms	Diagnostic method of choice	Findings
Solitary cyst	14%–30% F:M = 3:1	Fullness in abdomen Nausea and vomiting Hepatomegaly	US	Thin walls, smooth contours, anechoic mass Variable size
Adenoma	3–4 per 100,000 F>M 3rd–5th Decades Linked to OCP	Abdominal pain in 50% 10% Rupture Palpable mass in 30%	US/CT Biopsy advocated Technition-99 sulfur colloid scan	No definitive findings, single mass Hypovascular on arteriogram
Focal nodular hyperplasia	Unknown incidence F>M	10% only with abdominal pain	US/CT Biopsy advocated	No definitive findings Tumor usually > 5 cm Tumor usually solitary
Hemangioma	2%–7% F>M 3rd–5th Decades	Pain/discomfort Hepatomegaly RUQ mass	Arteriography IV timed sequence CT Biopsy not advocated	Vascular "puddling" on arteriogram
Hepatocellular carcinoma	1–7 per 100,000 M:F = 4–8:1 Associated with cirrhosis, HBV	Weakness/malaise Upper abdominal pain Mass in RUQ	CT-IV Biopsy advocated if patient is not a surgical candidate Serum AFP elevation diagnostic	No definitive findings
Metastatic cancer (colorectal)	30% Synchronous lesion	Hepatomegaly Asymptomatic (symptomatic patient, nonsurgical)	CT-portography Biopsy advocated	Hypovascular lesions

AFP—alpha-fetoprotein; CT—computed tomography; F—female; HBV—hepatitis B virus; IV—intravenous; M—male; OCP—oral contraceptive pill; RUQ—right upper quadrant; US—ultrasonography.

Focal Benign Liver Disease

The differentiation between malignant and benign lesions of the liver is a common clinical problem for the hepatobiliary surgeon. Certainly, advances in diagnostic imaging assist in this task. Adenomas, focal nodular hyperplasia, vascular abnormalities, granulomas, infarctions, or normal variations in liver anatomy can mimic malignant disease. Liver biopsy under laparoscopic guidance is highly effective in diagnosing these lesions when tissue is necessary for the diagnosis [9].

Diffuse Liver Disease

Liver biopsy is also performed to assess the parenchyma of the liver. This can be done to 1) diagnose primary liver disease (eg, Wilson's disease); 2) assess progression of disease or response to therapy; 3) diagnose the condition of the liver in metabolic disease (eg, glycogen storage disease, alcoholic cirrhosis); and 4) ascertain liver involvement in multisystem disease (eg, amyloidosis, sarcoidosis).

Although many of these diseases are considered diffuse liver disease, abnormalities of the liver parenchyma may not be distributed evenly throughout the liver, leading to sampling errors from blind biopsy [10,11]. Laparoscopy allows for biopsy of the most abnormal appearing tissue.

Imaging methods, including radionuclide scanning, ultrasonography, and CT, have poor sensitivity and specificity in the diagnosis of cirrhosis. Percutaneous liver biopsy for the diagnosis of cirrhosis had a false-negative rate of 24% in one study; laparoscopy and biopsy decreased this rate to 9% [12]. In addition to being more accurate, laparoscopy can direct biopsy of specific areas and differentiate foci of hepatocellular carcinoma from regenerating nodules [13].

Diagnosis of cirrhosis may be missed if needle biopsy of the liver is used. In a study of histologic findings obtained from laparoscopic needle biopsy of cirrhosis, the diagnosis was made in 68% of cases. The visual appearance of a diffusely nodular liver with a firm surface was more sensitive [14]. The combination of laparoscopic visualization and directed biopsy improves the diagnostic yield to 97.7% [15].

Table 15-3. Computed tomography–guided biopsy versus laparoscopic guided biopsy	
Advantages of computed tomography	**Advantages of laparoscopic**
Preferred for posterior and retroperitoneal lesions	Can visualize lesions as small as 1 mm in diameter
Can visualize whole liver	Can detect disease otherwise missed by computed tomography
Avoid complications associated with laparoscopy	Can be used to see, evaluate, and biopsy other tissues for cancer staging
Better for drainage of liver abscess	Larger tissue piece can be obtained if necessary
	Control of bleeding
Disadvantages of computed tomography	**Disadvantages of laparoscopic**
Resolution is 5–10 mm at best	Can see only 70% of the liver (even with 30° scope)
Misses lesions on the retroperitoneum and diaphragm	Cannot examine lesions deep in parenchyma
	Cannot be used to evaluate dome of liver, extreme right lateral area, and posterior areas
	Adhesions may limit examination

Surgical Technique

Figures 15-4 through 15-10 depict the surgical technique for laparoscopic liver biopsy.

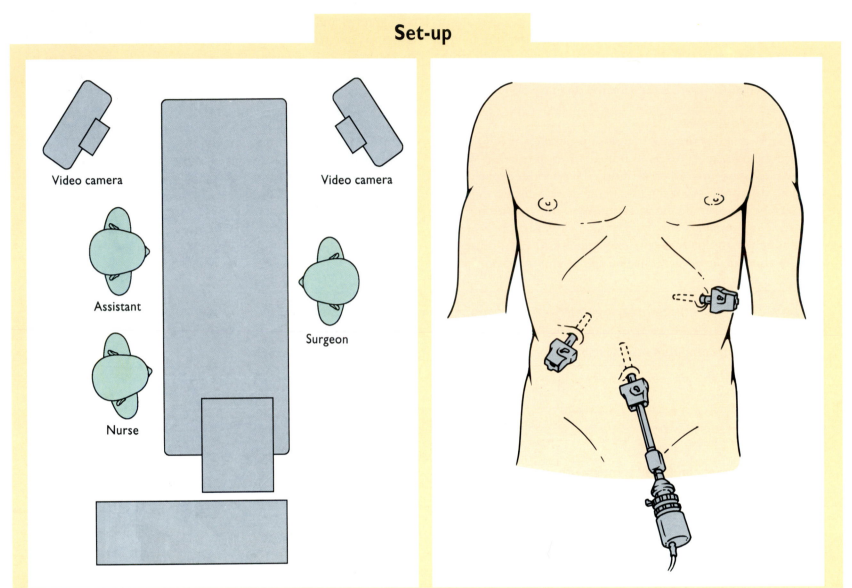

FIGURE 15-4.

The set-up for a laparoscopic liver biopsy is straightforward. The assistant operates the camera, while the surgeon uses a retracting/grasping device and a needle or pair of scissors to perform the biopsy.

FIGURE 15-5.

Three trocars are used for this operation, although it can be performed with only two. Besides the camera port, one port is placed in a position to gain good access to the abnormality in question. In this example, the abnormality is in the caudate lobe; thus, a trocar is placed in the left upper quadrant, in the anterior-axillary line, 5 to 7 cm below the costal margin. The addition of a third port allows use of retraction of the liver which facilitates the procedure. If a retraction device is used, a port sufficiently large to allow the passage of such an instrument should be placed; otherwise, 5-mm ports in addition to the camera port are usually adequate.

Procedure

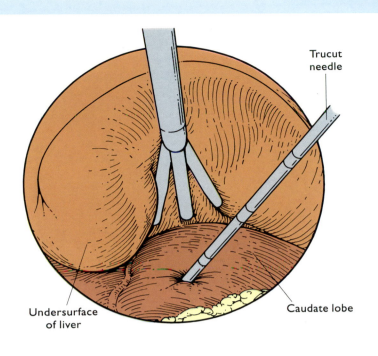

FIGURE 15-6.
With the aid of a fan retractor, the right lobe of the liver is lifted anteriorly and the undersurface of the liver is exposed. The abnormality in the caudate lobe is clearly visualized. The Trucut needle (Allegiance Heatlthcare Corps., McGraw Park, IL) is passed through the 5-mm port and positioned on the liver. Care and attention must be taken when performing this procedure to ensure that the tip of the needle is not placed beyond the liver; it is possible to inadvertently pass the needle too aggressively beyond the other side of the liver. This is a source of concern because complications resulting from this maneuver are often never visualized. One should always familiarize oneself with the mechanism of the needle being used to ensure as little disruption of the liver parenchyma as possible. Should excessive bleeding ensue, pressure or cautery applied directly to the site is usually adequate to stop the bleeding.

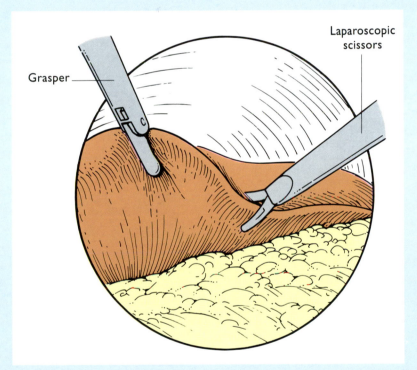

FIGURE 15-7.
A wedge biopsy of the liver can also be performed. Again the use of a second port greatly facilitates this procedure. The grasper is used to stabilize the liver, while scissors are introduced through a second port. The bleeding is usually not torrential, thus, cautery can be delayed until the specimen has been removed.

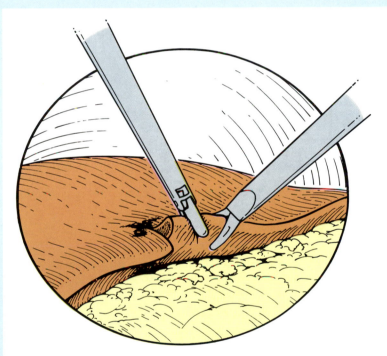

FIGURE 15-8.
The second arm of the wedge is made after the grasper has positioned the piece appropriately. Care should be exercised so that the specimen is not damaged as it is grasped.

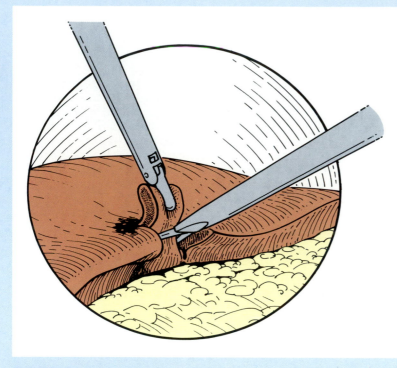

FIGURE 15-9.

The last portion of the capsule is cut and the specimen can be removed.

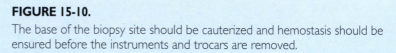

FIGURE 15-10.

The base of the biopsy site should be cauterized and hemostasis should be ensured before the instruments and trocars are removed.

Complications

Diagnostic laparoscopy is a straightforward procedure that carries a remarkably low morbidity and mortality. Postbiopsy bleeding is the single most serious complication (outside of the risks of laparoscopy), and it has been reported to occur at a frequency of less than 1%. Bile leaks are reported to occur in less than 0.1% of cases. Even more rare are cyst perforations, infection, and tumor implantation. The overall morbidity (complications requiring surgical intervention or prolonged hospital stay) and mortality are quoted as 0.46% and 0.53%, respectively

References

1. Schaffner F, Thung SN: Liver biopsy. In: *Bockus Gastroenterology*, edn 5. Edited by Haubrich WS, Schaffner F. Philadelphia: WB Saunders; 1995.

2. van Leeuwen DJ, Wilson L, Crowe DR: Liver biopsy in the mid-1990s: questions and answers. *Semin Liver Dis* 1995, 15:340–359.

3. Couinaud. *Le Foce Etudes Anatomique et Chirurgicales.* Paris: Masson; 1957.

4. Prior C, Kathrein H, Mikuz G, *et al.*: Differential diagnosis of malignant intrahepatic tumors by ultrasonically guided fine needle aspiration biopsy and by laparoscopic/intraoperative biopsy. A comparative study. *Acta Cytol* 1988, 32:892–895.

5. Leuschner M, Leuschner U: Diagnostic laparoscopy in focal parenchymal disease of the liver. *Endoscopy* 1992, 24:689–692.

6. Olthoff KM, Millis JM, Rosove MH, *et al.*: Is liver transplantation justified for the treatment of hepatic malignancies? *Arch Surg* 1990, 125:1261–1266.

7. Hogg L, Pack GT: Diagnostic accuracy of hepatic metastases at laparotomy. *Arch Surg* 1956, 72:251–252.

8. Ozarda A, Pickren J: The topographic distribution of liver metastases: its relation to surgical and isotope diagnosis. *J Nucl Med* 3:149–152.

9. Beck KL, ed.: *Color Atlas of Laparoscopy.* Philadelphia: W.B. Saunders; 1984.

10. Soloway RD, Baggenstoss AH, Schoenfield LJ, *et al.*: Observer error and sampling variability tested in evaluation of hepatitis and cirrhosis by liver biopsy. *Am J Dig Dis* 1971, 16:1082–1086.

11. Wondwosen A, Millen JC, Mezey E: Sampling variability of percutaneous liver biopsy. *Arch Intern Med* 1979, 139:667–699.

12. Nord HJ: Biopsy diagnosis of cirrhosis: blind percutaneous versus guided direct vision techniques: a review. *Gastrointest Endosc* 1982, 28:102–104.

13. Vilardell F: The value of laparoscopy in the diagnosis of primary cancer of the liver. *Endoscopy* 1977, 9:20–22.

14. Poniachik J, Bernstein DE, Reddy KR, *et al.*: The role of laparoscopy in the diagnosis of cirrhosis. *Gastrointest Endosc* 1996, 43:568–571.

15. Orlando R, Lirussi F, Okolicsanyi L: Laparoscopy and liver biopsy: further evidence that the two procedures improve the diagnosis of liver cirrhosis. A retrospective study of 1,003 consecutive examinations. *J Clin Gastroenterol* 1990, 12:47–52.

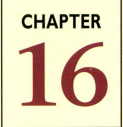
*L*aparoscopic Approach to Palliation of Periampullary Tumors

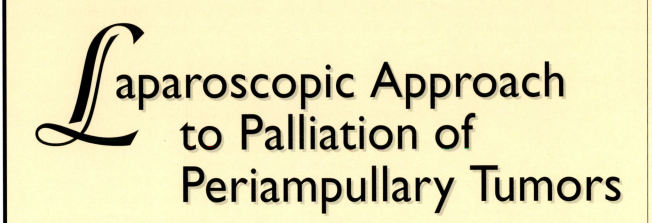

Lisa A. Clark

Theodore N. Pappas

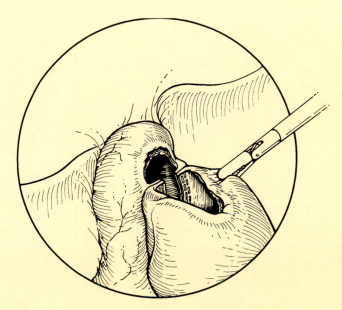

eriampullary tumors include neoplasms of the bile ducts, gallbladder, and pancreas. These tumors are unresectable at presentation in 70% to 90% of cases; as a result, optimal palliation with minimal procedure-related morbidity and mortality are the key goals [1]. Periampullary tumors create two clinical problems by virtue of their location and propensity to local spread: 1) jaundice from biliary obstruction and 2) nausea, vomiting, and poor nutrition caused by duodenal obstruction. As laparoscopic techniques have improved, so has our ability to offer minimally invasive means of palliation for these patients. This chapter discusses the background and approach to laparoscopic gastrojejunostomy and cholecystojejunostomy.

Anatomy

The stomach and jejunum are intraperitoneal components of the upper gastrointestinal tract that are separated by the duodenum. Anatomically, the stomach is divided into five regions: cardia, fundus, corpus, antrum, and pylorus (Figure 16-1). These areas aid the surgeon in the description, planning, and execution of gastric resections; with the exception of the pylorus, however, they do not correspond to functional regions. The major arterial supply to the stomach includes the left and right gastric arteries, which supply the lesser curvature; the left and right gastroepiploic arteries, which supply the greater curvature; the short gastric arteries, which supply the fundus; and the gastroduodenal artery, which supplies the pyloric region (Figure 16-2). Venous drainage of the stomach parallels the arterial system.

The common hepatic duct starts at the union of the right and left hepatic ducts (Figure 16-3). The junction of the cystic duct and the common hepatic duct is generally considered to be the beginning of the common bile duct. The upper limit of the normal length of this duct is 6 to 8 mm; after surgery, the upper limit is 10 to 12 mm. Intrahepatic and extrahepatic ducts generally lie anterior to their corresponding portal branches. The common bile duct, like all extrahepatic bile ducts, lies within the hepatoduodenal ligament and then passes behind the first part of the duodenum, through the head of the pancreas, and into the wall of the duodenum to form the ampulla of Vater.

The duodenum is a retroperitoneal portion of the upper gastrointestinal tract that begins immediately distal to the pylorus and extends to the ligament of Treitz. It assumes a characteristic C-loop configuration in situ and is divided into four segments. The head of the pancreas is situated within the C loop of the duodenum, and the confluence of the common bile and pancreatic ducts enters the intestinal tract in the second portion of the duodenum.

Although no anatomic structure indicates the terminus of the jejunum, it is generally accepted that it spans two-fifths of the distance from the ligament of Treitz to the ileocecal valve. The jejunum receives its blood supply via mesenteric vessels that originate from the superior mesenteric artery. The primary function of the jejunum is the absorption of nutrients generated by the digestive actions of the stomach, duodenum, pancreatic secretory products, and bile. Gastrojejunostomy is a feasible option because proximal gastrointestinal tract orientation, although redirected, is often fairly well preserved.

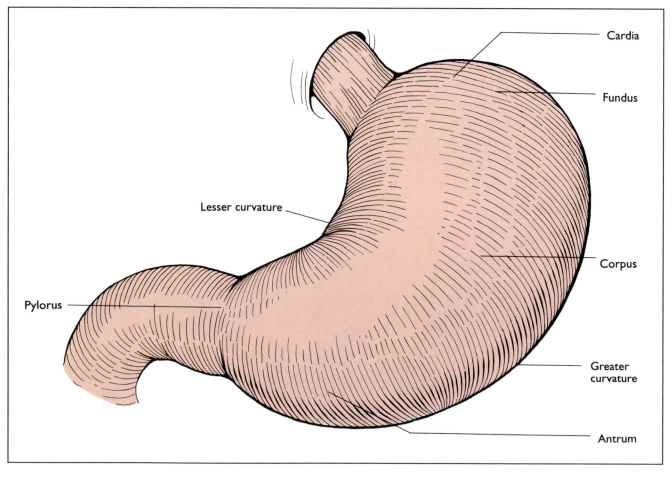

FIGURE 16-1.

The five regions of the stomach: cardia, fundus, corpus, antrum, and pylorus. The greater and lesser curvatures are also demonstrated.

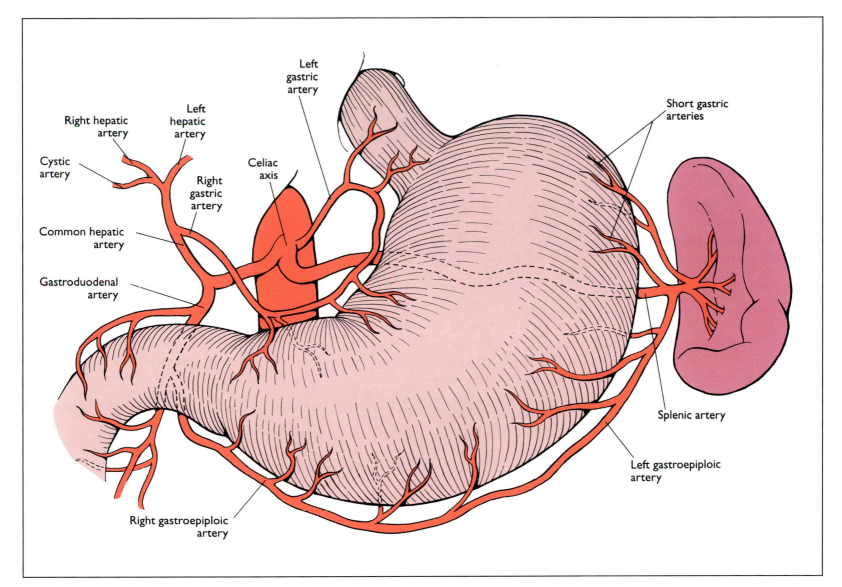

FIGURE 16-2.

The stomach is an extremely well-vascularized organ. The majority of arterial blood is supplied by four vessels: the right and left gastric arteries and the right and left gastroepiploic arteries. Simultaneous ligation of any three of these vessels usually does not affect gastric viability. The short gastric arteries also contribute to the stomach's blood supply.

FIGURE 16-3.

Relevant anatomy for cholecystojejunostomy.

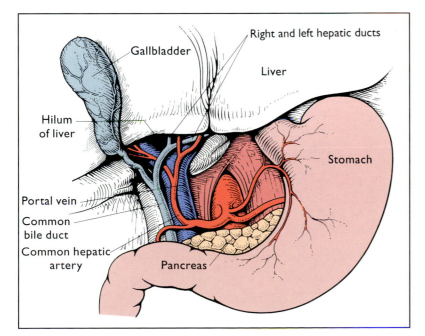

Laparoscopic Cholecystojejunostomy

Biliary obstruction is common in periampullary tumors. About 65% to 75 % of patients present with jaundice caused by tumor compression of the extrahepatic bile ducts [1]. With the advent of advanced endoscopic techniques, the management of malignant obstructive jaundice has changed over the past decade. Nonoperative biliary drainage techniques have replaced surgical drainage procedures as the mainstay for palliation of periampullary tumors. Nonoperative intervention was first developed via the transhepatic route [2]; however, with the development of larger channel, side-viewing endoscopes [3], biliary stent placement via the endoscope has provided good decompression with a much lower incidence of complications [4]. A randomized controlled trial has demonstrated a significantly lower complication rate with endoscopic stenting than with surgery [5], and wider-bore, expanding stents occlude less frequently, eliminating the need for repeated endoscopy [6].

These data support the routine use of endoscopy in the management of malignant biliary obstruction. Surgical biliary bypass should be reserved for younger, fitter patients who might survive more than 6 months or for those in whom endoscopic biliary stenting is not technically possible.

Surgical bypass can be accomplished via palliative pancreaticoduodenectomy (the Whipple procedure), choledochoduodenostomy, cholecystojejunostomy (CCJ), or choledochojejunostomy (CDJ). Palliative pancreaticoduodenectomy offers increased risk for complications without survival advantage and is not generally recommended. Choledochoduodenostomy sometimes does not provide acceptable palliation when the point of duodenal obstruction is more distal than the biliary anastomosis. Thus, the commonly preferred procedures are CCJ and CDJ. In a collective review of the two procedures in 461 patients, mean survival times for CCJ and CDJ were 5.2 and 7.4 months, respectively, and the procedure-related mortality rates were 19% and 25.3%, respectively [7]. Another series demonstrated that serum bilirubin concentrations returned to normal in 37.5% of patients with CCJ compared with 40.5% of patients with CDJ; the recurrence rate for jaundice was 8.3% after CCJ and 13.5% after CDJ [7].

These data have made CCJ an acceptable procedure provided that the cystic duct is patent and enters the common bile duct 2 to 3 cm away from the tumor mass. If any question arises about the patency of the cystic duct, intraoperative cholangiography should be performed. If the gallbladder is not present or is unsuitable for use, CDJ should be performed [8].

Surgical Technique

The set-up and technique for laparoscopic CCJ is depicted in Figures 16-4 through 16-17.

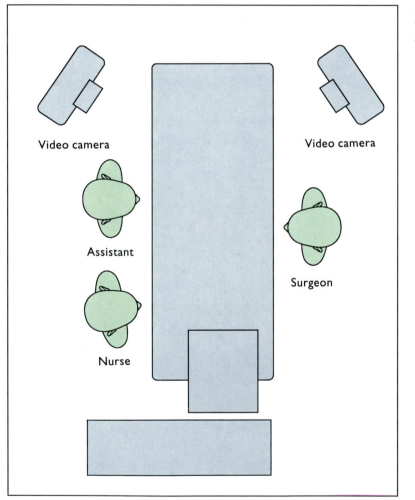

FIGURE 16-4.

The set-up for the laparoscopic cholecystojejunostomy is similar to the set-up for the laparoscopic Nissen fundoplication. The surgeon and assistants are as identified in this figure.

Video camera

Video camera

Assistant

Surgeon

Nurse

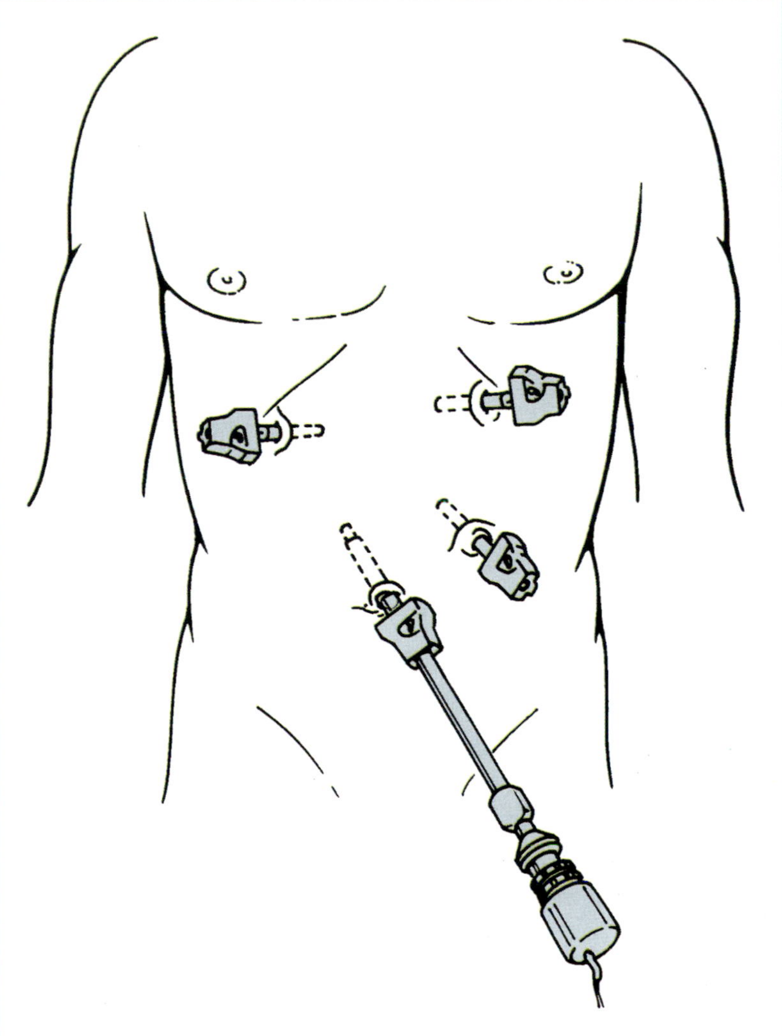

FIGURE 16-5.

Trocar placement. Trocars are placed as shown in the figure. After the umbilical port for the camera is placed, a 5-mm port is placed in the left upper quadrant, in the mid clavicular line, 5 to 10 cm below the costal margin. A 10-mm port is placed in the left upper quadrant of the abdomen in the anterior axillary line, at the costal margin. Finally, a 12-mm port is placed in the right upper quadrant, in the anterior axillary line, at the costal margin.

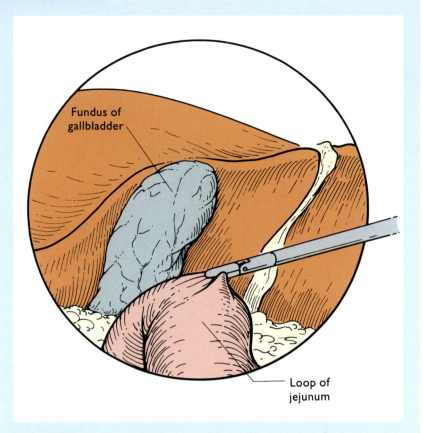

FIGURE 16-6.

Through the supraumbilical 5-mm port, a grasper is introduced into the abdomen and used to aid in a full visual inspection of the abdomen. Careful attention should be given to inspection for not only possible trocar injury but also for unsuspected pathology. More specifically, the area around the head of the pancreas and the duodenum should be inspected for tumor involvement; in cases where the tumor is large and the duodenum is involved, simultaneous performance of a gastrojejunostomy may be elected. Once it has been determined that a cholecystojejunostomy will be performed, the ligament of Treitz is identified, and the small bowel is followed and a portion of the bowel is selected and brought up to the fundus of the gallbladder in an antecolic fashion.

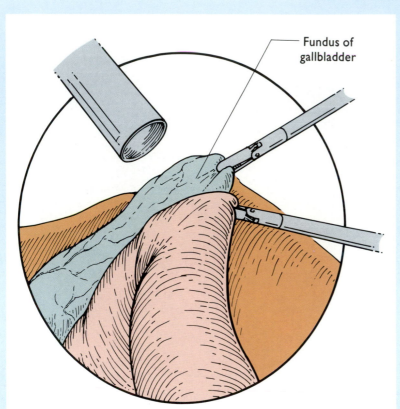

Fundus of gallbladder

FIGURE 16-7.
A second grasper is introduced through the left upper quadrant port, and the fundus of the gallbladder is gently grasped. The jejunum and gallbladder should be placed in a position to ensure that neither the gallbladder nor bowel is tented or stretched in this position.

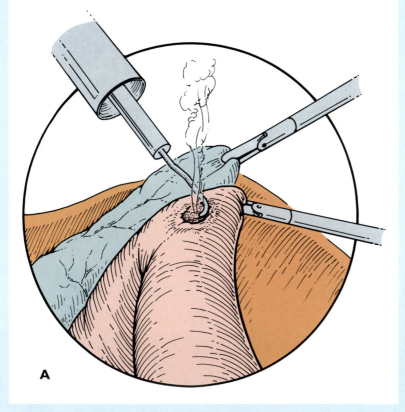

A

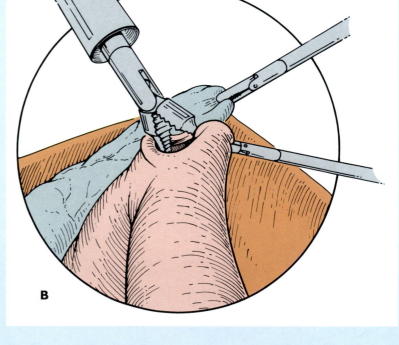

B

FIGURE 16-8.
A, A 5-mm cautery hook is placed through the 12-mm trocar placed in the right upper quadrant. The cautery hook is gently applied to the antimesenteric border of the jejunum and used to create a 5-mm opening in the bowel wall.

The end of the endoscopic stapler will be placed through this enterotomy. **B**, After the enterotomy has been made with the hook cautery, a grasper is placed into the abdomen and used to enlarge the enterotomy.

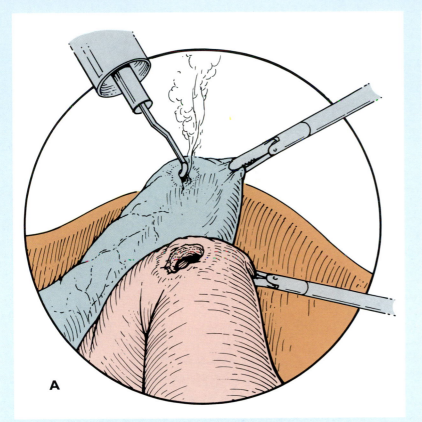

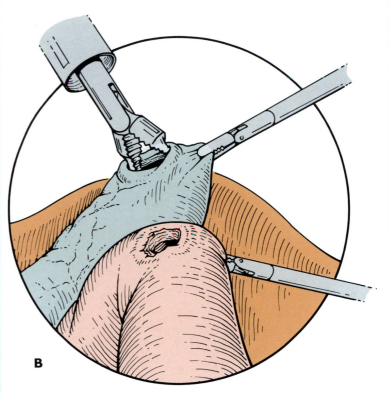

FIGURE 16-9.

A, In a fashion similar to that applied to the jejunum, a enterotomy is made in the fundus of the gallbladder.
B, A grasper is placed into the abdomen and used to enlarge the enterotomy.

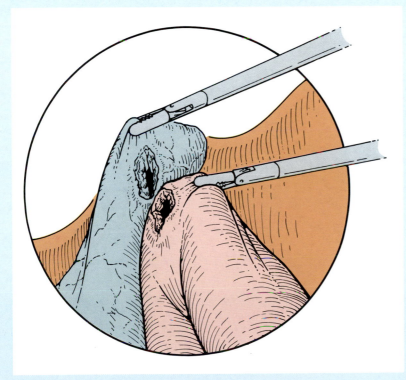

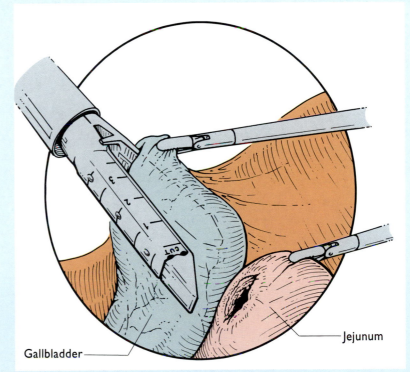

FIGURE 16-10.

The enterotomy and cholecystotomy are demonstrated as they are held in apposition. Note that the graspers used to hold each should not be removed until the stapler has been successfully placed.

FIGURE 16-11.

An endoscopic stapler is placed into the abdomen via the 12-mm port. The jejunum is retracted from the field of view while one blade of the stapler is inserted into the cholecystotomy.

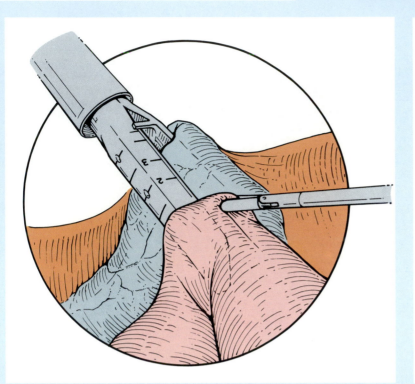

FIGURE 16-12.
The free blade of the stapler is then inserted into the jejunum via the enterotomy.

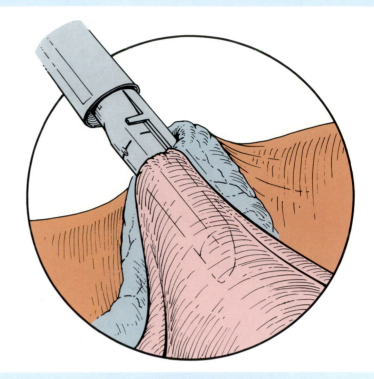

FIGURE 16-13.
Carefully, the stapler is closed. The stapler should not be fired until proper positioning and freedom from adjacent structures is verified.

FIGURE 16-14.
Using the two graspers from the supraumbilical and left upper quadrant ports, the head of the stapler and free jejunum are mobilized and inspected to ensure that no bowel, bile duct, or colon is entrapped when the stapler was closed. Once this is verified, the stapler can be fired. After firing the stapler, it is carefully removed so that the staple line is not disrupted.

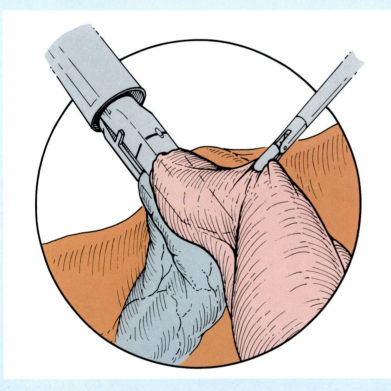

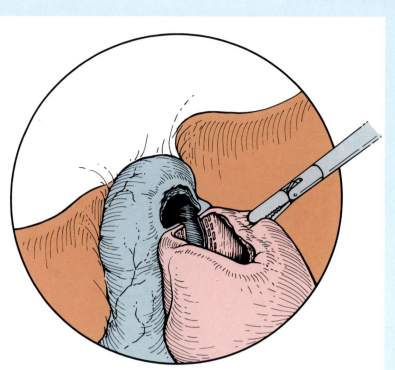

FIGURE 16-15.
After the stapler has been removed, the graspers are used to open the anastomosis and carefully inspect the staple line for integrity and hemostasis.

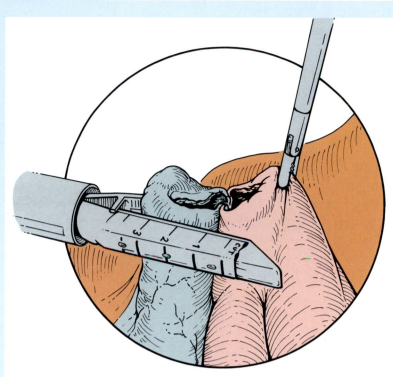

FIGURE 16-16.
The remaining defect is closed by transverse stapling of the anastomotic site.

FIGURE 16-17.
Remaining defect being closed.

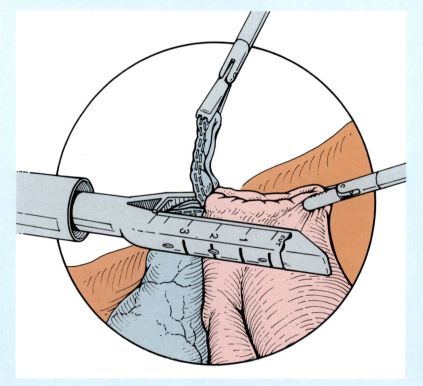

Postoperative Management

Feedings are advanced as soon as bowel function is demonstrated. A nasogastric tube is unnecessary.

Laparoscopic Gastrojejunostomy

The second clinical problem associated with unresectable periampullary tumors is nausea, vomiting, and poor nutrition caused by tumor compression of the duodenum. Symptomatic duodenal obstruction develops in at least 20% of patients with unresectable periampullary tumors [1]. The treatment of choice for this entity is gastrojejunostomy. This has traditionally been performed by using an open surgical approach but has recently been performed laparoscopically in patients who have not otherwise come to laparotomy and who are cared for in an institution with surgeons technically proficient in this procedure. In 1992, Brune and Schonleben reported their results of laparoscopic gastrojejunostomy in two patients with gastric outlet obstruction due to carcinoma of the pancreatic head [9]. Goh and coworkers [10] performed laparoscopic subtotal gastrectomy with Billroth II reconstruction for the treatment of chronic gastric ulcer in an elderly patient. As has been demonstrated with laparoscopic cholecystectomy and appendectomy, advocates of laparoscopic gastrojejunostomy have maintained that such benefits as decreased postoperative discomfort and shorter hospitalizations warrant wider application of this technique.

Surgical Technique

Figures 16-18 through 16-27 outline two techniques of laparoscopic gastrojejunostomy.

Set-up

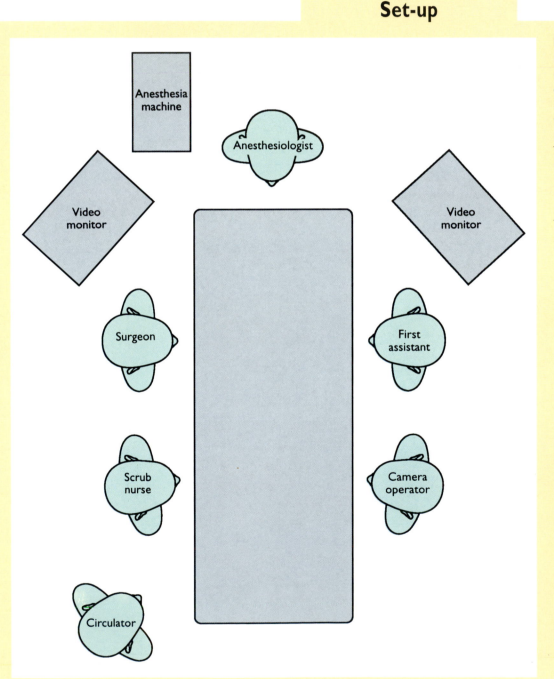

FIGURE 16-18.

Proper performance of laparoscopic procedures requires adequate preoperative planning so that each member of the operating team knows his or her function. Proper positioning of personnel and equipment is essential if the procedures are to be performed efficiently. This diagram depicts the location of each operating team member and major equipment. The surgeon and scrub nurse are to the right of the patient and the first assistant, and camera operator are to the patient's left. Note that video monitors are placed on both sides of the operating table so that all members of the operating team have an unobstructed view of the operation.

Set-up

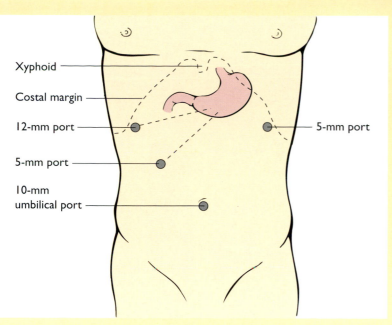

FIGURE 16-19.

An effective scheme for laparoscopic gastrojejunostomy trocar placement. A nasogastric tube and Foley catheter are placed after general anesthesia is induced so as to minimize the chance of stomach and bladder injury during trocar placement. The camera port is 10 mm and may be placed supra-, intra-, or infraumbilically. The peritoneal cavity is insufflated with CO_2. Exploratory laparoscopy is then performed. Some surgeons use exploratory laparoscopy before anticipated Whipple procedures. Laparoscopy permits biopsy of peritoneal implants or hepatic metastases not seen on computed tomography that may prove unresectability of disease. If a Whipple procedure is not indicated, laparoscopic gastrojejunostomy may then be performed. After adequate exploration of the peritoneal cavity is completed, the remaining trocars are placed under direct vision. Twelve-mm and 5-mm ports are placed in the right upper quadrant in such a manner that they form an isosceles triangle with the anticipated area of gastrojejunostomy serving as the vertex. A second 5-mm port is placed in the left upper quadrant for the first assistant.

Procedure

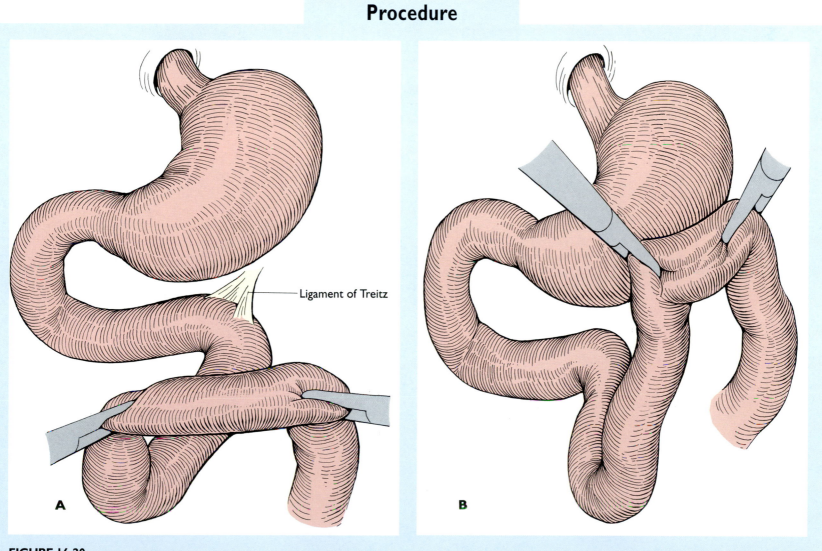

FIGURE 16-20.

A, Locate the ligament of Treitz and proceed distally along the jejunum until an adequate segment can be mobilized to the anterior surface of the stomach without tension. **B,** Care must be taken to properly orient the jejunum so that the mesentery is not twisted.

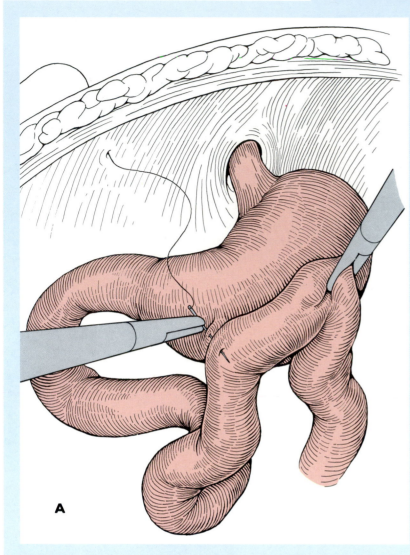

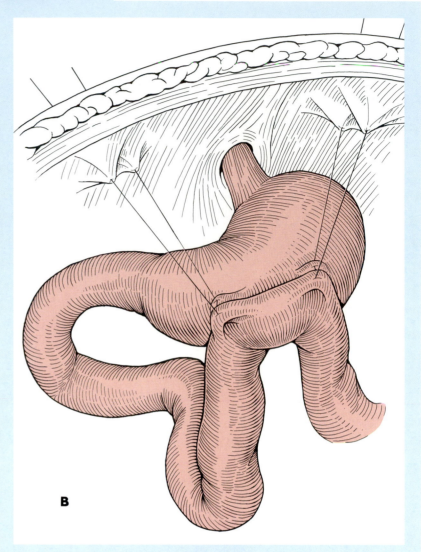

FIGURE 16-21.

A, After a segment of jejunum for anastomosis is selected, the orientation of jejunum and stomach is maintained by silk sutures that are passed through the abdominal wall with straight needles under direct vision. The straight needle is grasped with an endoscopic grasper or needle driver, passed through the seromuscular layers of the stomach and jejunum, and then driven out of the peritoneal cavity through the abdominal wall. **B**, These tagging sutures should be placed at least 6 cm apart so that a generous gastrojejunostomy is formed. Appropriate pressure is then applied to these sutures so that the stomach and jejunum are tented and the boundaries of the gastrojejunostomy are delineated.

Procedure

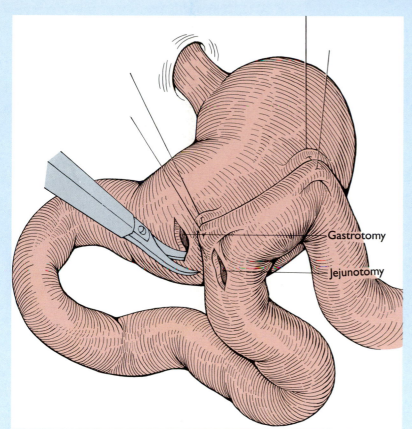

FIGURE 16-22.

Electrocautery is used to make a gastrotomy and a jejunotomy just large enough to accommodate the limbs of the endoscopic stapling device.

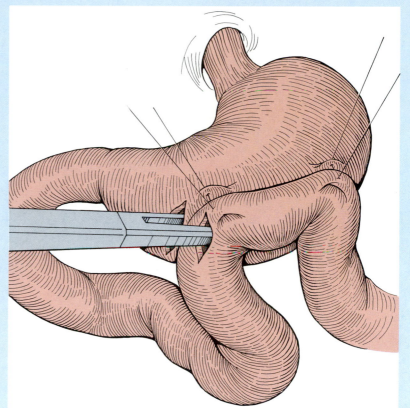

FIGURE 16-23.

An endoscopic stapler is passed through the 12-mm port. One limb is fed through the gastrotomy and the other through the jejunotomy. The device is fired enough times to make an anastomosis 60 to 90 mm long.

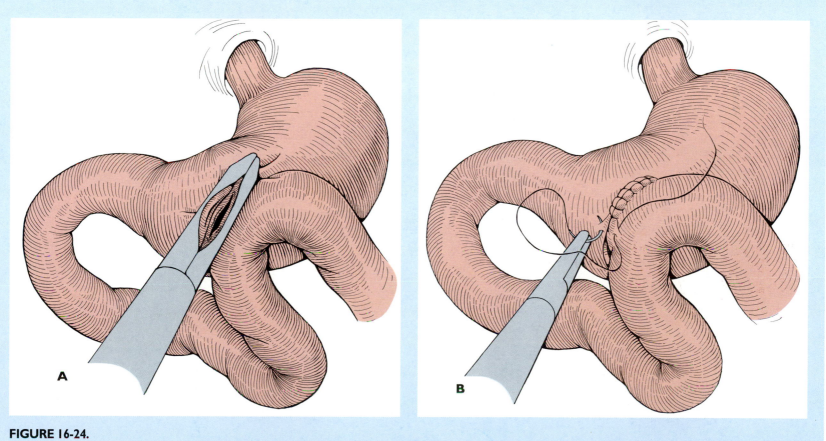

FIGURE 16-24.

The enterotomy that remains may be closed with **A**, an endoscopic stapler or **B**, silk sutures.

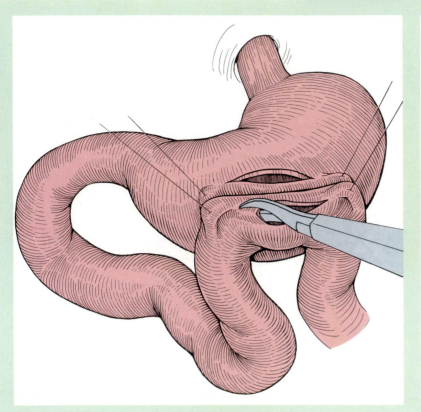

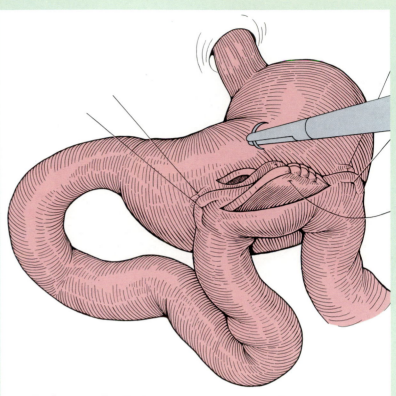

FIGURE 16-25.

An alternate method for laparoscopic gastrojejunostomy is a sewn anastomosis. Tenting of the stomach and jejunum is performed with straight needles as outlined in Figure 16-21. A long gastrotomy and corresponding jejunotomy are made between the tagging sutures.

FIGURE 16-26.

Full-thickness, interrupted sutures are placed along the posterior wall of the anastomosis. Intra- or extracorporeal knot-tying techniques may be used.

FIGURE 16-27.

The anastomosis is completed by placing interrupted sutures along the anterior edge of the anastomosis.

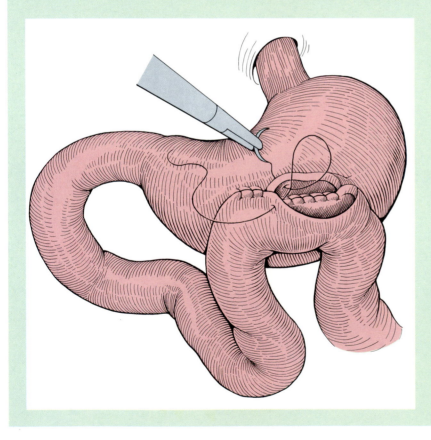

Postoperative Management

In younger patients without diabetes or significant gastric dilatation from obstruction, it is generally safe not to place a nasogastric tube. In patients with evidence of significant gastroparesis, however, it may be necessary to leave a nasogastric tube in place until gastric function returns. Pain after laparoscopic gastrojejunostomy is usually limited; however, any pain associated with unresected tumor will remain, and the patient may require more narcotics than would be expected from the procedure itself.

Results

In the past several years, many case reports have described small groups of patients who have undergone laparoscopic CCJ or laparoscopic gastrojejunostomy. These data, although limited, have revealed few complications and brief postoperative stay requirements [11–13].

In a case-control study, Bergamaschi and coworkers [14] recently reviewed patients with unresectable pancreatic cancer undergoing laparoscopic and open gastrojejunostomy. Patients undergoing open surgery and those having laparoscopic procedures did not significantly differ in terms of mortality, overall morbidity, operating time, time to intake of oral solid food, use of nonsteroidal anti-inflammatory drugs and opioids, delayed-return gastric emptying, postoperative hospital stay, survival, and further hospital stay before death. However, the patients undergoing the laparoscopic procedure had significantly less blood loss and fewer days in the hospital at the time of operation [14].

We have reviewed our own experience with biliary and gastric bypass in a group of 57 patients in whom this surgery was done during the past 4.5 years. We compared the patients undergoing laparoscopic CCJ and gastrojejunostomy with those undergoing open CCJ and gastrojejunostomy. Postoperative length of stay was similar in all four groups and was consistent with that published in the literature. No significant complications occurred in the laparoscopic group. One patient in the open group and no patients in the laparoscopic group died after surgery.

Conclusions

As laparoscopic surgeons become more skilled, the indications for laparoscopic surgery will continue to expand. At many medical centers, it is feasible to perform laparoscopic gastrojejunostomy and CCJ for palliation of unresectable periampullary tumors. Whether these procedures provide any tangible advantages to the open approach continues to be evaluated. Most certainly, however, a patient with a life span of a few months would benefit from the decreased length of stay and recuperation that the laparoscopic approach can provide.

References

1. Lillemoe KD, Sauter PK, Pitt HA, *et al.*: Current status of surgical palliation of periampullary carcinoma. *Surg Gynecol Obstet* 1993, 176:1–10.

2. Hatfield AWR, Tobias R, Terblanche J, *et al.*: Preoperative external biliary drainage in obstructive jaundice: a prospective controlled clinical trial. *Lancet* 1982, 2:896–899.

3. Chari RS, Meyers WC: The liver. In: *Current Practice of Surgery.* Edited by Levine BA, Copeland EM III, Howard RJ, Sugarman HJ, Warshaw AL. New York: Churchill Livingstone; 1993:1–41.

4. Speer AAG, Cotton PB, Russel RCG, *et al.*: Randomised trial of endoscopic versus percutaneous stent insertion in malignant obstructive jaundice. *Lancet* 1987, 2:57–62.

5. Smith AC, Dowsett JF, Hatfield AWR, *et al.*: A prospective randomized trial of by-pass surgery versus endoscopic stenting in patients with malignant obstructive jaundice [Abstract]. *Gut* 1989, 30:A1513.

6. Prat F, Chapat O, Ducot B, *et al.*: Predictive factors for survival of patients with inoperable malignant distal biliary strictures: a practical management guideline. *Gut* 1998, 42:76–80.

7. Singh SM, Reber HA: Surgical palliation for pancreatic cancer. *Surg Clin North Am* 1989, 69:599–611.

8. Tarnasky PR, England RE, Lail LM, *et al.*: Cystic duct patency in malignant obstructive jaundice. An ERCP-based study relevant to the role of laparoscopic cholecystojejunostomy. *Ann Surg* 1995, 221:265–271.

9. Brune IB, Schonleben K: Laparoskopische seit-zu-seit-gastro-jejunostomie, *Chirurg* 1992, 63:577–580.

10. Goh P, Tekant Y, Kum CK, *et al.*: Totally intra-abdominal laparoscopic Billroth II gastrectomy. *Surg Endosc* 1992, 6:160.

11. Shimi S, Banting S, Cuschieri A: Laparoscopy in the management of pancreatic cancer: endoscopic cholecystojejunostomy for advanced disease. *Br J Surg* 1992, 79:317–319.

12. Fletcher DR, Jones RM: Laparoscopic cholecystojejunostomy as palliation for obstructive jaundice in inoperable carcinoma of the pancreas. *Surg Endosc* 1992, 6:147–149.

13. Mouiel J, Katkhouda N, White S, *et al.*: Endolaparoscopic palliation of pancreatic cancer. *Surg Laparosc Endosc* 1992, 2:241–243.

14. Bergamaschi R, Marvik R, Thoresen JE, *et al.*: Open vs laparoscopic gastrojejunostomy for palliation in advanced pancreatic cancer. *Surg Laparosc Endosc* 1998, 8:92–96.

Laparoscopic Splenectomy

Paul J. Mosca
Steve Eubanks

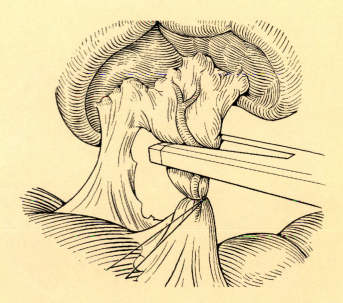

The spleen has been the focus of considerable intrigue and debate since the time of Aristotle, who more than 2000 years ago asserted that it is not essential for human existence. Over the past several centuries, this organ has come to the attention of surgeons primarily in the setting of trauma and hematologic diseases. Although of questionable veracity, the first account of a splenectomy described a procedure performed by Andriano Zaccarello of Italy in 1549 for splenomegaly in a young women, who went on to survive for 6 years after surgery [1]. The first splenectomy for trauma is credited to the British naval surgeon E. O'Brien, who in 1816 excised the protruding spleen from a Mexican tailor after he was stabbed; the patient recovered despite an associated renal injury [2]. The first authenticated successful splenectomy for splenic disease was performed by Jules Pean in 1867 to remove a massive splenic cyst from a 20-year-old woman [2].

By the middle of the 20th century, the pendulum had swung toward a fairly liberal application of splenectomy, particularly in cases of trauma. King and Shumacker's 1952 report [3] of overwhelming sepsis after splenectomy for congenital hemolytic anemia was among contributions that helped stimulate an interest in preserving a part of the spleen or the entire organ when feasible. Since that time, a trend toward splenic preservation has ensued. Nevertheless, there are several conditions for which splenectomy may be the most appropriate or only effective therapy. Because of the evolution of advanced laparoscopic techniques, many such patients for whom elective splenectomy is indicated may be managed entirely by the laparoscopic approach. The technique of laparoscopic splenectomy was first described in the literature in 1991 [4]. Since that time, numerous series have been reported, and the technique has been shown to be a safe alternative to open splenectomy in selected patients when performed by properly trained surgeons.

Anatomy and Physiology

The spleen is located in the left hypochondrium, bounded by the diaphragm superiorly, the left kidney posteriorly, and the gastric fundus and splenic flexure of the colon anteriorly (Figure 17-1). It lies deep to ribs 9 to 11. The spleen arises from a condensation of mesenchymal cells within the left dorsal mesogastrium by the fifth week of gestation. The dorsal mesogastrium suspends the developing stomach from the dorsal body wall and gives rise to the gastrosplenic ligament, which contains the short gastric vessels. Other major peritoneal attachments of the spleen include the splenocolic, splenophrenic, splenorenal, and phrenico-colic ligaments. The tail of the pancreas, which lies within the splenorenal ligament, terminates within 1 cm of the spleen in 73% of cases and contacts the spleen in 30% of cases [5]. The phrenico-colic ligament serves as a sling or brassiere-like structure for the lower pole of the spleen [5]. The combination of these extensive peritoneal attachments provides a unique suspensory mechanism to help protect this fragile organ. Failure of mesenchymal fusion results in the formation of accessory splenic tissue, which in approximately 80% of cases may be found within the splenic hilum or adjoining suspensory ligaments (Figure 17-2) [6]. In a series of 3000 consecutive autopsies, the incidence of accessory spleens was 10% [7], although the incidence is greater in patients with hematologic disease [8].

The arterial supply of the spleen originates from the celiac axis. The principal blood supply arises directly from the splenic artery, which typically travels along the superior border of the pancreas

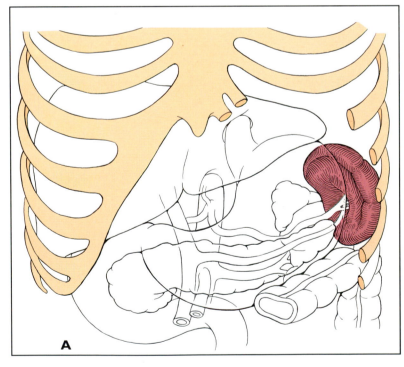

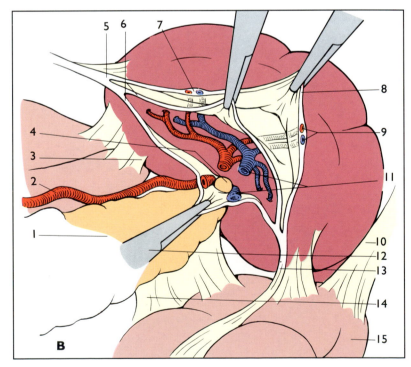

FIGURE 17-1.

A, Anatomic relationships of the spleen. **B**, Anatomy of the splenic hilus and ligamentous attachments: pancreas (*1*), splenic artery (*2*), splenophrenic ligament (*3*), pancreatic tail (*4*), gastrophrenic ligament (*5*), splenophrenic ligament (cut) (*6*), short gastric vessels (*7*), gastrosplenic ligament (*8*), left gas-troepiploic vessels (*9*), phrenicocolic ligament (*10*), splenic vein (*11*), pancreaticosplenic ligament (*12*), splenocolic ligament (*13*), pancreaticocolic ligament (*14*), and splenic flexure of colon (*15*). (*Adapted from* Seufert and Mitrou [6]; with permission.)

until it branches in or proximal to the splenic hilum. Two primary patterns of branching exist: magistral and distributed [9]. In the magistral pattern, occurring in about 30% of cases, the main splenic artery is long and divides near the hilum into three to four large, terminal branches, which enter the spleen over one-third to one-fourth of its medial surface. The distributed pattern, occurring in about 70% of cases, is characterized by six to 12 long branches originating between 3 and 13 cm from the hilum and entering the spleen over three-fourths of the medial facet [10]. These vessels branch into the trabecular connective tissue matrix and terminate as central arteries within the splenic pulp. Splenic outflow occurs through the splenic vein, which ultimately joins the superior mesenteric vein to form the portal vein.

Histologically, the spleen is composed of three regions: red pulp, white pulp, and the marginal zone. In the red pulp, the central arterioles either empty directly into venous sinuses (closed circulation) or enter splenic cords separated from the venous sinuses by fenestrated endothelium, constituting the open circulation [11]. The white pulp consists of lymphocytes, plasma cells, and macrophages and is associated with the central arteries as periarterial sheaths of T lymphocytes, as well as uniformly distributed nodules containing primary and secondary B lymphocyte follicles. The white pulp makes up 15% of the splenic mass and 25% of the body's lymphoreticular system [6]. The interface between the red and white pulp, termed the marginal zone, is populated primarily by B lymphocytes.

The spleen serves three primary roles: filtration, storage, and immunologic function. With a blood flow of approximately 300 mL/min, splenic filtration through the cords of Billroth is efficiently performed by reticular cells. Filtration involves the culling out of senescent cells, destruction (erythroclasis) of abnormal erythrocytes, and removal (pitting) of erythrocyte inclusion bodies. The spleen may contain approximately one-third of the body's platelet and granulocyte mass and thus serves as a repository for these cells under normal conditions [12]. In pathologic states, the spleen may sequester as much as 98% of the body's platelets [13].

The histologic organization of the spleen is well structured for immunologic processes, such as opsonization, phagocytosis, and presentation of foreign antigens. It is also paramount in the production of tuftsin and properdin, peptides that play important roles in the stimulation of phagocytosis by reticular cells and in the complement pathway [14,15]. The spleen is also a setting for the primary antibody response, resulting in the production of IgM class antibodies after initial exposure to a foreign antigen [16]. The spleen is the primary site for phagocytosis of polysaccharide-encapsulated bacteria. Thus, patients who have had a splenectomy and are infected with encapsulated pathogens are at risk for life-threatening sepsis. The overall risk for overwhelming postsplenectomy infection in adults after splenectomy is 0.28% to 1.9%; the risk is greater in infants, children, and persons whose indication for splenectomy is hematologic disease (as opposed to trauma) [17]. *Streptococcus pneumoniae* accounts for more than 50% of microbial isolates in postsplenectomy infections, followed by *Haemophilus influenzae* and *Neisseria meningitidis* [18]. Therefore, patients who have had a splenectomy should receive vaccination against *S. pneumoniae* with multivalent capsular polysaccharide. Although no human studies have confirmed an advantage to the practice, most surgeons prefer to administer the vaccine 1 to 2 weeks before surgery in elective cases. If the pneumococcal vaccine has not been given before surgery, however, it should be administered after surgery because patients who have had splenectomy may mount an antibody response of nearly the same magnitude as persons with normal splenic function [19]. The vaccination against *H. influenzae* and *N. meningitidis*, although not standard, is frequently administered to patients at risk for exposure to these pathogens. In addition, an oral antibiotic directed primarily toward *S. pneumoniae* is often given to patients at highest risk for severe infection, including children and immunocompromised patients, because the efficacy of vaccination is approximately 80% [18].

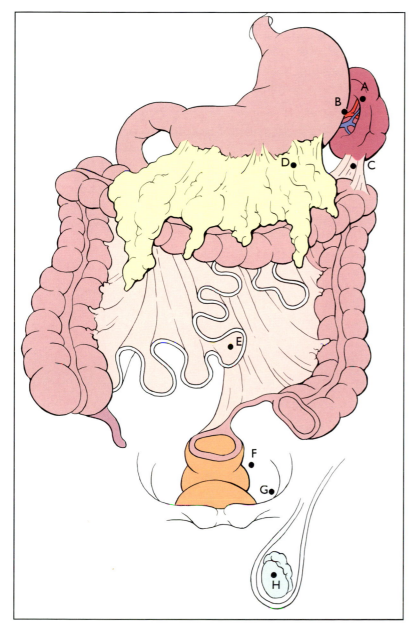

FIGURE 17-2.

Location of accessory splenic tissue. **A**, Splenic hilum. **B**, Splenic artery and tail of pancreas. **C**, Splenocolic ligament. **D**, Omentum. **E**, Mesentery. **F**, Presacral. **G**, Adnexal. **H**, Peritesticular. The splenic hilum, including the tail of the pancreas, contains two thirds of all accessory splenic tissue. (*Adapted from* Seufert and Mitrou [6]; with permission.)

Indications for Laparoscopic Splenectomy

In general, the indications for laparoscopic splenectomy are similar to those for elective open splenectomy. Use of laparoscopy, and particularly laparoscopic splenectomy, in cases of suspected or documented splenic trauma is an emerging yet controversial practice that is beyond the scope of this discussion. Most remaining indications for splenectomy may be grouped into three general categories (although there is some overlap): 1) hypersplenism, 2) neoplasms or space-occupying lesions, and 3) diagnosis and staging (Table 17-1).

After trauma, the most common condition for which splenectomy is performed is hypersplenism. This condition involves cytopenia of one or more peripheral blood elements with a normally compensating bone marrow; the cytopenia typically improves or resolves with splenectomy [20]. Hypersplenism may be primary, may be related to underlying splenic abnormality, or may be secondary to another type of lesion, such as an autoantibody or intrinsic erythrocyte abnormality (Table 17-1). Although hypersplenism is often accompanied by splenomegaly, the latter term simply refers to splenic enlargement and is not necessarily correlated with disease severity or urgency of splenectomy.

Immune thrombocytopenic purpura (ITP) is a disorder associated with the production of an IgG autoantibody against a platelet membrane protein (eg, glycoprotein IIb/IIIa [21]), causing platelets to be coated with antibody and destroyed in the spleen. Splenectomy is indicated when corticosteroids or intravenous gammaglobulin treatment does not control the disease or when patients require long-term steroid treatment to prevent relapse. In approximately 80% of patients, the platelet count increases adequately; this figure is closer to 90% in patients who have experienced a good response to corticosteroid treatment and 60% in those who have not [22,23]. The practice of thorough exploration for accessory spleens is particularly important in patients with ITP because this is a major cause of recurrence.

Splenectomy can also be beneficial in IgG-mediated (but not IgM-mediated) autoimmune hemolytic anemia, as well as the neutropenia of Felty's syndrome. Patients with anemia due to hereditary spherocytosis have defective erythrocyte cell membranes, resulting in inadequate deformability and consequent red cell trapping and destruction in the spleen. These patients (as well as patients with severe cases of elliptocytosis, a similar disorder) are cured by splenectomy.

Previously, splenectomy was used in patients with medically intractable thrombotic thrombocytopenic purpura (TTP). More recently, the practice of aggressive plasmapheresis has resulted in clinical improvement in many such patients. Consequently, only the occasional patient who does not respond to plasmapheresis requires splenectomy for treatment of this disorder.

The staging of Hodgkin's disease has traditionally been among the more common indications for splenectomy. Staging entails carefully exploring the peritoneal cavity; performing splenectomy; and obtaining biopsy specimens from the liver, lymph node, and iliac crest bone marrow. Because of the increasingly accurate staging by noninvasive techniques, such as modern computed tomography, and administration of effective chemotherapeutic regimens for a wider gamut of stages, surgical staging is no longer necessary in most patients. Surgical staging is now typically performed to evaluate for the presence or extent of infradiaphragmatic disease in asymptomatic patients with clinical stage I or II nodular sclerosing type Hodgkin's disease [24].

Hematologic disease is the most common category of disorders for which laparoscopic splenectomy has been performed (Table 17-2). However, laparoscopic splenectomy is used for a wide range of disorders, and further experience with the technique may show that it is appropriate for most of the same indications as open splenectomy.

Although splenectomy may improve thrombocytopenia in patients with hypersplenism secondary to cirrhosis and portal hypertension, splenectomy is generally not indicated in this setting because it can exacerbate the portal hypertension and may be associated with substantial morbidity or mortality. The preferred approach to such patients is portal decompression, which usually increases the platelet count [24].

Table 17-1. Indications for splenectomy

Hypersplenism
  Primary
    Hematologic cancer
      Lymphoma
      Leukemia
    Infiltrative diseases
      Sarcoidosis
      Gaucher disease
  Secondary
    Autoimmune cytopenias
      Immune thrombocytopenic purpura
      Autoimmune hemolytic anemia
      Felty's syndrome
      Thrombotic thrombocytopenic purpura
      HIV-associated thrombocytopenia
    Disorders of erythrocytes
      Hereditary spherocytosis or elliptocytosis
      Thalassemia
      Sickle-cell anemia
      Malaria
Neoplasms and space-occupying lesions
  Hodgkin's disease
  Non-Hodgkin's lymphoma
  Hairy cell leukemia
  Splenic cysts
  Splenic abscesses
Diagnosis and staging
  Hodgkin's disease
  Splenomegaly of unknown cause

The only absolute contraindications to laparoscopic splenectomy are contraindications to laparoscopic surgery: the need for a laparotomy, an inability to tolerate general anesthesia, dense adhesions or massive distension preventing access to the peritoneal cavity, and uncontrollable coagulopathy. Relative contraindications include massive splenomegaly and significant adhesive disease or inflammation in the left upper quadrant. The application of laparoscopic splenectomy during pregnancy should be approached with extensive preparation and extreme caution.

Surgical Technique

Preparation for laparoscopic splenectomy involves the same careful preoperative evaluation and planning used for any major surgery, with additional considerations. The patient should receive appropriate vaccines against encapsulated organisms at least 1 to 2 weeks before surgery if possible. Preoperative intravenous antibiotics are administered within 30 minutes of incision. Parenteral stress-dose steroids and blood products are administered in the standard fashion when indicated. Platelets are not transfused before surgery in cases of ITP because they may be rapidly destroyed; if platelets are needed in such patients, they are usually transfused after splenic artery ligation.

After induction of anesthesia, orogastric and urinary bladder catheters are inserted. The patient is positioned on the operating table in one of several positions, depending on the surgeon's preference. In initial reports of the technique, the patient was placed in a supine or lithotomy position [25]. Subsequently, the lateral position was described [26] and was considered to offer improved exposure of the splenic hilum. In the double-access position, the patient is placed in a supine (or lithotomy) position, the surgeon is positioned at the right side of the table (or between the legs), and the table is rotated toward the right side. This offers the ease of placement of trocars afforded by the supine position, as well as improved access to the hilum with the lateral position (Figure 17-3).

The peritoneal cavity is then accessed in the supraumbilical position by using an open technique, and the Hasson trocar is placed (alternatively, the surgeon may prefer the closed method). After establishment of a 15–mm Hg pneumoperitoneum, a 10-mm sheath remains situated at the umbilicus. By using a 30° or 45° angled laparoscope, the peritoneal cavity is inspected for occult abnormality and to assess technical feasibility. As shown in Figure 17-4, additional secondary ports are then placed in the subxiphoid and left midabdominal positions. A 12-mm operating port is placed in the left anterior axillary line in order to accommodate the endoscopic stapler or clip applier. All trocars should be placed at least about 4 fingerbreadths apart to reduce instrument crossing. Port positions may be modified based on the patient's body habitus, and additional ports may be inserted as indicated. The peritoneal cavity is carefully explored, with a search for accessory spleens.

With the table rotated to the right, the patient is placed in the reverse Trendelenburg position. The spleen is exposed in the left upper quadrant after medial retraction on the greater curvature of the stomach and elevation of the left lobe of the liver (Figure 17-5). Additional exposure is gained by mobilization of the splenic flexure of the colon. Accessory splenic tissue should be sought as the suspensory ligaments and hilar region are exposed before dissection.

The inferior pole of the spleen is mobilized by division of the generally avascular splenocolic ligament using the ultrasonic dissector or electrocautery scissors (Figure 17-6). The lateral splenorenal ligaments are divided in a similar manner. The inferior margin of the splenic hilum is then exposed with continued cephalad dissection and elevation of the inferior splenic pole. Vascular control may be obtained in several ways. The application of surgical clips may be helpful in the initial control of hilar vascular branches. Definitive proximal control is gained either

Table 17-2. Clinical experience with laparoscopic splenectomy

Study	Year	Patients, n	Most frequent indication, n	Operative time, min	Conversion to open procedure, %	Blood transfusions, %	Overall morbidity, %	Mortality, %	Mean length of stay, d
Gigot and coworkers [8]	1995	50	ITP, 31	203	10	16	22	2	5
Friedman and coworkers [27]	1997	63	ITP, 30	153	7	3.5	14	0	3.5
Glasgow and coworkers [28]	1997	52	ITP, 23	196	11	27	4	6	4.8
Poulin and Mamazza [29]	1998	51	ITP, 28	180	10	9	11	2	3
Targarona and coworkers [30]	1998	74	ITP, 37	157	6.7	20	17	0	4

ITP—idiopathic thrombocytopenic purpura.

by laparoscopy-assisted ligation of individual vessels or by application of the endoscopic vascular stapler (Figure 17-7). The splenic parenchyma will become discolored with progressive devascularization, confirming the adequate control of feeding vessels.

The short gastric vessels are encountered with cephalad dissection. These vessels may be managed with the ultrasonic dissector, individually ligated or clipped, or stapled en masse with the endoscopic stapling device (Figure 17-8). The splenophrenic and any remaining posterior attachments may now be divided with the ultrasonic dissector or cautery scissors.

The amputated spleen is positioned medially by using atraumatic grasping forceps, and the hilar vessels, pancreatic tail, and greater curvature of the stomach are inspected for hemostasis, evi-dence of injury, and the presence of accessory splenic tissue. The left upper quadrant is irrigated and aspirated dry. Drainage is generally not necessary unless a pancreatic tail injury is suspected.

A sterile plastic endoscopic specimen sac is inserted through the 12-mm port, and the spleen is gently manipulated into the bag (Figure 17-9). The mouth of the sac is closed by countertraction on the drawstrings. The enclosed spleen is then brought to the 12-mm port site. At this point, the spleen is usually morcellated by finger fracture within the bag and delivered through the 12-mm trocar site, which is enlarged as needed. Great care is taken to avoid spillage of splenic fragments into the peritoneal cavity, either around the mouth of the sac or by disruption of the sac, as this may result in splenosis. All 10-mm or larger fascial trocar defects are subsequently closed, and the skin edges are reapproximated.

Set-up

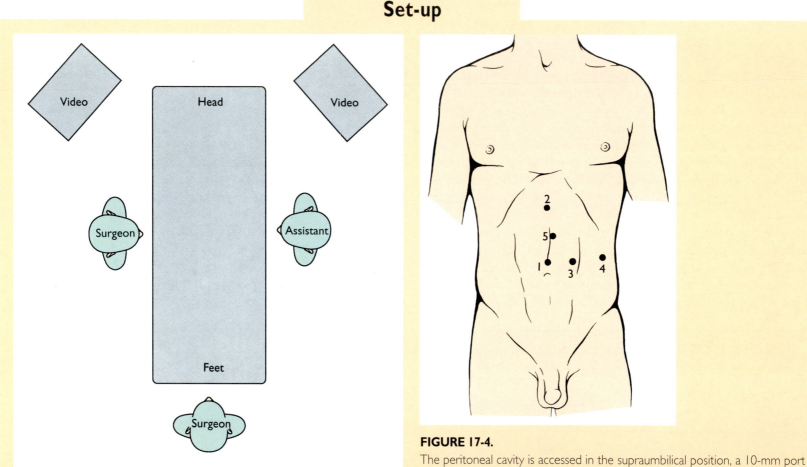

FIGURE 17-3.

Operative set-up for laparoscopic splenectomy. The video monitors are placed at the head of the operative table as for upper abdominal laparoscopy. The patient is placed on the operating table in the supine or low lithotomy position. The operating surgeon is positioned either to the patient's right side or in the double-access position with the surgeon at the bottom of the table/between the legs (both positions are shown).

FIGURE 17-4.

The peritoneal cavity is accessed in the supraumbilical position, a 10-mm port is placed (1), and a 15–mm Hg pneumoperitoneum is established. A 30° or 45° laparoscope is inserted through this port. The remaining ports are placed in either an "L" or a curvilinear configuration as follows: A 5- or 10-mm retraction port is placed in the subxiphoid position (2), and two operating ports are placed in the left anterior axillary line and left mid-abdomen as shown (3 and 4). A fifth port may be placed between the subxiphoid and supraumbilical ports if needed for additional retraction (5).

Procedure

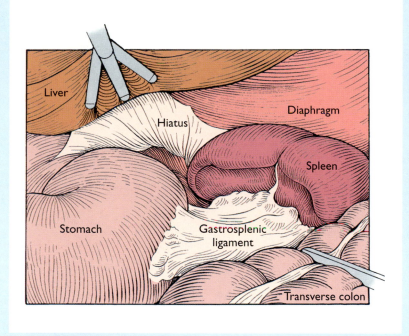

FIGURE 17-5.

The spleen is exposed by using medial retraction on the greater curvature, elevation of the left lobe of the liver, and caudad retraction of the splenic flexure. The suspensory ligaments and hilar region are carefully examined for accessory splenic tissue.

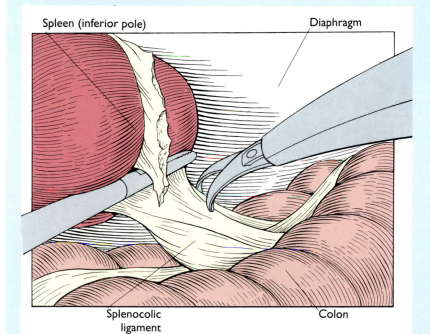

FIGURE 17-6.

The inferior pole of the spleen is mobilized by division of the splenocolic ligament, working in a cephalad direction.

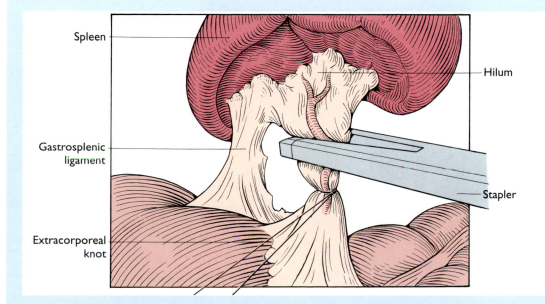

FIGURE 17-7.

The hilar vessels are then divided by double ligation of individual vessels and extracorporeal knot-tying or by application of the endoscopic vascular stapler.

Procedure

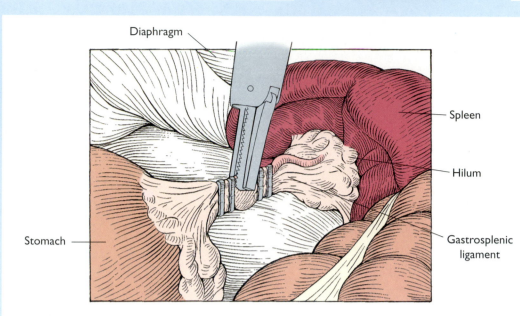

Diaphragm

Spleen

Hilum

Stomach

Gastrosplenic
ligament

FIGURE 17-8.

The short gastric vessels may be managed with the ultrasonic dissector, individually ligated or clipped, or stapled en masse in a single pedicle if technically suitable. The splenorenal and splenophrenic ligaments are then divided.

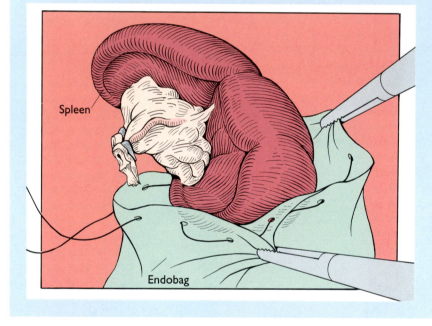

Spleen

Endobag

FIGURE 17-9.

The amputated spleen is placed in an endoscopic specimen sac, morcellated by finger fracture, and removed through a trocar incision, which is enlarged as needed.

Results

Approximately 1000 laparoscopic splenectomies have been reported in the literature to date; some of the largest reported series of patients undergoing laparoscopic splenectomy are summarized in Table 17-2. Hematologic disorders are the most common indications for laparoscopic splenectomy, and the most frequent indication within this group is ITP. In fact, laparoscopic splenectomy is probably the preferred technique for most patients with small to mildly enlarged spleens. Some fear that a high recurrence rate resulting from a failure to identify accessory spleens may represent a major limitation with this technique [31,32], but the long-term success rate will not be known for some time. In the series in Table 17-2, the rate of identification of accessory spleens reported ranged from 11.5% to 24% of patients, which is similar to rates reported in open splenectomy for hematologic disease [8].

Reported operative times among patients and institutions vary widely, but in experienced hands, the average operative time ranges

from about 2.5 to 3.5 hours (Table 17-2), typically requiring 20 minutes to 2 hours longer than open splenectomy [28,33–35]. Operative time generally decreases with experience, however, and eventually may even approach that for laparoscopic splenectomy [27]. The overall rate of conversion from laparoscopic to open splenectomy in experienced hands ranges from 7% to 11%. Operative blood loss, morbidity, and mortality are generally similar to or lower than with open splenectomy (Table 17-2). The duration of postoperative ileus is shorter following laparoscopic splenectomy than after open splenectomy, and the mean length of stay after successful laparoscopic splenectomy ranges from 3 to 5 days, typically about 4 days shorter than that for open splenectomy [27,28]. Although operative costs are higher for laparoscopic splenectomy, total hospital costs may not be significantly greater than for open splenectomy [28]. Success with laparoscopic splenectomy for children has been similar [37], although the cost-benefit ratio does not appear to be as favorable as that for adult patients [38].

Perhaps the most challenging cases with the largest blood loss are those in the setting of massive splenomegaly, as defined by an estimated weight of 1000 g or length of at least 20 cm. Massive splenomegaly is associated with a longer operative time and length of stay, and often necessitates a fascial incision for removal of the spleen, but it is not necessarily a contraindication to laparoscopic splenectomy [27,30]. If laparoscopic splenectomy is attempted in such patients, some have suggested preoperative angiographic embolization via the splenic artery in an effort to reduce intraoperative blood loss [27,29,39]. Other factors that may also predispose the patient to increased intraoperative bleeding include AIDS, lymphoma, splenic abscess and myelodysplasia [27].

Patients with hereditary spherocytosis may develop pigmented gallstones. For patients with both anemia and cholelithiasis due to hereditary spherocytosis, combined laparoscopic cholecystectomy and splenectomy has been reported [40,41]. Such experience suggests that selected patients with an indication for elective laparoscopic splenectomy and uncomplicated cholelithiasis of any cause may be candidates for this combined procedure.

Laparoscopic splenectomy thus appears to be the preferred surgical approach for many adults requiring surgery for hematologic disease, and possibly many other settings in which elective splenectomy is indicated. The short-term results using this approach are encouraging, and it is anticipated that the long-term success will be similar.

References

1. Coon WW: The spleen and splenectomy. *Surg Gynecol Obstet* 1991, 173:407–414.

2. Morganstern L: A history of splenectomy. In: *Surgical Diseases of the Spleen*. Edited by Hiatt JR, Phillips EH, Morgenstern L. Berlin: Springer-Verlag; 1997:7–9.

3. King H, Shumacker HB Jr: Splenic studies: I. Susceptibility to infection after splenectomy performed in infancy. *Ann Surg* 1952, 136:239–242.

4. Delaitre B, Maignien B: Splenectomie par voie laparoscopique. 1 Observation [letter]. *Presse Med* 1991, 20:2263.

5. Poulin EC, Thibault C: The anatomical basis for laparoscopic splenectomy. *Can J Surg* 1993, 36:484–488.

6. Seufert R, Mitrou P: The diseased spleen. In: *Surgery of the Spleen*. Edited by Reber HA. New York: Theme; 1986:27–32.

7. Halpert G, Gyorkey F: Lessons observed in accessory spleens of 311 patients. *Am J Clin Pathol* 1959, 32:165–168.

8. Gigot J-F, Legrand M, Cadiere G-B, *et al.*: Is laparoscopic splenectomy a justified approach in hematologic disorders? Preliminary results of a prospective multicenter study. *Int Surg* 1995, 80:299–303.

9. Ssoson-Jaroschewitsch A: Zur chirurgischen Anatomie des Milzhilus. *Z Gesamte Anat Abt* 1937, 84:218–224.

10. Michels NA: The variational anatomy of the spleen and splenic artery. *Am J Anat* 1942, 70:21–72.

11. Russell SJ, Richards JDM: Medical indications for splenectomy. *Br J Hosp Med* 1989, 42:120–128.

12. Aster RH: Pooling of platelets in the spleen. *J Clin Invest* 1966, 45:645–657.

13. Hill-Zobel RL, McCandless B, Kang A, *et al.*: Organ distribution and fate of human platelets: studies of asplenic and splenomegalic patients. *Am J Hematol* 1986, 3:231–238.

14. Constantopoulos A, Najjar VA, Wish JB: Defective phagocytosis due to tuftsin deficiency in splenectomized subjects. *Am J Dis Child* 1973, 125:663–665.

15. Frank EL, Neu HC: Postsplenectomy infection. *Surg Clin North Am* 1981, 61:135–155.

16. Sullivan JL, Ochs HD, Schiffmann G, *et al.*: Immune response after splenectomy. *Lancet* 1978, 1:178–181.

17. Lynch AM, Kapila R: Overwhelming postsplenectomy infection. *Infect Dis Clin North Am* 1996, 10:693–707.

18. Shaw JHF, Print CG: Postsplenectomy sepsis. *Br J Surg* 1989, 76:401–403.

19. Ruben FL, Hankins WA, Zeigler Z, *et al.*: Antibody responses to meningococcal polysaccharide vaccine in adults without a spleen. *Am J Med* 1984, 76:115–121.

20. Nieman RS: Pathology of the spleen. In: *Surgical Diseases of the Spleen*. Edited by Hiatt JR, Phillips EH, Morgenstern L. Berlin: Springer-Verlag; 1997:29–31.

21. Woods VL Jr, Oh EH, Mason D, *et al.*: Autoantibodies against the platelet glycoprotein IIb/IIIa complex in patients with chronic ITP. *Blood* 1984, 63:368–375.

22. Ahn YS, Harrington WJ: Treatment of idiopathic thrombocytopenic purpura. *Ann Rev Med* 1977, 29:299–309.

23. Harrington WJ Jr, Harrington TJ, Harrington WJ: Is splenectomy an outmoded procedure? *Adv Intern Med* 1990, 35:415–440.

24. Schwartz SI: Role of splenectomy in hematologic disorders. *World J Surg* 1996, 20:1156–1159.

25. Carroll BJ, Phillips EH, Semel CJ, *et al.*: Laparoscopic splenectomy. *Surg Endosc* 1992, 6:183–185.

26. Delaitre B: Laparoscopic splenectomy, the "hanged spleen" technique. *Surg Endosc* 1995, 9:528–529.

27. Friedman RL, Hiatt JR, Korman JL, *et al.*: Laparoscopic or open splenectomy for hematologic disease: which approach is superior? *J Am Coll Surg* 1997, 185:49–54.

28. Glasgow RE, Yee LF, Mulvihill SJ: Laparoscopic splenectomy: the emerging standard. *Surg Endosc* 1997, 11:108–112.

29. Poulin EC, Mamazza J: Laparoscopic splenectomy: lessons from the learning curve. *Can J Surg* 1998, 41:28–36.

30. Targarona EM, Espert JJ, Balague C, *et al.*: Splenomegaly should not be considered a contraindication for laparoscopic splenectomy. *Ann Surg* 1998, 228:35–39.

31. Gigot JF, Jamar F, Ferrant A, *et al.*: Inadequate detection of accessory spleens and splenosis with laparoscopic splenectomy. A shortcoming of the laparoscopic approach in hematologic disease. *Surg Endosc* 1998, 12:101–106.

32. Targarona EM, Espert JJ, Balaque C, *et al.*: Residual splenic function after laparoscopic splenectomy: a clinical concern. *Arch Surg* 1998, 133:56–60.

33. Brunt LM, Langer JC, Quasebarth MA, *et al.*: Comparative analysis of laparoscopic versus open splenectomy. *Am J Surg* 1996, 172:596–599.

34. Yee LF, Carvajal SH, de Lorimier AA, *et al.*: Laparoscopic splenectomy. The initial experience at University of California, San Francisco. *Arch Surg* 1995, 130:874–877.

35. Smith CD, Meyer TA, Goretsky MJ, *et al.*: Laparoscopic splenectomy by the lateral approach: a safe and effective alternative to open splenectomy for hematologic diseases. *Surgery* 1996, 120:789–794.

36. Friedman RL, Fallas MJ, Carroll BJ, *et al.*: Laparoscopic splenectomy for ITP. The gold standard. *Surg Endosc* 1996, 10:991–995.

37. Farah RA, Rogers ZR, Thompson WR, *et al.*: Comparison of laparoscopic and open splenectomy in children with hematologic disorders. *J Pediatr* 1997, 131:41–46.

38. Waldhausen JH, Tapper D: Is pediatric laparoscopic splenectomy safe and cost-effective? *Arch Surg* 1997, 132:822–824.

39. Poulin EC, Thibault C: Laparoscopic splenectomy for massive splenomegaly: operative technique and case report. *Can J Surg* 1995, 38:69–72.

40. Trias M, Targarona EM: Laparoscopic treatment of hereditary spherocytosis (splenectomy plus cholecystectomy). *J Laparoendosc Surg* 1994, 4:71–73.

41. Patton ML, Moss BE, Haith LR Jr, *et al.*: Concomitant laparoscopic cholecystectomy and splenectomy for surgical management of hereditary spherocytosis. *Am Surg* 1997, 63:536–539.

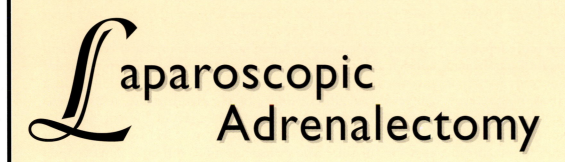

Laparoscopic Adrenalectomy

Andrew J. Lodge
Steve Eubanks

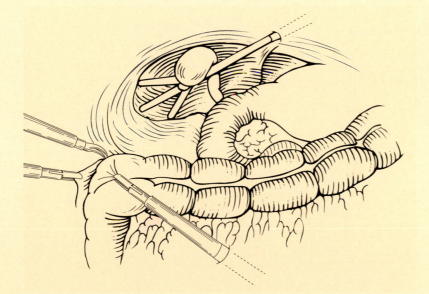

The adrenal glands are small paired glands located in the retroperitoneum just superomedial to the kidneys (Fig. 18-1). Their functions include production of aldosterone, cortisone, sex hormones, and epinephrine. Among the many conditions for which surgical removal of the adrenal gland is indicated are aldosteronoma, pheochromocytoma, carcinomas, sex hormone–producing tumors of the adrenal cortex, and larger nonfunctioning adrenal cortical adenomas. Unilateral adrenalectomy is generally well tolerated because normal function can be sustained by one adrenal gland. Bilateral adrenalectomy is sometimes indicated.

Laparoscopic adrenalectomy is a relatively new procedure, first described in 1992 [1]. Although the indications for laparoscopic adrenalectomy compared with the open procedure have not been clearly delineated, the laparoscopic approach is becoming accepted as the procedure of choice for many adrenal lesions [2–5]. Most of the conditions necessitating adrenalectomy are well suited to a laparoscopic approach because the tumors are small and the visualization afforded by laparoscopy is in many ways superior to that achieved with the open approach. The usual benefits of laparoscopic surgery (less postoperative pain and shorter hospital stays) can also be expected after adrenalectomy. In many cases, patients may be discharged the day after surgery.

Several anatomic issues are important when adrenalectomy is being considered. The first is the retroperitoneal location of the adrenal glands. Both retroperitoneal and transabdominal approaches to removal of the adrenal gland have been described. Most surgeons performing laparoscopic adrenalectomy, including those at our institution, favor the transabdominal approach. The benefits of this approach include a larger working space, easier conversion to an open procedure if necessary, and higher success rates for the removal of larger tumors.

A second issue is the difference in anatomy between the right and left sides that gives rise to specific concerns depending on the side of the adrenal lesion. On the right side, the greatest danger lies in the proximity of the gland to the inferior vena cava and the corresponding short length of the adrenal vein. On the left side, the venous anatomy is less treacherous, but exposure of the gland is usually more difficult. This chapter first discusses laparoscopic right adrenalectomy and then addresses left adrenalectomy, with the intention of highlighting the important differences.

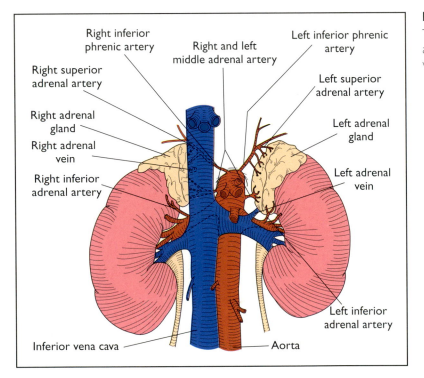

FIGURE 18-1.

The anatomy of the adrenal glands and their relationship to the kidneys, aorta, and inferior vena cava. Note the proximity of the right adrenal gland to the vena cava and its short main adrenal vein. (*Adapted from* [11]; with permission).

Setup

In addition to the standard equipment used for other laparoscopic general surgical procedures, some special equipment is helpful for adrenalectomy: a right-angle dissector, a liver retractor, and some type of bag retrieval system for the specimen. Another useful device is the harmonic scalpel.

Figure 18-2 shows the operating room setup for laparoscopic adrenalectomy. The surgeon may stand on either the contralateral or ipsilateral side. The assistant stands across from the surgeon, and the scrub nurse stands next to the assistant. The camera operator is on the surgeon's left, across from the scrub nurse. Two monitors are used, one on either side of the patient above the level of the shoulders.

The patient is initially positioned supine, and the targeted side is elevated 30° to 45° on a padded roll or beanbag. Anesthesia is induced, and a Foley catheter is inserted. Additional monitoring equipment is used according to the patient's diagnosis and comorbid conditions. Because deep venous thrombosis and pulmonary embolism have been reported in many patients in a large series [2], sequential compression devices for the lower extremities are routinely used.

Set-up

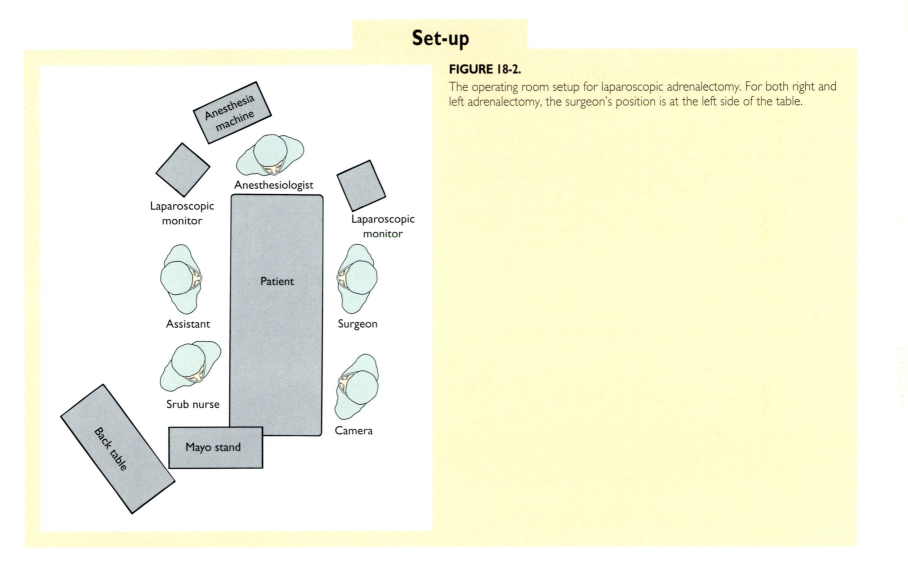

FIGURE 18-2.

The operating room setup for laparoscopic adrenalectomy. For both right and left adrenalectomy, the surgeon's position is at the left side of the table.

Procedure

Right Adrenalectomy

Positioning and Preparation

The position of the patient is changed from supine to right side up with an angle of 30° to 45°. The position is maintained with appropriate cushioning or a beanbag. An axillary roll is placed under the left axilla, and the right arm is positioned across the chest and held in place on cushions or a padded, elevated armboard. The operating table should then be flexed slightly at the patient's waist. The abdomen and flank are prepared; the sterile preparation solution should be applied as far posteriorly as possible because the sterile field should extend to the posterior axillary line. The sterile field should also extend well across the midline, to below the level of the iliac crests inferiorly and to the level of the xiphoid superiorly. After a standard laparotomy drape is put in place, the patient is rotated to the right; this change in position flattens the abdomen and makes the initial port insertion easier.

Port Placement

Figure 18-3 shows the port placement for right adrenalectomy. An open approach is used to insert a 10-mm port for the camera in the midline between the umbilicus and the xiphoid. A 30° laparoscope is used, and an initial abdominal exploration should be undertaken. The remainder of the ports are inserted through small skin incisions under direct vision. A port is placed in the midline just below the xiphoid for a liver retractor. For the assistant, a 5-mm port is sometimes placed, also in the midline, between the camera and the subxiphoid port. A retractor through the subxiphoid port is then used to elevate the liver so that the anatomy can be assessed. On the basis of this assessment, the surgeon places two additional ports in the right abdomen. These ports are generally in the mid-abdomen at about the level of the

umbilicus and should be spaced far enough apart to avoid interference of the instruments with one another. At least 5 cm is necessary, and 8 cm is desirable. The port in the most lateral position should be placed approximately in the anterior axillary line. The port to be used by the surgeon's dominant hand is 10 mm, and the other is 5 mm.

Dissection

While the assistant elevates the liver, the surgeon assesses the anatomy. If the hepatic flexure of the colon overlies the right adrenal gland, some mobilization of the hepatic flexure is necessary. The assistant achieves this by placing the hepatic flexure under medial and caudal tension using a blunt grasper with his or her left hand. The surgeon uses his or her left hand to apply lateral countertension, and uses a dissecting instrument, preferably the harmonic scalpel, to divide the lateral peritoneal attachments and a portion of the gastrocolic ligament (Fig. 18-4). In this manner, the superior pole of the right kidney, the duodenum, and the adrenal gland are exposed. In some cases, visualization of the adrenal gland may be hampered by a particularly fatty retroperitoneum. In these situations the difference in color between the adrenal gland (bright yellow) and the retroperitoneal fat (pale yellow) helps to distinguish the gland.

The dissection of the adrenal gland itself begins at the inferior edge. The dissection is then taken in a superior and lateral direction (Fig. 18-5). The harmonic scalpel is again useful for this dissection. Vessels, particularly at the inferior pole, are individually ligated with clips and divided as necessary. In this manner, the lateral edge of the gland is mobilized. The surgeon then posteriorly dissects the gland free in a medial direction. After the posterior dissection is complete, the medial edge of the gland is dissected free from the lateral surface of the inferior vena cava. It is important that the surgeon and assistant apply appropriate tension and countertension to facilitate the

Procedure

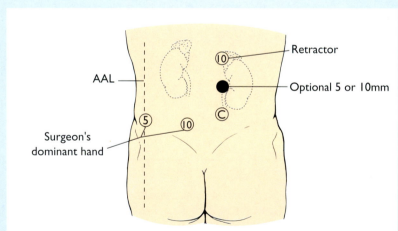

FIGURE 18-3.

Port position for right adrenalectomy. The surgeon works via two ports in the right mid-abdomen, at least one of which is 10 mm. The other (for the non-dominant hand) may be 5 mm. The assistant places two ports in the midline: one in the subxiphoid area for a liver retractor and one between the camera port and the subxiphoid port. The camera is placed in the midline in a supraumbilical location. AAL—anterior axillary line.

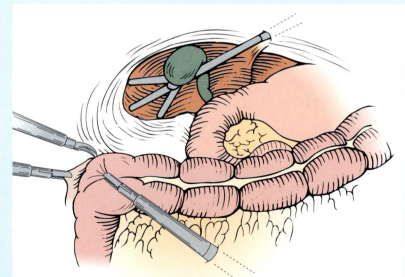

FIGURE 18-4.

The hepatic flexure is mobilized to expose the retroperitoneal location of the adrenal gland. The assistant provides inferior and medial traction on the colon. The surgeon provides countertraction and divides the lateral peritoneal attachments and a portion of the gastrocolic ligament, if necessary, with the cautery/scissors or the harmonic scalpel. (*Adapted from* [11]; *with permission.*)

dissection and avoid major vascular injury (Fig. 18-6). During this portion of the dissection, the main right adrenal vein should be identified. This structure is circumferentially dissected free by using a right-angle dissector. The vein is divided between silk ligatures, and the knots are tied extracorporeally (Fig. 18-7).

Dissection of the right adrenal gland is completed after the vein is divided by taking the remaining medial and superior attachments. Minor vessels should be ligated with clips and divided as appropriate. Once completely free, the gland is placed in a plastic retrieval bag and brought out through one of the 10-mm port sites. This incision frequently has to be extended in order to remove the specimen.

The larger incision is closed in layers by using heavy absorbable or nonabsorbable monofilament suture. The adrenal bed is then inspected for hemostasis. The site is irrigated with saline solution if necessary, and the field is aspirated dry. The remaining ports are removed under direct vision to confirm hemostasis. Before removal, the 10-mm port sites are closed by using a laparoscopic closure device and heavy polyglycolic acid suture. The pneumoperitoneum is completely evacuated, and the camera site is closed with a figure-eight suture made with heavy absorbable suture material. The skin incisions are irrigated and closed with fine absorbable subcuticular sutures.

Procedure

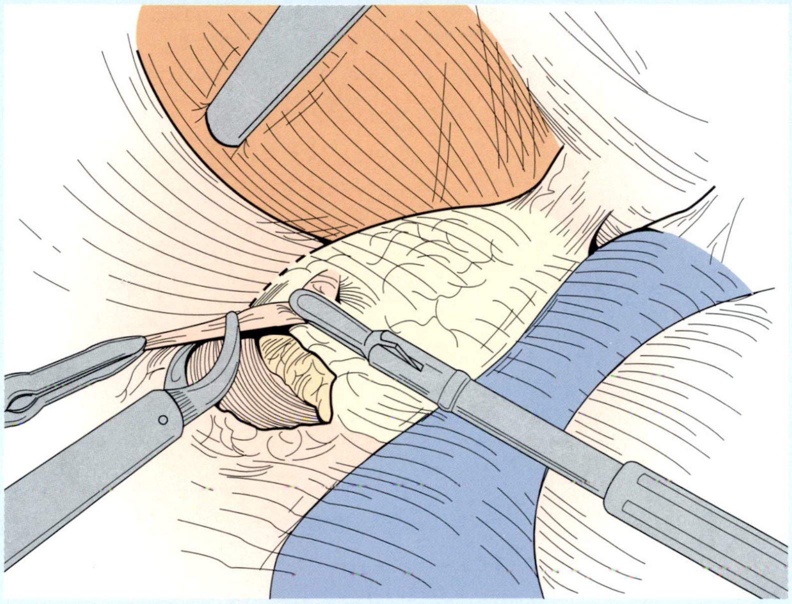

FIGURE 18-5.

Dissection of the right adrenal gland begins at the inferior edge and is taken in a superior and lateral direction (*dashed line*). The assistant can then use a grasper to elevate this dissected edge of the gland, providing posterior and medial exposure. The surgeon then performs the posterior dissection. Much of this portion of the mobilization is best performed with the harmonic scalpel. The occasional inferior vessels may require ligation and division. (*Adapted from* [11]; with permission.)

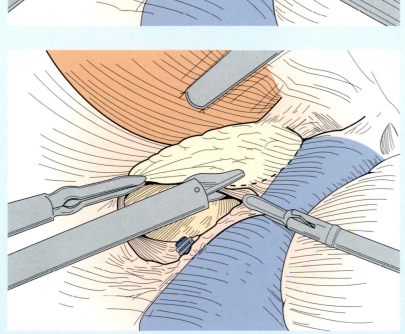

FIGURE 18-6.

Once the gland is mobilized laterally and posteriorly, the medial portion of the dissection is begun to expose the right adrenal vein. The line of dissection is shown by the *dashed line*. Again, the harmonic scalpel is useful for this portion of the operation. (*Adapted from* [11]; with permission.)

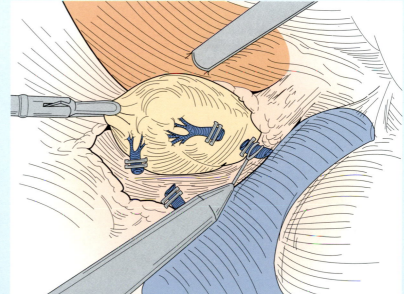

FIGURE 18-7.

Once the vein is exposed (a process facilitated by lateral retraction of the adrenal gland), it is circumferentially dissected with a right-angle dissector. The adrenal vein is ligated with silk ligatures or clips. A large cuff should be left on the side of the vena cava. Inferior and lateral retraction is then placed on the gland to facilitate the completion of the medial and superior dissection. If additional venous branches from the vena cava or inferior phrenic vessels are encountered, they must be ligated and divided. Once completely dissected free, the adrenal gland is placed in a retrieval bag and removed via one of the larger port sites. (*Adapted from* [11]; with permission.)

Left Adrenalectomy

Position and Preparation

Positioning of the patient for laparoscopic left adrenalectomy mirrors that for the opposite side. The patient is placed with the left side elevated approximately 30° to 45°. Although the orientation of the ports is slightly different, the surgeon and assistant may choose not to change sides of the table. Sterile preparation and draping are similar to that for the opposite side.

Port Placement

Figure 18-8 shows port placement for left adrenalectomy. The camera port placement is identical to that for the right side. The subxiphoid port may be 5 mm. A 10-mm port is again placed for use by the surgeon for the dissecting instrument and clip applier. Two ports are placed at the level of the umbilicus in the left mid-abdomen between the anterior axillary line and the camera.

Set-up

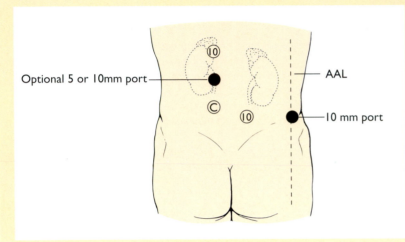

FIGURE 18-8.

Port position for left adrenalectomy. This mirrors the port position for the right side. The ports should generally lie on the circumference of a circle centered on the target gland and again should be spaced adequately to prevent interference of the instruments. AAL—anterior axillary line.

Dissection

To expose the left adrenal gland, the splenic flexure of the colon is mobilized. The assistant begins this dissection by placing the proximal descending colon under lateral tension, and the surgeon incises the lateral peritoneal attachments. The dissection proceeds proximally toward the splenocolic ligament (Fig. 18-9). Once this structure is reached, the assistant uses the shaft of a second grasper to elevate the lower pole of the spleen to place the ligament under tension. This maneuver must be performed with caution to avoid troublesome bleeding from the spleen. The harmonic scalpel is useful during this portion of the dissection. The splenic flexure should be mobilized sufficiently to expose the superior pole of the left kidney. The lateral attachments to the spleen are divided to allow the spleen to fall medially.

With the assistant maintaining retraction of the spleen and splenic flexure to expose the retroperitoneum, the surgeon locates the gland above and slightly medial to the superior pole of the kidney. Because the gland may be somewhat buried in the retroperitoneal fat, the color distinction is again useful. Just as for the right side, the lateral aspect of the adrenal gland is dissected free first (Fig. 18-10). The inferior edge follows. The main left adrenal vein is found along this edge as it courses caudally toward the renal vein and should be isolated, ligated with sutures (as on the right side) or clips, and divided. The gland can then be elevated and the posterior attachments divided. The medial side of the gland is dissected, and the main arterial supply is located, clipped, and divided (Fig.18-11). Once the main vascular supply is taken, the superior aspect of the gland is freed and the specimen is removed from the abdomen in a retrieval bag. Closure is identical to that described for the right side.

Procedure

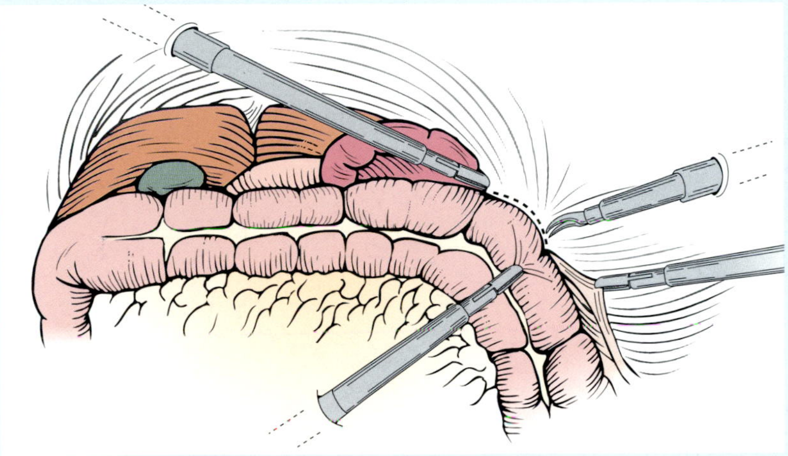

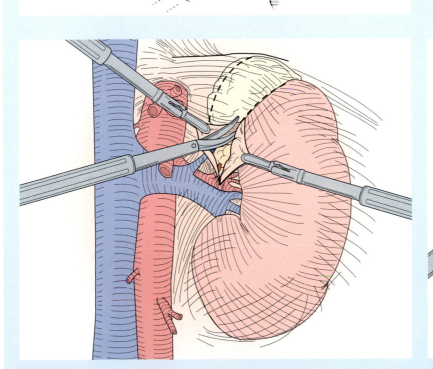

FIGURE 18-9.

The splenic flexure of the colon must be mobilized to expose the retroperitoneum and the left adrenal gland. The course of dissection is shown by the *dashed line*. As is done for the procedure on the right side, the surgeon and assistant maintain tension and countertension as the splenocolic ligament is divided. (*Adapted from* [11]; with permission.)

FIGURE 18-10.

The assistant provides exposure by elevating the spleen with the body of one blunt grasper and depressing the colon with another. The retroperitoneum is then opened, and the gland is located within the retroperitoneal fat by its distinct color. The location of the superior pole of the kidney provides guidance. Again, the gland is first dissected free along its lateral and inferior surfaces. (*Adapted from* [11]; with permission.)

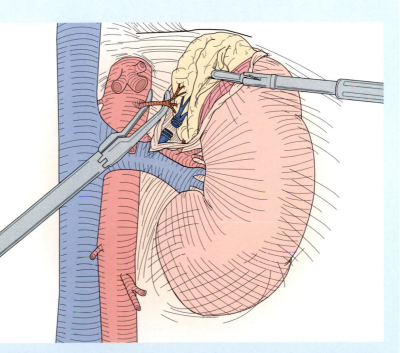

FIGURE 18-11.

Inferior veins encountered should be dissected free and divided. At this point, the assistant can place tension on the gland as the surgeon completes the posterior, medial, and superior aspects of the dissection. Vessels, particularly the arterial supply to the adrenal gland that comes in a medial to lateral direction, should be divided between clips where appropriate. (*Adapted from* [11]; with permission.)

Alternative Procedure

Just as there are alternate methods for open adrenalectomy, a variety of laparoscopic procedures have also been reported. The original description of laparoscopic adrenalectomy by Gagner involves a lateral transperitoneal approach [1,6]. In this procedure, the patient is placed in the lateral decubitus position and four trocars are used. Figure 18-12 shows the room setup, and Figure 18-13 depicts trocar placement. A Veress needles is used to create the pneumoperitoneum, and a 30° laparoscope is used as in the anterior approach. One disadvantage to the lateral approach is that it is not well suited to bilateral adrenalectomy.

An alternative to transperitoneal laparoscopic adrenalectomy is the retroperitoneal approach. Kelly [7] and Mercan [8] and their coworkers have described this approach. Three or four trocars are used, and the retroperitoneal space is developed by using either insufflation or a balloon dissector. In Fernandez-Cruz and coworker's randomized prospectivetrial [9], the anterior and retroperitoneal approach did not differ in terms of operative time or postoperative recovery, but CO_2 insufflation had slightly more pronounced effects in the transperitoneal group. Both procedures were deemed appropriate and safe, and the retroperitoneal approach had a potential advantage in patients with a history of abdominal surgery.

In a nonrandomized study, Baba and coworkers [10] described two retroperitoneal approaches—a posterior lumbar approach and a lateral flank approach—and compared both with the transperitoneal anterior approach. The posterior lumbar approach involves three 11-mm ports with an additional 5-mm port used to retract the kidney if necessary (Fig. 18-14). This approach has the theoretical advantage of allowing control of the blood supply to the adrenal gland before manipulation of a pheochromocytoma. Port placement for the lateral flank approach is similar to that for the lateral transperitoneal approach (Fig. 18-15). Findings in this study included shorter operating time and less blood loss for both retroperitoneal approaches; the posterior lumbar approach had the additional advantage of generally involving one less port.

Alternative Procedure

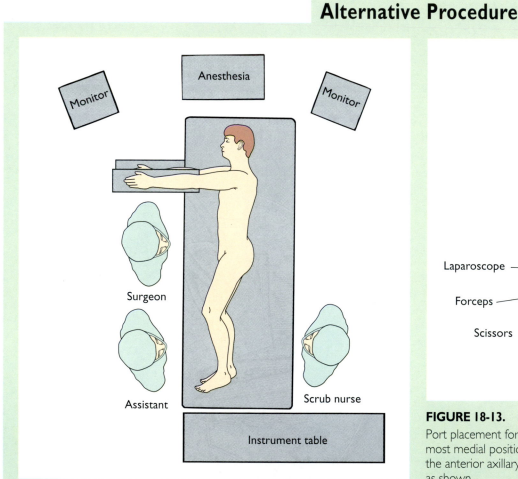

FIGURE 18-12.

The operating room setup for lateral transperitoneal laparoscopic adrenalectomy. The surgeon and assistant are on the same side of the table, and the assistant operates the camera. The patient is in the straight lateral decubitus position.

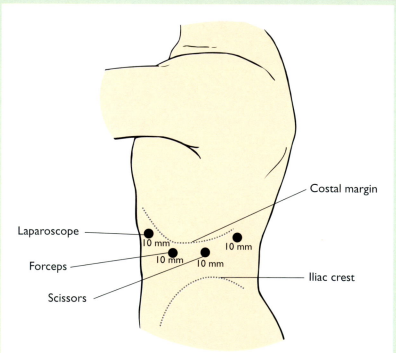

FIGURE 18-13.

Port placement for lateral transperitoneal left adrenalectomy. The port in the most medial position is used for the camera and is placed approximately in the anterior axillary line. The other ports, all 10 mm, are spaced and positioned as shown.

Alternative Procedure

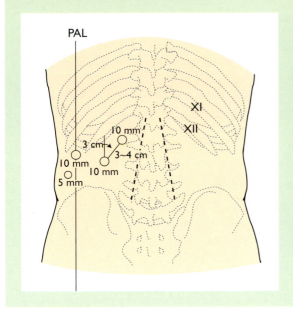

FIGURE 18-14.

Port placement for the posterior lumbar (retroperitoneal) approach to adrenalectomy. The patient is in the prone position, with the table somewhat jack-knifed. Three 10-mm ports are placed as shown. The ports are spaced more closely than in the other approaches. An additional 5-mm port is placed only if necessary.

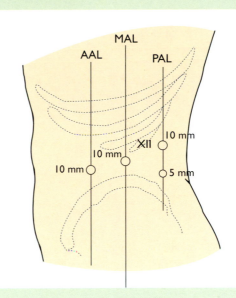

FIGURE 18-15.

Port position for the lateral retroperitoneal approach to laparoscopic adrenalectomy. The patient is placed in the straight lateral decubitus position. Three 10-mm ports are placed as shown. An additional 5-mm port is generally placed in the posterior axillary line (PAL). AAL—anterior axillary line; MAL—middle axillary line.

Results and Conclusions

It has become clear that laparoscopic adrenalectomy can be performed safely and that outcomes are good in terms of effectiveness of treatment, at least for benign adrenal disease [2]. A variety of laparoscopic approaches may be taken depending on individual surgeon preference and the circumstances of each particular case. Although initial reports demonstrated significantly longer operation times than with the open approach, duration of surgery has decreased with experience. Comparison with open adrenalectomy has shown laparoscopic adrenalectomy to be cost-effective. Because of this benefit and the shorter postoperative recovery times, laparoscopic adrenalectomy has been heralded as a new standard of care for benign adrenal lesions [5].

References

1. Gagner M, Lacroix A, Bolte E: Laparoscopic adrenalectomy in Cushing's syndrome and pheochromocytoma [Letter]. *N Engl J Med* 1992, 327:1033.
2. Gagner M, Pomp A, Heniford BT, *et al.*: Laparoscopic adrenalectomy: lessons learned from 100 consecutive procedures. *Ann Surg* 1997, 226:238–46, discussion 246–247.
3. Hansen P, Bax T, Swanstrom L: Laparoscopic adrenalectomy: history, indications, and current techniques for a minimally invasive approach to adrenal pathology. *Endoscopy* 1997, 29:309–314.
4. Horgan S, Sinanan M, Helton WS, *et al.*: Use of laparoscopic techniques improves outcome from adrenalectomy. *Am J Surg* 1997, 173:371–374.
5. Jacobs JK, Goldstein RE, Geer RJ: Laparoscopic adrenalectomy. A new standard of care. *Ann Surg* 1997, 225:495–501, discussion 501–502.
6. Gagner M: Laparoscopic adrenalectomy. *Surg Clin North Am* 1996, 76:523–537.
7. Kelly M, Jorgensen J, Magarey C, *et al.*: Extraperitoneal 'laparoscopic' adrenalectomy. *Austr N Z J Surg* 1994, 64:498–500.
8. Mercan S, Seven R, Ozarmagan S, *et al.*: Endoscopic retroperitoneal adrenalectomy. *Surgery* 1995, 118:1071–1075, discussion 1075–1076.
9. Fernandez-Cruz L, Saenz A, Benarroch G, *et al.*: Laparoscopic unilateral and bilateral adrenalectomy for Cushing's syndrome. Transperitoneal and retroperitoneal approaches. *Ann Surg* 1996, 224:727–734, discussion 734–736.
10. Baba S, Miyajima A, Uchida A, *et al.*: A posterior lumbar approach for retroperitoneoscopic adrenalectomy: assessment of surgical efficacy. *Urology* 1997, 50:19–24.
11. Wake Forest University Website, *Online Surg Atlas*: http:\\www.bgsm.edu/surg-sci/atlas/text/prices.htlm

Thoracoscopic Pericardiectomy

William R. Burfeind, Jr
Thomas A. D'Amico

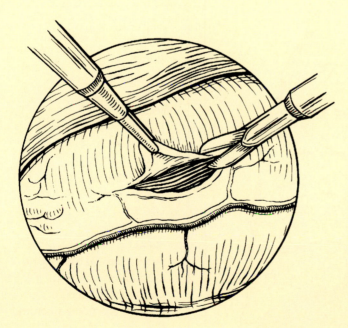

Multiple surgical options are available when the pericardium is being approached. Traditional methods include a left thoracotomy, a median sternotomy, and a subxiphoid approach. The development of video-assisted endosurgical equipment has led to the successful application of thoracoscopy to pericardial resection in effusive disease.

Anatomy

The parietal pericardium consists of dense collagen and elastin fibers with an inner serous layer composed of a single layer of mesothelial cells. The parietal pericardium is a sac-like structure that surrounds the heart and fuses to the adventitia of the proximal great vessels (Figure 19-1). The visceral pericardium covers the surface of the heart and consists of a thin layer of fibrous tissue covered by mesothelium. The parietal and visceral pericardium are continuous at the sites of attachment to the proximal great vessels. Ligaments fix the pericardium anteriorly to the sternum, posteriorly to the spine, and inferiorly to the diaphragm. The phrenic nerve and pericardiacophrenic artery course along the lateral aspect of both sides of the pericardium. Normally, the pericardium contains up to 50 mL of serous fluid.

The pericardium reduces friction between the heart and surrounding tissues and fixes the heart within the mediastinum. Experimental evidence reveals that the pericardium performs important physiologic functions that include equalization of hydrostatic forces, limitation of cardiac distension, and diastolic hemodynamic coupling [1].

Pathophysiology

Pericardial effusions may develop after acute pericarditis and trauma. The most common types of pericardial effusions include neoplastic, idiopathic, infectious, and traumatic. A complete list is presented in Table 19-1. Acute inflammation in the pericardium results in increased vascular permeability and fibrin deposition. Fibrous adhesions and exudation are typical. Complications of fibrosis (constriction) and effusions (tamponade) may develop.

Pericardial tamponade develops if the accumulation of fluid causes a rise in intrapericardial pressure (normal = -5 to +5 cm H_2O). This rise in pressure depends on the volume of effusion and the rate at which it accumulates. Over the long term, large volumes (1500 mL) may collect without hemodynamic compromise. However, the acute accumulation of as little as 150 to 250 mL of pericardial fluid may cause acute pericardial tamponade (Figure 19-2). Elevated intrapericardial pressures decrease ventricular filling, decrease stroke volume, and thereby reduce cardiac output. The reduced stroke volume is compensated by increased heart rate and sympathetic tone. When these compensatory mechanisms fail, systemic perfusion decreases and cardiogenic shock follows.

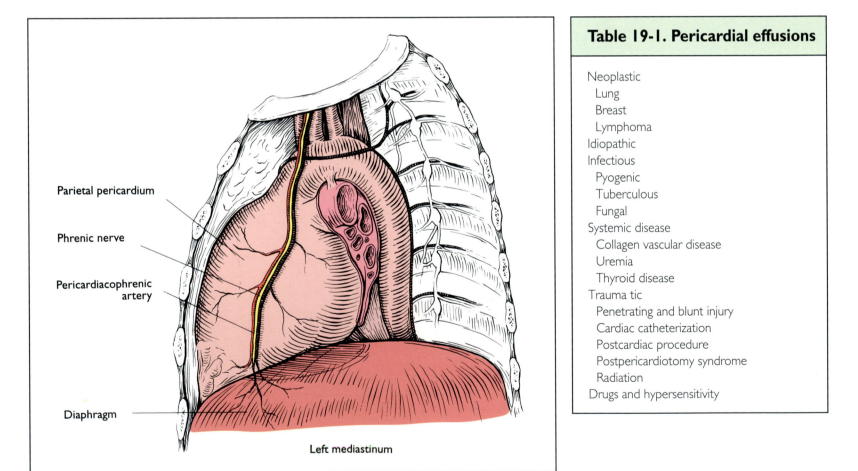

Table 19-1. Pericardial effusions

Neoplastic
  Lung
  Breast
  Lymphoma
Idiopathic
Infectious
  Pyogenic
  Tuberculous
  Fungal
Systemic disease
  Collagen vascular disease
  Uremia
  Thyroid disease
Trauma tic
  Penetrating and blunt injury
  Cardiac catheterization
  Postcardiac procedure
  Postpericardiotomy syndrome
  Radiation
Drugs and hypersensitivity

Parietal pericardium

Phrenic nerve

Pericardiacophrenic artery

Diaphragm

Left mediastinum

FIGURE 19-1.

Anatomy of the pericardium. The pericardium, phrenic nerve, and pericardiacophrenic artery are shown within the mediastinum.

Presentation and Differential Diagnosis

Acute pericarditis is characterized by chest pain, a pericardial friction rub, and electrocardiogram (ECG) changes. Chest pain varies in location and may be exacerbated by supine position and deep inspiration. The pericardial friction rub classically has three components that correspond with atrial systole, ventricular systole, and ventricular filling during diastole. The ECG changes are described in four stages. Stage 1 consists of ST-segment elevation in all leads except AVR and V1. Stage 2 is characterized by normalization of ST segments and T-wave flattening. Later, in stage 3, the T waves become inverted. In stage 4, the T waves normalize. Acute pericarditis is usually self-limiting. However, hemodynamic complications may develop in the form of cardiac tamponade from a pericardial effusion, constriction from fibrosis, or both.

The onset of cardiac tamponade may be sudden or insidious. The signs of tamponade include distended neck veins, distant heart sounds, and hypotension (Table 19-2). This triad of symptoms is known as Beck's triad [2]. Tamponade is also characterized by a pulsus paradoxus that is an inspiratory fall in arterial systolic blood pressure greater than 10 mm Hg. Cyanosis, tachycardia, and tachypnea may also be present. In general, signs of cardiogenic shock predominate. The ECG may show electrical alternans, a phasic alteration in the amplitude of the R wave. The chest radiograph may show an enlarged cardiac silhouette. Invasive monitoring reveals rising central venous pressure with decreased cardiac output and mean arterial pressure.

Echocardiography is the most sensitive test for the diagnosis of a pericardial effusion. It may also reveal findings of early cardiac tamponade. Increased respiratory variation in valvular flow, diastolic right ventricular collapse, and loss of normal inspiratory inferior vena cava collapse are sensitive indicators of cardiac tamponade.

The differential diagnosis of cardiac tamponade includes other major disorders of the chest that cause shock and hypotension (Table 19-3). These include tension pneumothorax, hemothorax, acute myocardial infarction, congestive heart failure, pulmonary embolism, superior vena cava syndrome, and constrictive pericardial disease.

Surgical Indications

Surgical drainage of a pericardial effusion is indicated when medical management fails to control the effusion or a specific diagnosis is required to direct therapy. Early physical signs of tamponade may be present or may be demonstrated by echocardiography. The objectives of surgical therapy are to drain the effusion, prevent recurrence, and provide a specific diagnosis.

Surgical approaches to the pericardium include right or left anterior thoracotomy, a subxiphoid approach, and thoracoscopy. A subxiphoid pericardial window can be performed under local anesthesia and is usually well tolerated. This technique is an excellent therapeutic option for many patients, but it should not be used when the underlying disease process may lead to constrictive pericardial disease (eg, in patients with tuberculosis, *Haemophilus influenzae* infection, or radiation pericarditis). In addition, because the pericardial resection is limited with the subxiphoid approach, recurrence rates are as high as 10% to 18% [3–5]. A thoracotomy allows for a more thorough pericardial resection and a decreased incidence of recurrent effusions [3]. However, this approach is more invasive and involves the added morbidity of general anesthesia.

A thoracoscopic approach provides access for an extended pericardial resection while simultaneous access to lung and pleural abnormalities while avoiding a formal thoracotomy.

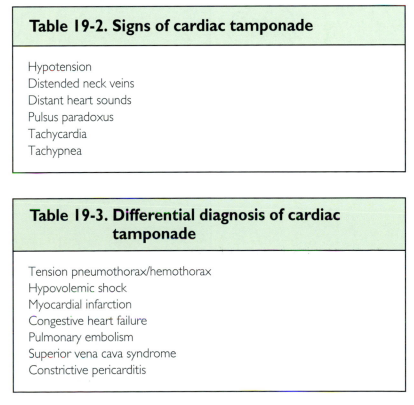

FIGURE 19-2.

Experimental cardiac tamponade produced by injection of saline into the pericardium. As the volume of pericardial fluid increases, mean arterial pressure falls and right atrial and pericardial pressures rise. BP—blood pressure. (*From* Fowler [8]; with permission.)

Table 19-2. Signs of cardiac tamponade
Hypotension
Distended neck veins
Distant heart sounds
Pulsus paradoxus
Tachycardia
Tachypnea

Table 19-3. Differential diagnosis of cardiac tamponade
Tension pneumothorax/hemothorax
Hypovolemic shock
Myocardial infarction
Congestive heart failure
Pulmonary embolism
Superior vena cava syndrome
Constrictive pericarditis

Postoperative pain would be expected to be less than with a thoracotomy [6], although general anesthesia and single-lung ventilation are still necessary. If tamponade physiology is present, pericardiocentesis should be performed before the induction of general anesthesia.

In summary, the subxiphoid approach has the advantages of allowing the use of a local anesthetic, not requiring single-lung ventilation, and not requiring that the patient be turned laterally. The subxiphoid approach is limited by the fact that other chest abnormalities will be missed and that the recurrence rate for pericardial effusion is higher than with the thorascopic approach. The thoracoscopic approach has the advantages of allowing for a more thorough pericardial resection and facilitating the ability to perform concomitant diagnostic and therapeutic procedures, such as drainage of pleural effusion, decortication, lung biopsy, or pleural biopsy. The disadvantages of thoracoscopy include the need for general anesthesia, selective ventilation, lateral positioning, and decompression of the pericardial space before induction in unstable patients.

Surgical Technique

Figures 19-3 through 19-8 depict the surgical technique for thoracoscopic pericardiectomy.

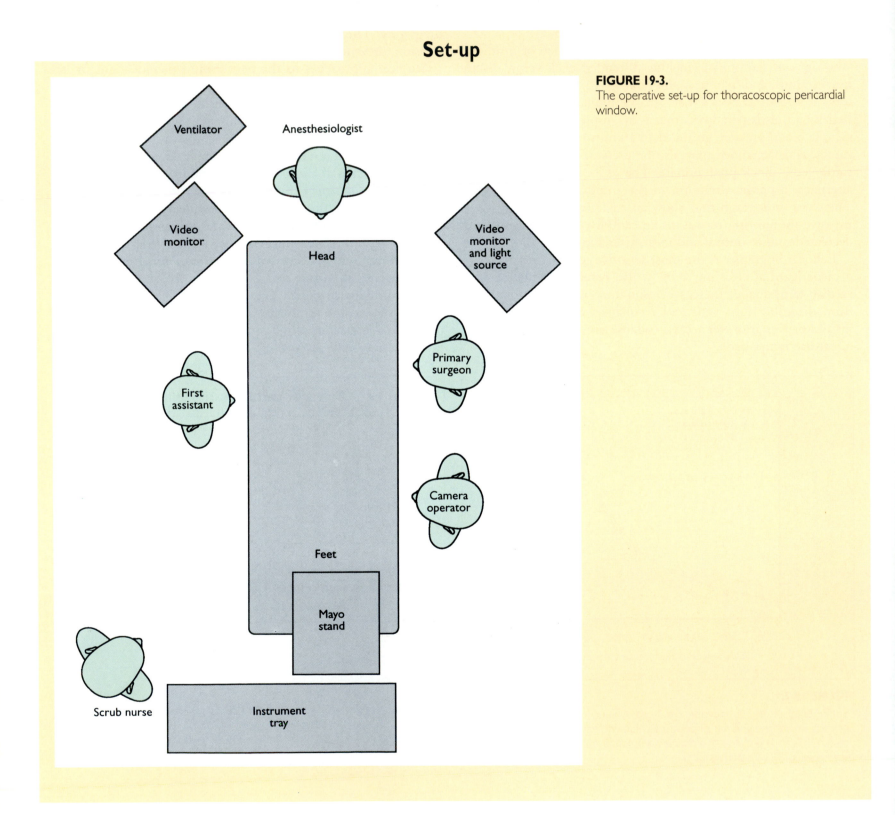

Set-up

FIGURE 19-3.
The operative set-up for thoracoscopic pericardial window.

Procedure

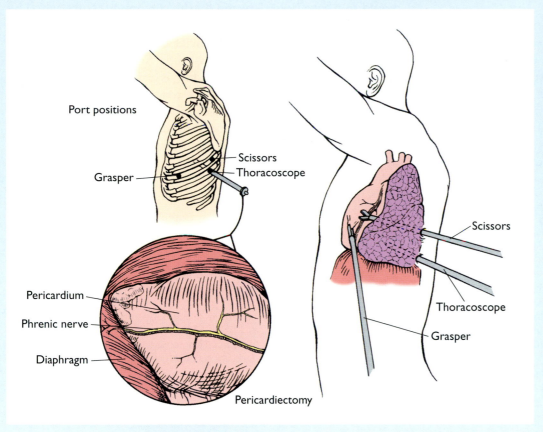

FIGURE 19-4.
The patient is intubated with a dual-lumen endotracheal tube for single-lung ventilation. A Foley catheter and nasogastric tube are inserted. If significant tamponade is present, pericardiocentesis should be performed before the induction of anesthesia. The patient is placed in the left lateral position and single-lung ventilation is established. Access to the thoracic cavity is gained by blunt dissection over the 8th rib (7th interspace) in the midscapular line posteriorly. A 10-mm port is inserted and the thoracoscope introduced. The chest cavity is explored. Two 5-mm ports are inserted under direct vision into an interspace higher (6th) in the midscapular line and in the anterior axillary line. A grasper and scissors are introduced.

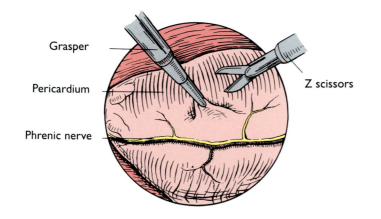

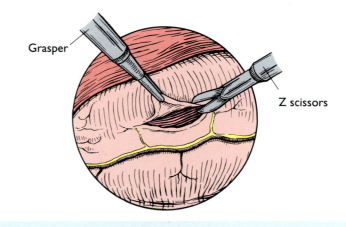

FIGURE 19-5.
The pericardium and phrenic nerve are identified. The pericardium anterior to the phrenic nerve is grasped and incised. Care is taken to avoid injury to underlying cardiac structures.

FIGURE 19-6.
The anterior pericardium is widely excised. If posterior loculated fluid collections exist, a posterior resection of pericardium may also be performed.

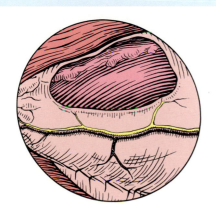

FIGURE 19-7.
The pericardium is removed. The area of resection is inspected for adequate hemostasis.

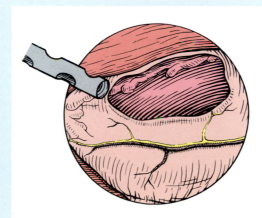

FIGURE 19-8.
A 28- or 32-French chest tube is placed and angled toward the pericardium. Port sites are inspected for hemostasis and the thoracoscope is withdrawn.

Results

Results of thoracoscopic pericardial resection have been encouraging. Hazlerigg and coworkers [7] reported on thoracoscopic pericardiectomy in 35 patients. Malignant effusions accounted for just over half (52%) of their patients. No patients died during surgery, and hospital stay averaged 4.6 days. No recurrent effusions had occurred by 9 months of follow-up.

Liu and coworkers [9] had similar results in 28 patients who underwent thoracoscopic pericardiectomy. In 60% of their patients, pleuropulmonary abnormalities were diagnosed that would not have been detected by the subxiphoid approach. The authors suggest that the ability to manage pleuropulmonary disorders simultaneously was beneficial to patients who presented with both abnormalities.

Thoracoscopic pericardial window is a new alternative to thoracotomy and the subxiphoid approach. This technique produces a wide pericardial resection and avoids the morbidity associated with open thoracotomy. Initial reports are encouraging and reveal a low incidence of recurrent pericardial effusions on short-term follow-up.

References

1. Spodick DH: The normal and diseased pericardium: current concepts of pericardial physiology, diagnosis and treatment. *J Am Coll Cardiol* 1983, 1:240.
2. Beck CS: Two cardiac compressor triads. *JAMA* 1935, 104:714.
3. Piehler JM, Pluth JR, Schaff HV, *et al.*: Surgical management of effusive pericardial disease: influence of extent of pericardial resection on clinical course. *J Thorac Cardiovasc Surg* 1985, 90:506.
4. Naunheim KS, Kesler KA, Fiore AC, *et al.*: Pericardial drainage: subxiphoid vs. transthoracic approach. *Eur J Cardiothorac Surg* 1991, 5:99–104.
5. Sugimoto JT, Little AG, Ferguson MK, *et al.*: Pericardial window; mechanisms of efficacy. *Ann Thorac Surg* 1990, 50:442–445.
6. Landreneau RJ, Hazlerigg SR, Mack MR, *et al.*: Postoperative pain related morbidity; video-assisted thoracic surgery versus thoracotomy. *Ann Thorac Surg* 1993, 56:1285–1289.
7. Hazlerigg SR, Mack MJ, Landreneau RJ, *et al.*: Thoracoscopic pericardiectomy for effusive pericardial disease. *Ann Thorac Surg* 1993, 56:792–795.
8. Fowler NO: Physiology of cardiac tamponade and pulsus paradoxus. *Med Conc Cardiovasc Dis* 1978, 47:109.
9. Liu HP, Chang CH, Lin PJ, *et al.*: Thoracoscopic management of effusive pericardial disease: indications and technique. *Ann Thorac Surg* 1994, 58:1695–1697.

CHAPTER 20

Thoracoscopic Pulmonary Resection

G. Chad Hughes

David H. Harpole, Jr

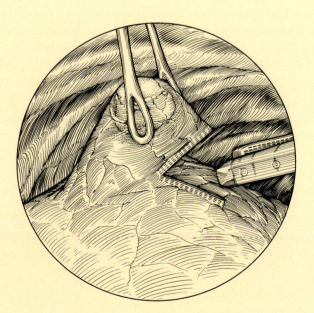

Thoracoscopy was first performed by Jacobaeous in 1910 [1] to divide pleural adhesions. However, because of limited instrumentation and poor visualization, this technique received little enthusiasm over the subsequent 80 years [2]. With the introduction of solid-state video technology in the late 1980s, thoracoscopy (now called video-assisted thoracic surgery [VATS]) has become an essential technique for the diagnosis and management of numerous clinical problems in general thoracic surgery [3]. This chapter describes the use of VATS for pulmonary wedge resection of the indeterminate pulmonary nodule.

Management of a Solitary Pulmonary Nodule

The differential diagnosis of a solitary pulmonary nodule, usually found incidentally on plain chest radiography, is listed in Table 20-1. Most of these nodules are benign; only 5% ultimately prove to be malignant. However, when resection is indicated because of size or rapid growth, approximately 40% of *resected* nodules are malignant. Therefore, the decision to perform a biopsy or resect a pulmonary nodule is of critical importance.

In any patient with a newly detected pulmonary nodule, a thorough history should emphasize tobacco use as well as exposure to chemicals, asbestos, or coal mining. Symptoms such as shortness of breath, chest pain, cough, hemoptysis, or weight loss may be elicited. Physical examination obligates careful palpation for cervical, clavicular, and axillary adenopathy and thorough auscultation of all lung fields. The probability of malignancy is low in patients younger than 30 years of age and is significantly greater in patients older than 50 years of age.

Old radiographs must be sought aggressively. If possible, comparison of the current chest radiograph with previous ones may provide immediate diagnostic and prognostic information. Lesions larger than 3 cm in diameter, regardless of other features or time course, are usually malignant. With nodules smaller than 3 cm in diameter, radiographic characteristics such as smooth contour, diffuse calcification, or popcorn calcification suggest benign tumors. Tumor doubling time, defined by the period in which tumor volume (not diameter) has increased twofold, provides the most reliable means of distinguishing between malignant and benign lesions. Malignant nodules double in volume over a period of weeks to months. By contrast, benign nodules may double over several years or remain unchanged in size. A solitary pulmonary nodule that is smaller than 3 cm and is radiographically unchanged over 2 years of documented observation may be considered a benign lesion; no further diagnostic work-up is required. Chest radiography should be performed annually as follow-up for these patients.

If these clinical and radiographic indicators are vague or suggest malignancy, further diagnostic measures are required immediately. This evaluation should begin with computed tomography (CT) of the chest, liver, and adrenal glands. With distant metastasis, extensive mediastinal adenopathy, involvement of the trachea, or tumor in the contralateral bronchus or lymph nodes, the cancer is considered inoperable and the prognosis is usually grave. Additional criteria for lung cancer inoperability are listed in Table 20-2.

In the absence of definitive clinical and radiologic findings consistent with a benign lesion, histologic diagnosis of an indeterminant pulmonary nodule is essential. Fiberoptic bronchoscopy is often performed as the next step in the diagnostic work-up. However, although bronchoscopy is necessary to identify endobronchial lesions, bronchoscopic biopsy is an unreliable technique for obtaining histologic diagnosis. Transthoracic needle aspiration (TTNA) is performed under fluoroscopic guidance with risks that include pneumothorax, bleeding, air leak, and infection. With malignancy, TTNA has a reported sensitivity ranging from 64% to 97%, whereas a benign diagnosis is only 14% specific.

A negative biopsy result obtained via TTNA does not rule out malignancy. Therefore, direct biopsy via thoracotomy or VATS is required in either case when TTNA results are "negative" or positive for malignancy. Thus, TTNA is reserved for only circumstances in which disease is considered inoperable (*see*

Table 20-1. Differential diagnosis of pulmonary nodule
Arteriovenous malformation
Hamartoma
Hematoma
Infection
Fungal (eg, *Histoplasma, Coccidioides, Aspergillus species*)
Pneumonia
Pulmonary abscess
Tuberculosis
Neoplasia
Benign
Adenoma
Mesothelioma
Papilloma
Malignant
Adenocarcinoma
Carcinoid
Large-cell carcinoma
Mesothelioma
Secondary malignancy (metastatic from nonlung primary)
Small-cell carcinoma
Squamous-cell carcinoma
Pulmonary infarction

Table 20-2. Criteria for lung cancer inoperability
Horner's syndrome (except superior sulcus tumors)
Contralateral disease
Distant metastasis
Involvement of the trachea
Tumor in contralateral main bronchus
Contralateral lymph node metastasis
Superior vena caval obstruction
Bloody pleural effusion
Malignant cells in pleural effusion

Table 20-2) and tissue diagnosis is desired for palliative radiation therapy or chemotherapy.

In the absence of inoperable disease, open lung biopsy should be performed on all pulmonary nodules suspicious for malignancy. Preoperative work-up (Table 20-3) should consist of bronchoscopy to identify endobronchial extension of tumor or extrinsic bronchial compression that may influence pulmonary function. CT of the chest and upper abdomen with intravenous contrast and lung field windows should then be performed. This will precisely define the dimensions and location of the pulmonary mass and identify hilar or mediastinal adenopathy as well as contralateral disease. This study should also be extended to the liver and adrenal glands to rule out distant metastases. If any neurologic abnormalities are detected by history or physical examination, head CT should also be performed. Likewise, radionuclide bone scans should be obtained only when symptoms, signs, or laboratory findings of possible bony involvement are present. After these studies are completed, pulmonary function testing is necessary to determine the available pulmonary reserve after a potential wedge resection, lobectomy, or possibly pneumonectomy. Patients are excluded from pneumonectomy if the FEV_1 (forced expiratory volume in 1 second) is predicted to be less than 1.0 L after resection of the pulmonary nodule. However, thoracoscopic lung resection can be safely performed on patients with FEV_1 less than 1.

All patients requiring open lung biopsy should be considered for VATS. As listed in Table 20-4, VATS wedge resection offers several advantages over conventional thoracotomy. These include enhanced visualization, decreased postoperative pain, and minimal cosmetic impairment, as well as the potential for decreased hospital length of stay and earlier return to work. The most significant disadvantage of VATS compared with thoracotomy for pulmonary resection remains the loss of direct tactile feedback for the surgeon.

Inclusion criteria for VATS wedge resection are listed in Table 20-5. In general, VATS wedge resection can be performed in most patients with noncalcified nodules less than 3 cm in diameter. Resection by VATS of lesions located in the outer one third of the lung is easily accomplished with little risk for injury to segmental vessels or bronchi. Computed tomography aids greatly in localizing the nodule and is generally the only localizing study required. If pathologic examination of the frozen section yields a diagnosis of malignancy, then lobectomy (by VATS technique or open thoracotomy) is required for even a small T1 lesion. This possibility must be discussed in detail with the patient before surgery. The Lung Cancer Study Group [4] compared wedge resection versus lobectomy for T1N0 lesions in a randomized trial and found an increased rate of local recurrence in the limited-resection group. Wedge resection is a compromise acceptable only for patients who cannot otherwise tolerate a larger operation because of limited pulmonary reserve [5].

Anatomy

The anatomy of the lung is defined by the branching of each bronchus (Table 20-6 and Figure 20-1). Each lobe is supplied

---

Table 20-3. Preoperative work-up of pulmonary nodule

Bronchoscopy
Computed tomography
Pulmonary function testing
Mediastinoscopy

Table 20-4. Advantages of video-assisted thoracic surgery for pulmonary resection

Enhanced visualization of entire thorax
Decreased postoperative pain
Decreased wound complications
Decreased incidence of post-thoracotomy pain syndrome
Hastened recovery of pulmonary mechanics
Minimal cosmetic impairment
Decreased hospital length of stay and earlier return to work

Table 20-5. Inclusion criteria for video-assisted thoracic surgery wedge resection

Noncalcified, <3 cm in diameter
Location in outer third of lung parenchyma
Absence of endobronchial extension

Table 20-6. Pulmonary lobar and segmental anatomy

	Left lung			Right lung	
Lobes	Divisions	Segments		Lobes	Segments
Upper	Superior	Apical-posterior		Upper	Apical
		Anterior			Posterior
	Lingular	Superior			Anterior
		Inferior		Middle	Lateral
					Medial
Lower		Superior		Lower	Superior
		Anteromedial			Medial basal
		Lateral basal			Anterior basal
		Posterior basal			Lateral basal
					Posterior basal

by divisions of the main bronchus. Each segment is supplied by divisions of the lobar branches. The pulmonary artery divides to the left of the ascending aorta. The right branch courses behind the ascending aorta, whereas the left branch runs through the concavity of the aortic arch. In their respective hila, each pulmonary artery gives off a large first branch or anterior trunk, supplying one or more of the segments of the upper lobe. Further branching occurs parallel to bronchial divisions. The pulmonary veins arise from pulmonary capillary plexi at the alveoli. Venules run in the interlobular spaces and form the trunks of the pulmonary veins. Two main trunks are derived from each lung, one superiorly and one inferiorly, and enter the posterior aspect of the left atrium. Bronchial arteries perfuse the lung parenchyma and are derived directly from the aorta or aortic intercostal vessels. They may number from one to three and accompany the bronchioles to the lung lobules. Below the root of the lung, the pulmonary ligaments are created by the two layers of pleura that form a distinct band that attaches from the inferior aspect of the pericardium to the inferior portion of the mediastinal surface of the pleura.

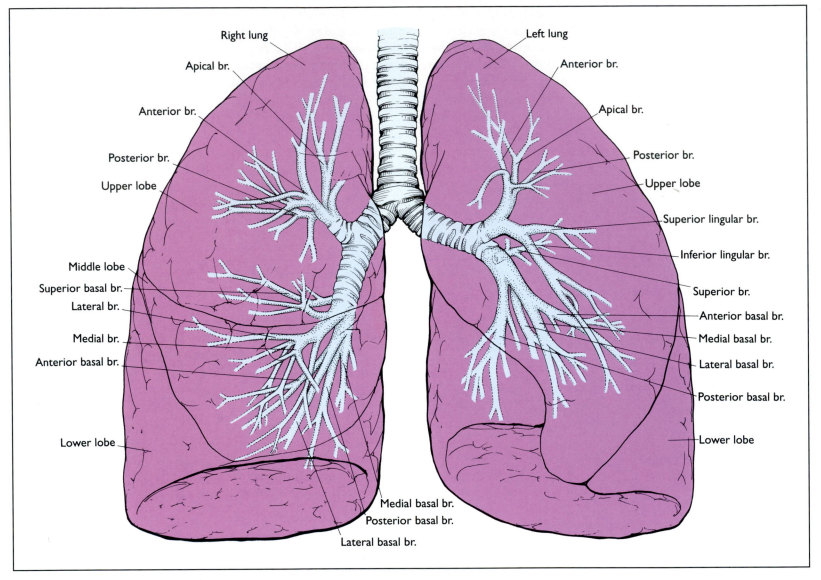

FIGURE 20-1.

Pulmonary anatomy. The topical surface of the lungs and the bronchial tree are illustrated. The right lung is composed of three lobes. The oblique (major) fissure separates the lower lobe from the upper and middle lobes, and the horizontal (minor) fissure separates the upper from the middle lobe. The left lung is composed of two lobes separated by the oblique (major) fissure. A thorough knowledge of the topical features of the lung as they relate to the underlying anatomic structures is essential to successful use of video-assisted thoracic surgery for pulmonary resections. br—bronchus.

Surgical Technique

Figures 20-2 through 20-12 depict the surgical technique for VATS. Wedge resection of a left upper lobe nodule is used as the demonstration example.

Set-up

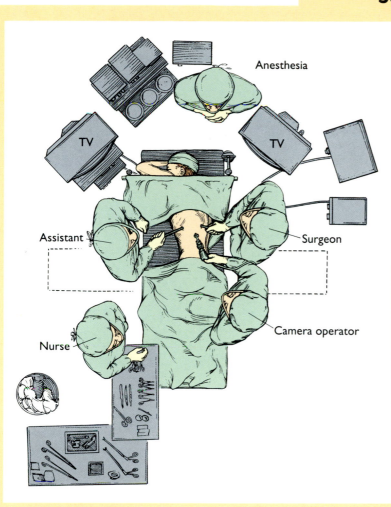

Anesthesia

TV

TV

Assistant

Surgeon

Camera operator

Nurse

FIGURE 20-2.

Operating room equipment and set-up for video-assisted thoracic surgery (VATS). Specialized equipment useful for VATS includes thoracic trocars or ports, optical systems (angled scope), fan retractor, thoracoscopic lung clamp, endoscopic staplers, and the endoscopic ultrasound probe. Thoracoscopic ports are useful for smooth movement of the video camera during VATS but are not essential. Often, standard thoracotomy instruments can be used through small open incisions. After the patient is placed in the lateral decubitus position and a double-lumen endotracheal tube is properly placed, the appropriate lung should be excluded from mechanical ventilation while the surgeons are scrubbing. This will allow adequate time for total lung deflation and absorption atelectasis. Insufflation is rarely necessary for VATS. If lung decompression is inadequate, insufflation may be introduced to the set-up. In these cases, insufflation pressure should be limited to no more than 10 mm Hg and patients should be carefully monitored for signs of impaired venous return and decreased cardiac output. In the operating room set-up, the position of the surgeon and assistants are the same as with an open thoracotomy. Video displays are positioned in a direct line between the operators and the surgical target. For upper thoracic lesions, video displays are usually positioned on opposite sides at the head of the table and at the foot of the table for lower thoracic lesions. VATS provides visualization of thoracic anatomy through a smaller, magnified, field of vision. Thus, orientation of the operative field as seen on the video display is essential. The two fields of vision recommended for VATS are obtained with the videoscope inserted through the posterior port or the inferior port. As viewed from the posterior port, the thoracic anatomy can be seen in the same orientation as that of the operating surgeon during an open thoracotomy. With left-chest thoracoscopy viewed on a standard video display, anterior structures appear at the top, posterior structures at the bottom, inferior structures to the left, and superior structures to the right. To achieve better visualization of the apical structures of the chest, the videoscope can be inserted through a port positioned inferiorly at the midaxillary line. In this orientation, apical structures appear at the top of the screen, inferior structures at the bottom, anterior structures to the left, and posterior structures to the right.

Set-up

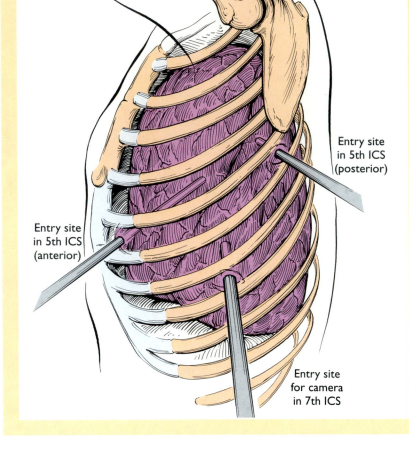

Entry site in 5th ICS (posterior)

Entry site in 5th ICS (anterior)

Entry site for camera in 7th ICS

FIGURE 20-3.

Port placement is of critical importance to successful video-assisted thoracic surgery (VATS) resection and is dictated by the location of the lesion to be resected. Ports should be positioned to create a "baseball diamond," in which the video camera is home plate relative to the pulmonary abnormality, which is located at second base. Working ports for retraction, grasping, and stapling are inserted at first and third bases. Wide port placement provides more room for effective retraction and adequate room to maneuver instruments. The initial port is inserted by using an open technique. The skin incision is made to accommodate the video camera and port (usually 10 mm), and the intercostal muscles are separated under direct vision by using a tonsil clamp down to the parietal pleura. The pleura is penetrated sharply and a finger is then inserted to confirm a circumferential space for insertion of the trocar and video camera. ICS—intercostal space.

Procedure

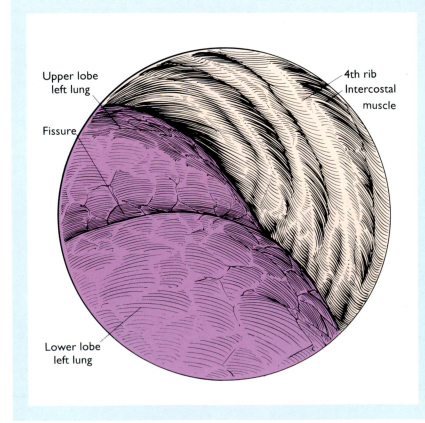

Upper lobe left lung

Fissure

4th rib Intercostal muscle

Lower lobe left lung

FIGURE 20-4.

Initial thoracoscopic exploration. Once the first trocar has been successfully introduced, the thoracic cavity is explored by using the video camera. Lung surfaces should be examined carefully for trocar injury as well as dimpling or retraction of the visceral pleura, which may indicate the exact location of pulmonary disease. Additional time should be directed at examination of the mediastinum for nodal abnormality. Additional ports are inserted transthoracically under direct vision with the video camera. Successful creation of the baseball diamond is facilitated by external palpation of the chest wall in relation to the abnormality to be removed.

Procedure

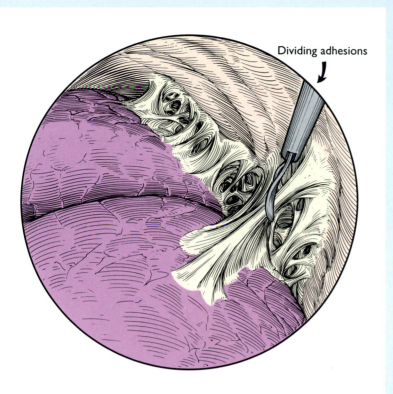

Dividing adhesions

FIGURE 20-5.

Takedown of pleural adhesions. Pleural adhesions are occasionally encountered upon insertion of the initial trocar and video camera. In this circumstance, endoscopic scissors may be inserted immediately next to the video camera in order to create enough free pleural space for placement of additional ports. These adhesions are usually taken down sharply with scissors connected to the electrocautery while cutting. Care must be taken to avoid tearing lung parenchyma or creating excessive bleeding.

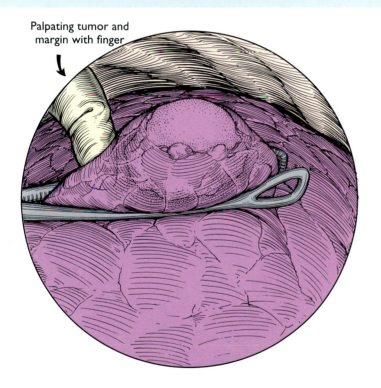

Palpating tumor and margin with finger

FIGURE 20-6.

Finger palpation of pulmonary mass. Localization of pulmonary nodules by using video-assisted thoracic surgery (VATS) requires extensive preoperative planning. As described earlier, computed tomography is essential to identify the position of the nodules in question. Peripheral one-third nodules that are 1 cm or larger in diameter are easily located thoracoscopically by using the video camera only. Nodules that are less than 1 cm in diameter or are located deep in the visceral pleura usually require additional techniques for intraoperative localization and subsequent resection. A nodule may be palpated by using a blunt instrument to observe visual changes in the contour of the lung surface as the instrument is used to gently compress areas of lung tissue. Direct finger palpation of lung tissue may also be done by grasping lung tissue with a ring forceps, Babcock clamp, or lung clamp and moving it to the chest wall where an index finger can be inserted through a trocar site. Lung tissue may also be digitally palpated between two fingers inserted through adjacent trocar sites.

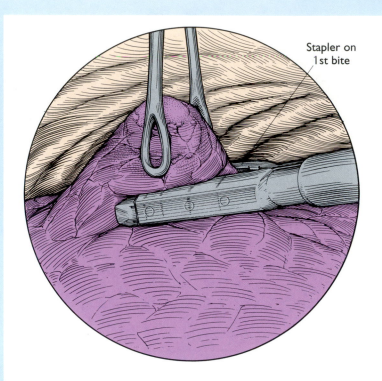

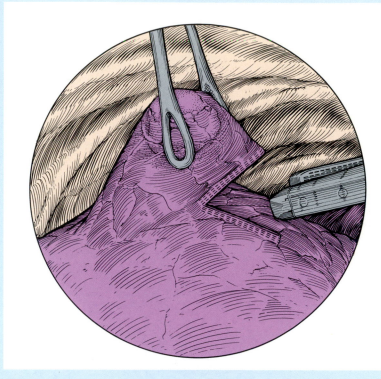

FIGURE 20-7.

Grasping of the nodule and initial placement of the stapler. After localization of the pulmonary nodule, an endoscopic stapler is used to resect the specimen. In most cases, the diseased area can be grasped with an instrument such as a ring forceps, Babcock clamp, or lung clamp to create a leading edge for insertion of the stapler. If the nodule is located on a flat surface not amenable to insertion into the narrow jaws of the endoscopic stapler, laser techniques may be used to create a leading edge of lung tissue for stapling.

FIGURE 20-8.

Wedge resection staple line. After the staple load is fired and the jaws of the instrument are opened, the staple line should be inspected for proper staple closure, bleeding, and air leak.

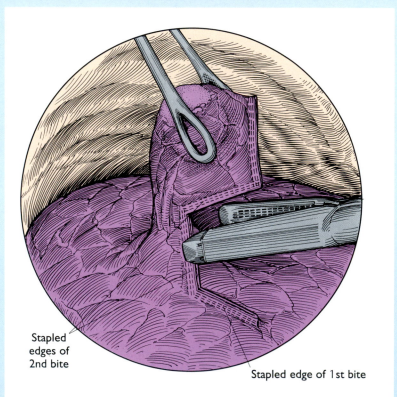

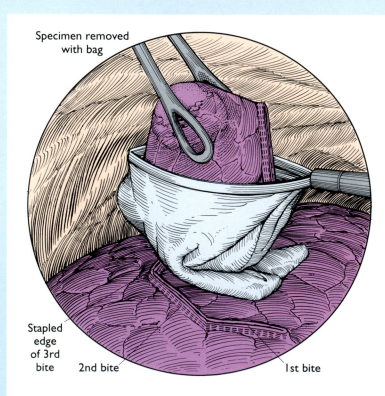

FIGURE 20-9.

Final staple load. Several staple loads are often required to resect a single specimen. With each firing, the specimen should be repositioned to facilitate smooth entry of the lung tissue into the jaws of the stapler.

FIGURE 20-10.

Placement of specimen into protective sleeve. To minimize the potential for local contamination of the trocar sites with possible cancer, the specimen should be placed in a protective sleeve by using an endoscopic bag or a simple glove before removal from the chest.

Procedure

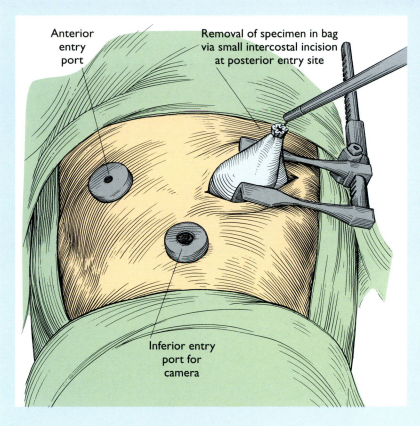

Anterior entry port

Removal of specimen in bag via small intercostal incision at posterior entry site

Inferior entry port for camera

FIGURE 20-11.

Utility thoracotomy and removal of specimen. A small utility thoracotomy slightly smaller than the length of the resected specimen may be required to facilitate removal of the specimen from the chest. The posterior port is recommended as the appropriate site if necessary.

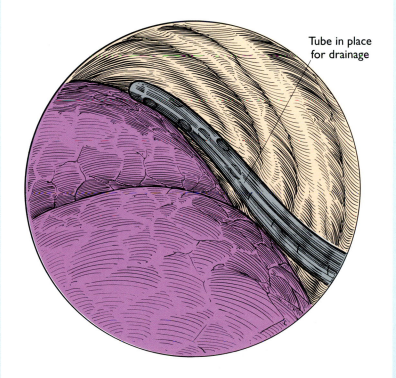

Tube in place for drainage

FIGURE 20-12.

Chest tube placement. After removal of the specimen, the chest should then be thoroughly reexamined with the video camera. The chest cavity should be partially filled with saline solution and the lungs inflated to examine the staple lines for air leaks or bleeding. A chest tube is then inserted through the most inferior port and directed to the apex under direct vision and connected to 20 cm H_2O suction after the trocar sites are closed.

Results

The results of VATS for the management of an indeterminate pulmonary nodule are summarized in Table 20-7. Overall, approximately one-third of patients undergoing VATS wedge resection ultimately required conversion to open thoracotomy. In most cases, conversion was done to perform a formal cancer operation when pathologic examination of the frozen section of the nodule yielded a diagnosis of malignancy. Additional indications for conversion to open thoracotomy are listed in Table 20-8.

Thoracoscopic wedge resection is essentially 100% sensitive and specific for the diagnosis of cancer and has minimal associated mortality [8]. The most commonly reported complications have been prolonged air leak, atelectasis, pneumothorax, pneumonia, and atrial arrhythmias [6–11]. Each has been seen in fewer than 2% of patients. Additional complications reported with VATS are listed in Table 20-9. Length of stay after VATS wedge resection has ranged from 2 to 5 days [6–11].

Table 20-7. Results of thoracoscopic wedge resection

Study	Year	Patients, n	Conversion, %*	Comments
Hazelrigg and coworkers [6]	1993	891	32.6	Mean hospital stay, 5 days
Allen and coworkers [7]	1993	118	45.8	No deaths; 6.3% complication rate
Mack and coworkers [8]	1993	242	12.8	No deaths; 3.6% complication rate
Landreneau and coworkers [9]	1993	74	35.1	No deaths; 6.2% complication rate
Santambrogio and coworkers [10]	1995	22	22.7	No deaths or complications
Allen and coworkers [11]	1996	352	22.2	2% mortality rate; 7.7% complication rate
Mean			28.5	

*Includes conversion to open thoracotomy because of technical reasons, including inability to locate nodule, and conversions necessitated by pathologic examination that revealed carcinoma.

Table 20-8. Indications for conversion to open thoracotomy

Pathologic examination of resected specimen reveals malignancy
Excessive adhesions (pleural space obliterated)
Uncontrolled bleeding
Trocar damage to intercostal bundle
Equipment malfunction
Inability to localize nodule
Hypoxemia or hypercapnia

Table 20-9. Complications of thoracoscopic pulmonary resection

Atrial arrhythmia	Atelectasis
Pneumothorax	Inadequate margins of resection
Persistent air leak	Lung injury
Hemorrhage	Intercostal neurovascular bundle injury
Air embolism	Equipment malfunction
Diaphragmatic perforation	Infection

References

1. Jacobaeus HC: Ueber die Möglichkeit die Zystoskopie bei untersuchung seröser höhlungen anzuwenden. *München Med Wochenschr* 1910, 57:2090–2092.
2. Bloomberg AE: Thoracoscopy in perspective. *Surg Gynecol Obstet* 1978, 147:433–443.
3. The 1st International Symposium on Thoracoscopic Surgery: Proceedings. San Antonio, Texas, January 22-23, 1993. *Ann Thorac Surg* 1993, 56:603–806.
4. Ginsberg RJ: The role of limited resection in the treatment of early stage lung cancer. *Lung Cancer* 1994, 11(Suppl 2):35.
5. Kaiser LR, Shrager JB: Video-assisted thoracic surgery: the current state of the art. *AJR Am J Roentgenol* 1995, 165:1111–1117.
6. Hazelrigg SR, Nunchuck SK, LoCicero J III: Video assisted thoracic surgery study group data. *Ann Thorac Surg* 1993, 56:1039–1043.
7. Allen MS, Deschamps C, Lee RE, *et al.*: Video-assisted thoracoscopic stapled wedge resection for indeterminate pulmonary nodules. *J Thorac Cardiovasc Surg* 1993, 106:1048–1052.
8. Mack MJ, Hazelrigg SR, Landreneau RJ, *et al.*: Thorascopy for the diagnosis of the indeterminate solitary pulmonary nodule. *Ann Thorac Surg* 1993, 56:825–832.
9. Landreneau RJ, Hazelrigg RS, Mack MJ, *et al.*: Postoperative pain-related morbidity: video-assisted thoracic surgery versus thoracotomy. *Ann Thorac Surg* 1993, 56:1285–1289.
10. Santambrogio L, Nosotti M, Bellaviti N: Videothoracoscopy versus thoracotomy for the diagnosis of the indeterminate solitary pulmonary nodule. *Ann Thorac Surg* 1995, 59:868–870.
11. Allen MS, Deschamps C, Jones DM, *et al.*: Video-assisted thoracic surgical procedures: the Mayo experience. *Mayo Clin Proc* 1996, 71:351–359.

Thoracoscopic Lung Volume Reduction

Ashish S. Shah
R. Duane Davis, Jr
David H. Harpole, Jr

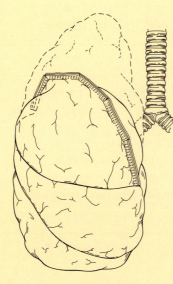

The surgical approach to end-stage pulmonary disease has progressed dramatically over the past decade and is driven by the nearly 14 million patients in the United States afflicted with emphysema [1]. In 1957, Otto Brantigan reported his experience with lung resection as a treatment for emphysema [2]. The method was abandoned until work performed by Cooper and coworkers in the 1990s generated renewed interest in therapeutic lung volume reduction. Stimulated by his growing experience with lung transplantation for emphysema, Cooper demonstrated objective improvements in pulmonary function among 20 patients who underwent lung resection for volume reduction with diffuse disease [3]. Since that report, work has continued to refine operative techniques, mechanisms of postoperative benefit, and most important, identification of patients who may predictably benefit from the procedure. Coincident with this development, video-assisted thoracoscopic techniques have gained many advocates and applications. Modern lung volume reduction surgery was initially performed via a median sternotomy, followed by unilateral thoracoscopic approaches, and ultimately a bilateral simultaneous thoracoscopic procedure.

Pathophysiology

The derangements of chronic obstructive pulmonary disease (COPD) have been well described and essentially involve the destruction of pulmonary parenchyma and the abnormal enlargement of airspaces distal to the terminal bronchioles. The disease results in a loss of compliance and elastic recoil in the lung, with resulting decline of one second forced-expiratory volume (FEV_1) and an increase in dead space ventilation. On gross examination, the lung may manifest this destruction and air trapping as discrete bulla and blebs. Typical bullous disease is seen at the apical regions of either lung, but emphysema also produces diffuse disease. Progressive, debilitating dyspnea and chronic hypoxia are common and inevitable consequences [4]. Current therapeutic options for select patients with severe, refractory COPD are lung transplantation and lung volume reduction surgery (LVRS) [5].

Lung volume reduction surgery is based on the idea that elimination of diseased regions of lung will restore functional pulmonary capacity in the remaining tissue. The true functional impact of LVRS is not yet fully understood, but studies have documented postoperative improvements in FEV_1, functional residual capacity, pulmonary chest wall mechanics, and most important, exercise tolerance and dyspnea [1,6–8].

Patient Selection

Proper patient selection remains a controversial and evolving issue. However, work in the past several years and the National Emphysema Treatment Trial have outlined relative inclusion and exclusion criteria (Table 21-1). Patients are considered candidates for LVRS only if they have severe dyspnea that is refractory to medical therapy, and a diagnosis of COPD confirmed by computed tomography. All of these parameters are subject to continued investigation and may vary by institution.

Preoperative Evaluation

Patients should undergo complete pulmonary function testing, electrocardiography, measurement of arterial blood gases, 6-minute walk test, chest radiography, chest computed tomography, and ventilation/perfusion (V/Q) scanning .

Table 21-1. Relative inclusion and exclusion criteria for lung volume reduction surgery

Inclusion criteria	Exclusion criteria
Chronic obstructive pulmonary disease refractory to medical therapy	Cigarette use within preceding 3 to 6 months
FEV_1 <35%	Severe obesity or cachexia (weight <80% or >120% of ideal body weight)
Age <70 years	Severe pulmonary hypertension (mean pressure >30–35 mm Hg)
	Hypercapnia ($PaCO_2$ ≥50 mm Hg)
Ability to complete postoperative rehabilitation	Severe hypoxia (O_2 requirement >4 L/min)
	Prednisone use ≥20 mg/d
	Previous major pulmonary resection
	Unstable angina

Procedure

Figures 21-1 through 21-7 depict the surgical technique for bilateral video-assisted thoracoscopic LVRS.

Set-up

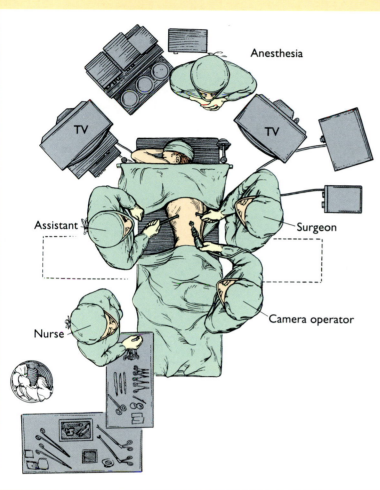

FIGURE 21-1.

Operative set up for video-assisted lung volume reduction surgery. As is done for traditional video-assisted lung resections, the patient is placed in the lateral position, with both arms positioned as shown. Double-lumen endotracheal intubation is performed with invasive monitoring, including Swan-Ganz catheterization and an arterial line.

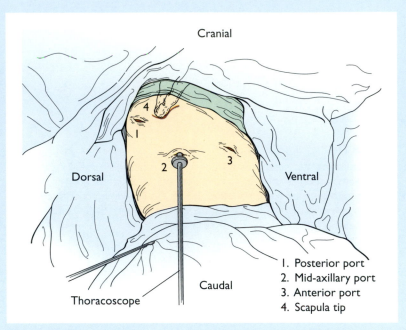

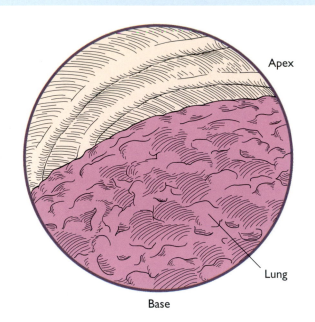

FIGURE 21-2.

Trocar positions are determined by the location of the disease. An initial port should be placed first in the 5th to 7th intercostal space along the mid-axillary line. Typical port positions for an apical resection are shown.

1. Posterior port
2. Mid-axillary port
3. Anterior port
4. Scapula tip

Cranial

Dorsal

Ventral

Caudal

Thoracoscope

Apex

Lung

Base

FIGURE 21-3.

A camera is then placed through the initial port; upon entering the chest, the lung is allowed to deflate. Under direct vision, a second port is then placed posteriorly and adhesions are then gently lysed. Particular attention is paid to the apex, where filmy adhesions are commonly encountered. Any large bullae should be identified. The resection goal for typical disease is approximately 50% of the upper lobe or 20% to 30% of the entire lung.

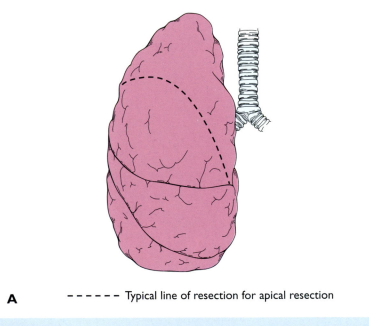

A – – – – – Typical line of resection for apical resection

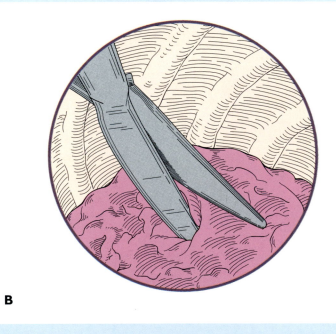

B

FIGURE 21-4.

The line of resection is further defined and may be improved by incision of the bulla, often revealing a demarcation. Other maneuvers, such as forced air trapping via the endotracheal tube may be used. Preoperative imaging may also be done to guide resections. In patients with diffuse disease, electrocautery may help demarcate the proposed line of resection.

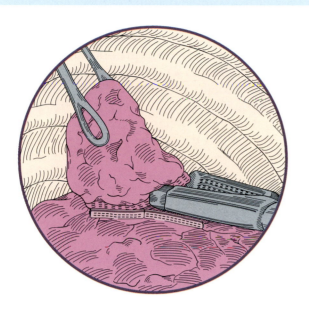

FIGURE 21-5.

Resection with an Endo-GIA (45-60) reinforced staple line is then performed lateral to medial, across the lung. This may be done from medial to lateral if necessary. In addition, basilar disease may be approached similarly. Apical resections for diffuse disease should be performed in a curvilinear fashion rather than transversely.

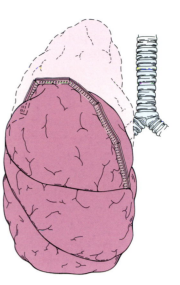

FIGURE 21-6.

The completed staple line. The resected specimen is brought out through the chest wall via a lateral port. If a large space remains or air leaks persist, a pleural tent may be performed. By using the electrocautery, an incision is made in the parietal pleura; it is then dissected off the chest wall by using a sponge stick.

FIGURE 21-7.

Two chest tubes are placed through the anterior ports and directed anteriorly and posteriorly. Attention is then turned to the contralateral side and resection is performed in a similar fashion.

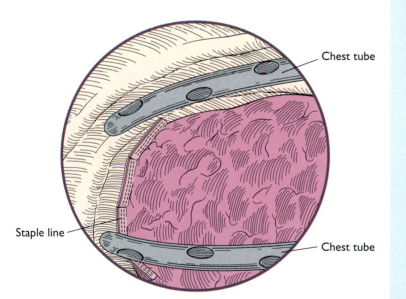

Chest tube

Staple line

Chest tube

Alternate Procedure

Lung volume reduction surgery may be performed in the supine position, obviating the need to reposition the patient. Other buttressing materials, such as polytetrafluoroethylene, may be used to reinforce the staple line.

Results

Reported perioperative mortality rates have ranged from 0.0% to 9.0% for patients undergoing bilateral thoracoscopic LVRS [9–11]. Pulmonary failure, pneumonia, air leaks, and prolonged stays in the intensive care unit and hospital are common postoperative complications [9–11]. Postoperative pulmonary rehabilitation is a necessary part of recovery and may be intimately tied to a sustained functional benefit [12].

The thoracoscopic approach to LVRS appears to have many advantages over median sternotomy. The thoracoscopic approach allows better visualization of the lower, posterior lung segments. Patients undergoing this type of surgery may also have a lower incidence of postoperative respiratory failure and early mortality [10]. In addition, the VATS approach may be associated with shorter hospital stays and lower rates of other respiratory complications [11]. The National Emphysema Treatment Trial should help to clarify the utility and cost-effectiveness of both approaches.

Functional benefits of LVRS remain a controversial and vexing subject. Many theories have been proposed and continue to be examined to explain the observed clinical improvement. LVRS may variably improve V/Q matching, chest-wall mechanics, and pulmonary elastic recoil. To date, no true consensus has emerged on the mechanism of functional improvement. No objective measure of pulmonary function has correlated with improvement in symptoms, but it appears clear that FEV_1, functional residual capacity, and exercise tolerance increase by at least 30% from preoperative values. Overall, 50% to 75% of patients appear to benefit from LVRS either subjectively or objectively at 1 year [1]. Although preoperative inspiratory resistance may be inversely related to outcome [13], no other preoperative study has been reported to have predictive value for postoperative improvement. Further studies will address not only these questions, but also the durability of improvement and identification of patients who will truly benefit from this innovative technique.

References

1. Fein AM: Lung volume reduction surgery: answering crucial questions. *Chest* 1998, 113:277s–282s.

2. Brantigan O, Muller E: Surgical treatment of pulmonary emphysema. *Am Surg* 1957, 23:789–804.

3. Cooper JD, Trulock EP, Triantafillou AN, *et al.*: Bilateral pneumonectomy (volume reduction) for chronic obstructive pulmoanry disease. *J Thorac Cardiovasc Surg* 1995, 109:106–119.

4. Cotran RS, Kumar V, Robbins SL: The respiratory system. In: *Robbins Pathologic Basis of Disease.* 1989: 766–770.

5. Mault JR: Surgical management of pulmonary emphysema. In: *Sabiston Textbook of Surgery* 1997:1838–1844.

6. Scuirba FC, Rogers RM, Keenan, *et al.*: Improvement of pulmonary function and elastic recoil after lung reduction surgery for diffuse emphysema. *N Engl J Med* 1996, 334:1095–1099.

7. Gelb AF, Brenner M, McKenna RJ, *et al.*: Serial lung function and elastic recoil 2 years after lung volume reduction surgery for emphysema. *Chest* 1998, 113:1497–1506.

8. Scharf SM, Rossoff L, McKeon K, *et al.*: Changes in pulmonary mechanics after lung volume reduction surgery. *Lung* 1998, 176:191–204.

9. Sabanathan A, Sabanathan S, Shah R, *et al.*: Lung volume reduction surgery for emphysema. A review. *J Cardiovasc Surg* 1998, 39:237–243.

10. Kotoloff RM, Tino G, Bavaria, *et al.*: Bilateral lung volume reduction surgery for advanced emphysema: a comparison of median sternotomy and thoracoscopic approaches. *Chest* 1996, 110:1399–1406.

11. Roberts JR, Bavaria JE, Wahl P, *et al.*: Comparison of open and thoracoscopic bilateral volume reduction surgery: complications analysis. *Ann Thorac Surg* 1998, 66:1759–1766.

12. Pulmonary rehabilitation for patients with advanced lung disease. *Clin Chest Med* 1997, 18:521–534.

13. Ingenito EP, Evans RB, Loring SH, *et al.*: Relation between preoperative inspiratory lung resistance and the outcome of lung volume reduction surgery for emphysema. *N Engl J Med* 1998, 338:1181–1185.

*T*horacoscopic Splanchnicectomy

G. Chad Hughes
Henry L. Laws
Kevin P. Landolfo

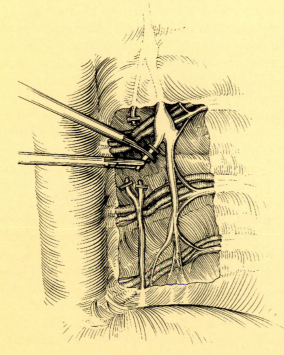

The management of pain in patients with chronic abdominal disease remains a difficult clinical challenge. Upper abdominal pain caused by primary or metastatic cancer of the liver, stomach, and gallbladder, as well as benign and malignant disease of the pancreas, is often severe and intractable. The concept of visceral sensation remained controversial until 1911, when Hearst [1] demonstrated that pain could be induced by balloon distention of the intestinal tract. With the subsequent acceptance of this concept, efforts were directed at defining the nature and location of pain perception in various intra-abdominal viscera [2].

This increased understanding of visceral pain sensation led to the observation that patients undergoing sympathectomy for treatment of essential hypertension had attenuated or ablated visceral pain sensation [3]. The anatomic explanation for this finding was a common pathway for the visceral afferents and the thoracic sympathetics. A clinical application was presented in 1945 when Mallet-Guy and coworkers [4] reported on a small series of patients with chronic pancreatitis treated by unilateral (left) splanchnicectomy. Their operative approach was a modification of that initially described by Peet [5], in which a lumbar incision was made with subsequent removal of a portion of the

twelfth rib. An extrapleural dissection allowed exposure of the lower thoracic ganglia and intervening trunk. The greater splanchnic nerve and celiac ganglion, as well as postganglionic branches were resected. Further experience and long-term follow-up by Mallet-Guy have continued to demonstrate that this procedure is both safe and relatively effective [6,7].

Rienhoff and Baker [8] were the first American investigators to report the use of splanchnic section for the control of chronic abdominal pain. They used a transthoracic approach; subsequently, both unilateral and bilateral thoracic as well as abdominal incisions to allow division of the visceral afferents have been described [9–12].

A novel approach to splanchnic denervation was devised by one of the authors of this chapter (Henry L. Laws, in conjunction with H. Harlan Stone). In this approach, a thoracoscopic technique is used to facilitate unilateral transthoracic exposure and division of the visceral afferents. The procedure was first performed at Duke University Medical Center in 1991 and has been widely used to treat chronic abdominal pain [13–21]. Thoracoscopic splanchnicectomy offers a relatively simple and effective method for the complete division of visceral afferent pathways in patients with chronic abdominal pain caused by a variety of benign and malignant disorders.

Anatomy

Traditionally, neuroanatomists have described the autonomic nervous system as an efferent system that supplies the heart, glands, and smooth muscle with efferent innervation. At the same time, afferent sensory fibers from the viscera are carried by the sympathetic nerves and white rami. Pain impulses arising within the abdominal cavity may reach the central nervous system by one or a combination of channels: 1) the sympathetic nerves (main pathway), 2) the somatic nerves innervating the body wall and diaphragm, and 3) the parasympathetic nerves (minor importance). However, these visceral afferent nerve fibers that transmit pain should not be thought of as part of the autonomic nervous system. Visceral innervation is mediated by mixed nerves with distinct sympathetic or parasympathetic efferent motor and visceral afferent sensory components [22]. The viscerosensory nerve fibers, both myelinated and nonmyelinated, run in the autonomic trunks and pass through the ganglia without synapses to reach their cells in the posterior root ganglia (Fig. 22-1).

Three nerves, present bilaterally, constitute the entire viscerosensory supply of the abdominal organs (Figs. 22-2, 22-3). The first is the greater splanchnic nerve, which is made up of rami leaving the fifth through the ninth ganglia of the paravertebral chain. The nerve descends on the lower thoracic vertebrae to penetrate the crus of the diaphragm and ends in the celiac ganglia around the origin of the celiac axis from the aorta. The celiac or solar plexus is the central distributing center for both

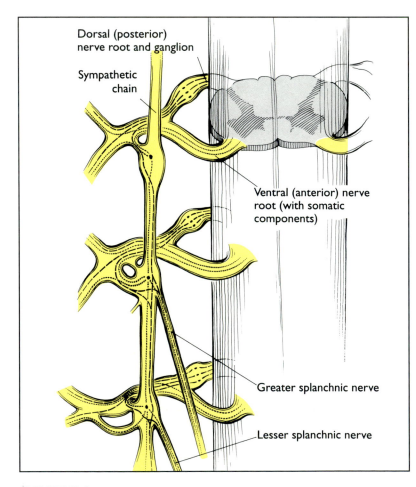

FIGURE 22-1.

The visceral afferent fibers as they arise from the spinal cord.

Dorsal (posterior) nerve root and ganglion

Sympathetic chain

Ventral (anterior) nerve root (with somatic components)

Greater splanchnic nerve

Lesser splanchnic nerve

the splanchnic nerves and the vagi. The plexus constitutes a network of nerve fibers around the aorta at the origin of the celiac axis, the superior mesenteric, and the renal arteries. The lesser splanchnic nerve originates from the tenth and eleventh thoracic ganglia and travels posterior to the greater nerve in the thoracic cavity. After piercing the crus of the diaphragm, it enters both the celiac and adrenocortical ganglion. The third nerve, denoted

the least splanchnic nerve, arises from the twelfth thoracic paravertebral ganglia (may not be visualized thoracoscopically), lies posterior to the lesser splanchnic nerve, and ends in the renal ganglion. These fibers, with or without the sympathetic chain, may be divided bilaterally with little morbidity, and division of these nerves effectively interrupts viscerosensory afferents from the intra-abdominal organs.

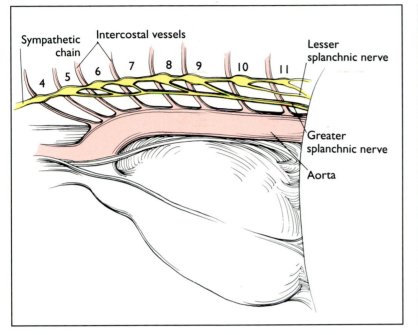

FIGURE 22-2.

Anatomic configuration of the visceral afferent fibers as seen in the left hemithorax.

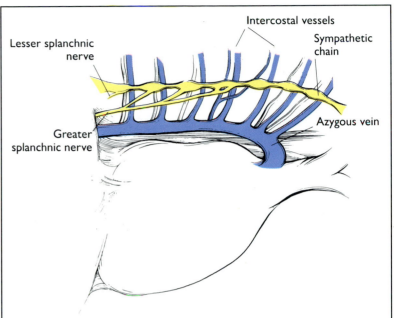

FIGURE 22-3.

The anatomic configuration of the visceral afferents as seen in the right hemithorax.

Surgical Technique

Figures 22-4 through 22-8 depict the surgical technique for thoracoscopic splanchnicectomy.

Set-up

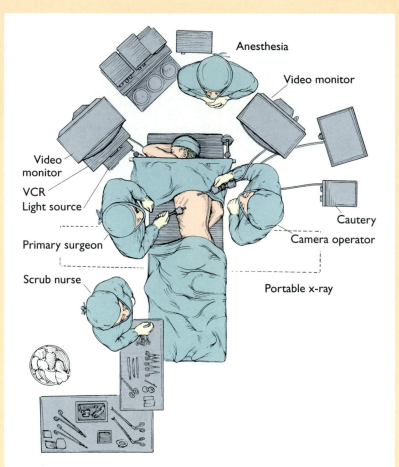

Anesthesia

Video monitor

Video monitor

VCR
Light source

Primary surgeon

Scrub nurse

Cautery

Camera operator

Portable x-ray

FIGURE 22-4.

Operative set-up for left thoracoscopic splanchnicectomy. Preoperative antibiotics are administered in routine fashion. A double-lumen endotracheal tube allows for single-lung ventilation on the nonoperative side. The patient is placed in the right lateral decubitus position on the operating table (for a left splanchnic section) with appropriate cushioning at contact points, the axilla, and between the legs. The positions of the surgeon and first assistant are shown.

Procedure

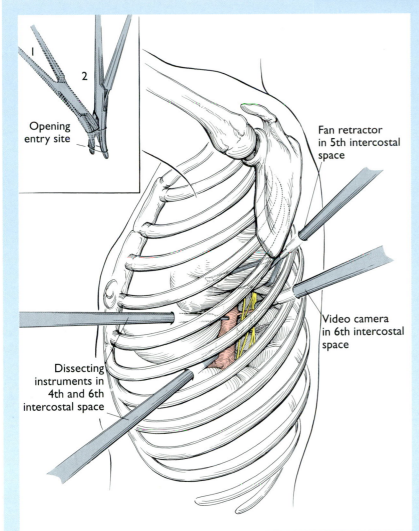

FIGURE 22-5.

The left lung is deflated before instrumentation. Insufflation of the chest is rarely necessary. The first trocar (10 mm) is placed by using blunt dissection through the chest wall in the manner shown to avoid injury to underlying thoracic structures (*inset*). This trocar will serve as the camera port and should be positioned two interspaces below the tip of the scapula. The remaining three trocars are placed under direct vision after insertion of the camera and inspection of the hemithorax for incidental findings. The operating trocars (5 mm and 10 mm) are placed in the 4th and 6th intercostal spaces and located in the anterior and mid-axillary lines, respectively. The larger trocar site is necessary to allow passage of a clip applier to facilitate nerve division. The last trocar (10 mm) is placed slightly posterior to the tip of the scapula, through which a fan retractor is placed to retract the left lower lobe of the lung. The surgeon then passes a grasper and scissors through the operating ports.

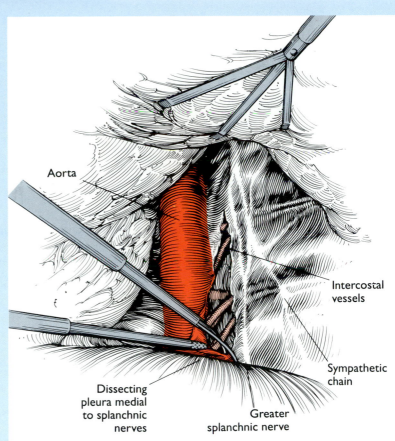

FIGURE 22-6.

The lung is retracted superiorly for exposure and the sympathetic chain (seen overlying and just anterior to the vertebral column), the greater, lesser, and least (may not always be seen) splanchnic nerves are visualized posterior to the aorta and beneath the parietal pleura. A vertical incision of the parietal pleura is made between the aorta and the sympathetic chain and blunt dissection is used to clearly define the visceral branches. A window in the parietal pleura is created by incising the pleura as shown, with care to avoid the intercostal vessels during the dissection. Once dissection is complete, surgical clips should be applied to each branch sequentially. As the nerve fibers become less distinct at the level of the diaphragm, the objective should be to clear all branches between the sympathetic chain and aorta. The sympathetic chain itself may also be divided.

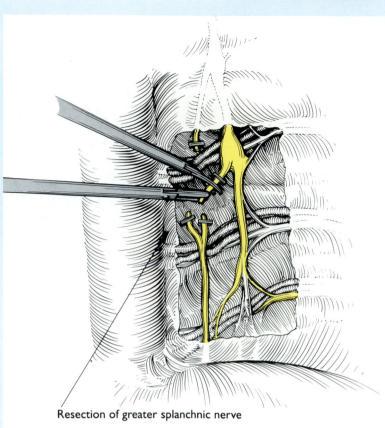

Resection of greater splanchnic nerve

FIGURE 22-7.

The completed dissection allows application of clips and partial resection of each nerve. Clips should be applied away from the intercostal vessels to avoid inadvertent trauma.

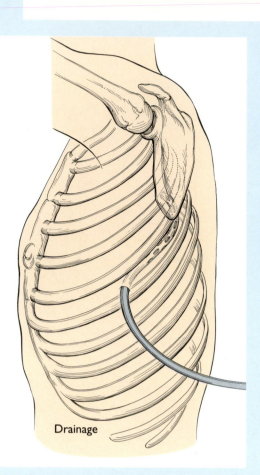

Drainage

FIGURE 22-8.

The trocars are then removed and a small chest tube (20 French) is placed through the anterior trocar site and placed to underwater seal. The lung is then reinflated and the trocar sites closed with sutures.

Results

Pain control is an important component of therapy in patients with benign or malignant chronic abdominal disease, especially when the disease is not otherwise amenable to surgical correction. Analgesics, the mainstay of therapy, often become less effective with time, and opiate addiction may become a significant problem. One option is chemical splanchnicectomy via a percutaneous celiac ganglion blockade. However, this approach is effective in only half of treated patients and has a relatively short duration of action [22–26].

Surgical denervation of the visceral organs via division of their afferent connections to the central nervous system is another alternative in the treatment of chronic abdominal pain. Early reports described left or bilateral splanchnicectomy coupled with celiac ganglionectomy or sympathectomy, with or without division of the vagi [27–31]. Good to excellent pain relief was obtained in up to 60% of cases. In 1990, Stone and Chauvin [32] reported the use of a transthoracic approach to splanchnicectomy. More recently, thoracoscopic techniques have been used to achieve similar exposure without formal thoracotomy (Table 22-1) [13–21]. These reports have described patients with advanced gastric, pancreatic, hepatic, and gallbladder cancers, as well as chronic pancreatitis. Reported success rates have ranged from 60% to 100% of patients with good to excellent pain relief. No deaths have been reported, and morbidity has generally been limited to transient mild postoperative hypotension and easily controlled intercostal neuralgia. This hypotension has been attributed to splachnic vasodilation after nerve transection and is also seen after chemical splanchnicectomy. Caution must be used to avoid injury to the hemiazygous vein or intercostal vessels lying close to the splanchnic nerves. Pain relief has been immediate in all patients. Good to excellent results appear to be somewhat more common for patients with cancer than in those with chronic pancreatitis. The side chosen for splanchnicectomy should depend on the site of the patient's pain. Those with central or left-sided symptoms are treated with left splanchnicectomy, whereas those with right-sided pain recieve right splanchnicectomy. If pain recurs, contralateral nerve resection can be performed. Some authors advocate performing a percutaneous celiac block before surgery to select patients who might benefit from the procedure [16,18].

In conclusion, thoracoscopic splanchnicectomy offers an alternative to open thoracotomy or lumbar incisions for the division of visceral afferents to the pancreas and other abdominal viscera. Accumulating experience with this procedure indicates that it is an effective and safe approach to the surgical management of chronic abdominal pain of either a benign or malignant nature.

Table 22-1. Results of thoracoscopic splanchnicectomy

Author	Patients, n	Indication	Patients with Good to Excellent Pain Relief, %
Cuschieri and coworkers [13]	8	Pacreatic cancer (n=3)	100
		Chronic pancreatitis (n=5)	60
Lin and coworkers [14]	14	Unresectable upper abdominal cancer	86
Takahashi and coworkers [15]	3	Pancreatic cancer	100
Maher and coworkers [18]	15	Chronic pancreatitis	79
Kusano and coworkers [19]	9	Chronic pancreatitis	67
Noppen and coworkers [20]	8	Chronic pancreatitis	63
Le Pimpec Barthes and coworkers [21]	20	Pancreatic cancer	80

References

1. Hearst AF: On the sensibility of the alimentary canal in health and disease. *Lancet* 1911, i:1051.

2. Ray BS, Neill CL: Abdominal visceral sensation in man. *Ann Surg* 1947, 126:709–722.

3. Bingham JR, Ingelfinger FJ, Smithwick RH: The effects of sympathectomy on abdominal pain in man. *Gastroenterology* 1950, 15:18–31.

4. Mallet-Guy PA, Jeanjean R, Sevvettaz P: Distant results in the treatment of chronic pancreatitis by unilateral splanchnicectomy. *Lyon Chir* 1945, 40:293–314.

5. Peet MM: Splanchnic section for hypertension: a preliminary report. *Univ Hosp Bull* 1935, 1:17–18.

6. White TT, Lawinski M, Poland D, Stacher G: Treatment of pancreatitis by left splanchnicectomy and celiac ganglionectomy. *Am J Surg* 1966, 112:195–199.

7. Mallet-Guy PA: Late and very late results of resections of the nervous system in the treatment of chronic relapsing pancreatitis. *Am J Surg* 1983, 145:224–228.

8. Rienhoff WF, Baker BM: Pancreolithiasis and chronic pancreatitis: preliminary report of a case of apparently successful treatment by transthoracic sympathectomy and vagotomy. *JAMA* 1947, 134:20–21.

9. Smithwick RH: Discussion of paper of A.O. Whipple. *Ann Surg* 1946, 124:1006.

10. De Takats G, Walter LE: The treatment of pancreatic pain by splanchnic nerve section. *Surg Gynecol Obstet* 1947, 95:742–746.

11. McDonough FE, Heffernon EW: Chronic relapsing pancreatitis. *Surg Clin North Am* 1948, 28:733–740.

12. Connolly JE, Richards VR: Bilateral splanchnicectomy and lumbodorsal sympathectomy for chronic relapsing pancreatitis. *Ann Surg* 1950, 131:58–63.

13. Cushieri A, Shimi SM, Crosthwaite G, *et al.*: Bilateral endoscopic splanchnicectomy through a posterior thoracoscopic approach. *J R Coll Surg Edinb* 1994, 39:44–47.

14. Lin CC, Mo LR, Lin YW, *et al.*: Bilateral thoracoscopic lower sympathetic-splanchnicectomy for upper abdominal cancer pain. *Eur J Surg Suppl* 1994, 572:59–62.

15. Takahashi T, Kakita A, Izumika H, *et al.*: Thoracoscopic splanchnicectomy for the relief of intractable abdominal pain. *Surg Endosc* 1996, 10:65–68.

16. Strickland TC, Ditta TL, Riopelle JM: Performance of local anesthesic and placebo splanchnic blocks via indwelling catheters to predict benefit from thoracoscopic splanchnicectomy in a patient with intractable pancreatic pain. *Anesthesiology* 1996, 84:980–983.

17. Olak J, Gore D: Thoracoscopic splanchnicectomy: technique and case report. *Surg Laparosc Endosc* 1996, 6:228–220.

18. Maher JW, Johlin FC, Pearson D: Thoracoscopic splanchnicectomy for chronic pancreatitis pain. *Surgery* 1996, 120:603–609.

19. Kusano T, Miyazato H, Shiraishi M, *et al.*: Thoracoscopic thoracic splanchnicectomy for chronic pancreatitis with intractable abdominal pain. *Surg Laparosc Endosc* 1997, 213–218.

20. Noppen M, Meysman M, D'Haese J, *et al.*: Thoracoscopic splanchnicolysis for the relief of chronic pancreatitis pain: experience of a group of pneumologists. *Chest* 1998, 113:528–531.

21. Le Pimpec Barthes F, Chapuis O, Riquet M, *et al.*: Thoracoscopic splanchnicectomy for control of intractable pain in pancreatic cancer. *Ann Thorac Surg* 1998, 65:810–813.

22. White JC, Sweet WH, eds.: *Pain: Its Mechanism and Neurosurgical Control.* Springfield, Il: Charles C. Thomas Publisher; 1955.

23. Copping J, Willix R, Kraft R: Palliative chemical splanchnicectomy. *Arch Surg* 1969, 98:418–420.

24. Gorbitz C, Leavens ME: Alcohol block of the celiac plexus for control of upper abdominal pain caused by cancer and pancreatitis. *J Neurosurg* 1971, 34:575–579.

25. Haaga JR, Kori SH, Eastwood DW, Borkowski GP: Improved technique for CT-guided celiac ganglia block. *Am J Radiol* 1984, 42:1202–1204.

26. Hegedus V: Relief of pancreatic pain by radiography-guided block. *Am J Radiol* 1979, 133:1101–1103.

27. Rack FJ, Elkins CW: Experiences with vagotomy and sympathectomy in the treatment of chronic pancreatitis. *Arch Surg* 1950, 61:937–943.

28. Heisy WG, Dohn DF: Splanchnicectomy for the treatment of intractable abdominal pain. *Cleve Clin Quart* 1967, 34:9–25.

29. Hurwitz A, Gurwitz J: Relief of pain in chronic relapsing pancreatitis by unilateral sympathectomy. *Arch Surg* 1950, 61:372–378.

30. Sadar ES, Cooperman AM: Bilateral thoracic sympathectomy-splanchnicectomy in the treatment of intractable pain due to pancreatic carcinoma. *Cleve Clin Quart* 1974, 41:185–188.

31. White TT, Lawinski M, Stacher G, *et al.*: Treatment of pancreatitis by left splanchnicectomy and celiac ganglionectomy. *Am J Surg* 1966, 112:195–198.

32. Stone HH, Chauvin EJ: Pancreatic denervation for pain relief in chronic alcohol associated pancreatitis. *Br J Surg* 1990, 77:303–305.

*L*aparoscopic Exposure of the Lumbosacral Spine for Discectomy and Fusion

G. Robert Stephenson, Jr

Jeffrey H. Lawson

Fredrick Brody

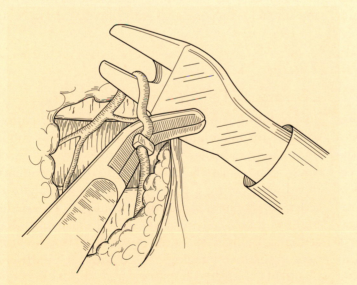

Laparoscopic techniques have advanced over the past 10 years and now include minimally invasive approaches to the lumbosacral spine. This chapter focuses on the development of the anterior laparoscopic approach to the lumbosacral spine for discectomy and spinal fusion. This approach to the lower spine is technically challenging because of the surrounding vascular, neurologic, and visceral structures. Therefore, it is generally recommended that only surgeons with extensive experience in advanced two-handed laparoscopy attempt these procedures.

According to statistics from the National Institutes of Health, approximately 400,000 lumbosacral spinal operations are performed annually in the United States. Several minimally invasive approaches to the lumbosacral spine have been developed to decrease patient morbidity and length of hospital stay [1,2]. These approaches include laparoscopic, endoscopic, percutaneous, and mini discectomy techniques. Although all of these techniques generally decrease postoperative pain and length of hospital stay, only the laparoscopic and endoscopic approaches allow instrumentation of the spine for fusion. The anterior laparoscopic exposure is the most common lumbosacral technique used by the general surgeon. Therefore, this chapter focuses on this approach.

Obenchain performed the first partial discectomy using a laparoscopic exposure in 1991 [3]. Currently, the anterior laparoscopic technique provides exposure for a diverse array of spinal procedures, including discectomy and fusion. However, these procedures have been performed for only about 8 years; thus, the long-term efficacy of this approach compared with that of the standard techniques is not yet available. Both laparoscopic and open techniques are associated with similar rates of morbidity and mortality. All patients undergoing a laparoscopic approach to spinal surgery require long-term postoperative follow-up to allow critical comparison of these new techniques with the standard open procedures.

Advantages of the Anterior Laparoscopic Approach

The anterior laparoscopic approach to the lumbosacral spine has several distinct advantages over the more commonly used posterior approach. The anterior approach avoids cutting through the posterior musculature or ligaments and does not violate the vertebral canal. As a result, the anterior approach produces less postoperative chronic pain and epidural fibrosis. The laparoscopic approach also produces significantly less acute postoperative pain and reduces the postoperative use of narcotics. For a one-level spinal fusion at the L5-S1 disc interspace, the laparoscopic approach is associated with a shorter length of hospital stay and faster return of bowel function; these translate into an overall reduction in hospital costs.

Complications of the Anterior Laparoscopic Approach

The anterior laparoscopic approach is associated with an overall morbidity rate of 5%. The incidence of a major vascular injury is less than 1% in most published series. When the L5-S1 interspace is being approached, the common iliac veins and arteries

must be retracted laterally to fully expose the intervertebral disc. In published series, the most commonly injured vessel is the right internal iliac vein. The median sacral vessels must also be identified and ligated with clips or cauterized with bipolar forceps. When the dissection is carried cephalad, the iliolumbar veins and segmented vessels must also be identified and ligated. Excessive dissection over the sacral prominence can cause troublesome bleeding from the presacral venous plexus. In addition, the parasympathetic nerve chain lies along the prevertebral fascia in a longitudinal fashion. This entire structure should be bluntly mobilized with minimal cautery to avoid parasympathetic nerve injury, which in men can cause retrograde ejaculation. Access to the L1-L2 through L4-L5 disc interspaces requires dissection between the psoas and the abdominal aorta. Along with avoiding aortic injury, the lumbar nerve plexus and ureter must be carefully identified and preserved. Injury to the lumbar plexus as it courses through the psoas muscle can produce neuropathy and chronic pain. Despite these risks, these approaches can be performed safely in most patients if the surgeon providing the exposure is an experienced laparoscopist who is attentive to the risks and familiar with this anatomy.

The most common reason for reoperation after laparoscopic spinal fusion is inadequate discectomy that presents as recurrent pain or radiculopathy and usually requires a posterior stabilization or an open approach for resolution. Another disadvantage of the anterior laparoscopic approach is that the L1-L5 interspace can be approached only from the left side, making some parts of the discs difficult to access. Most published series show excellent clinical results in terms of symptom relief, hospital stay, and return to work. However, randomized controlled trials with long-term data on patient outcome and cost-effectiveness are required to adequately validate the laparoscopic approach to discotomy and spinal fusion compared with the standard open approach.

Patient Selection

Laparoscopic Lumbar Discectomy

The indications for laparoscopic lumbar discectomy are similar to those for microlumbar discectomy. Patients should have predominately radicular leg pain associated with back pain. On physical examination, patients should have evidence of radiculopathy, including a positive result on a straight-leg-raise test, reflex asymmetry, and sensory changes. The patient's clinical findings should also correlate with an ipsilateral disc herniation at the appropriate spinal level, which is best identified by magnetic resonance imaging. If extruded or mildly migrated disc fragments are seen, the patient may still be a candidate for the laparoscopic approach. However, migrated fragments below the level of the disc space are difficult to extract using a laparoscopic approach. An attempt at nonoperative management (physical therapy, analgesic agents, and anti-inflammatory medications) should have failed.

Laparoscopic Lumbosacral Spine Fusion

Patients selected for laparoscopic spine fusion should have a well-documented history of lower back pain commonly associated with leg pain. Nonoperative therapy lasting at least 3 months should also have failed. A pathologic lesion at the L5-S1 disc interspace should be evident and should correlate with a positive provocative computed tomographic diskogram. Many of these patients will also benefit from wearing an orthotic firm brace. Ideally, patients should not be obese and should have documentation of their vascular anatomy, including the bifurcation of the common iliac artery and vein cephalad to the L5-S1 disc interspace. A relative contraindication for this procedure is a history of multiple intra-abdominal procedures or pelvic procedures associated with multiple adhesions and potential distortion of retroperitoneal pelvic structures.

Selection of Approach

The anterior laparoscopic approach is the only minimally invasive anterior approach to the L5-S1 interspace. As mentioned above, the retroperitoneum ends at the pelvic rim, making this disc space difficult to visualize through retroperitoneal endoscopy. For the L1-L2 to L4-L5 interspaces, an anterior laparoscopic approach or an endoscopic approach may be used. The techniques for anterior laparoscopic spinal fusion are fairly standardized and are discussed below. In recent years, however, endoscopic techniques through the retroperitoneum have also proven beneficial. Because the L5-S1 interspace cannot be accessed by retroperitoneal endoscopy, the anterior laparoscopic approach may be preferred in patients requiring fusions at multiple levels in the lumbosacral spine, including the L5-S1 interspace. Most important, regardless of the approach selected, the surgeon performing a minimally invasive spinal exposure must be familiar with the techniques and anatomy involved.

Equipment and Instrumentation

Along with the standard laparoscopic instrumentation, this procedure requires a high-quality video system for identification of small vascular structures sequestered in the retroperitoneal fat. Either a 45° or 30° angled telescope is recommended for adequate visualization of the disc space.

Surgical Technique

Figures 23-1 through 23-7 depict the surgical technique for anterior exposure and fusion of the lumbar spine. The technique presented below is a direct modification of the work described by Sachs and Schwaitzberg [4].

Set-up

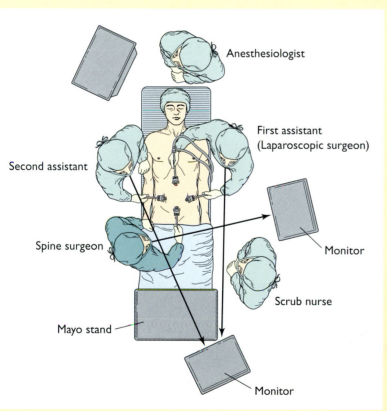

FIGURE 23-1.

Operating room setup for this procedure. The patient is placed in the supine position with slight flexion of the hips and knees. After induction of general anesthesia, a nasogastric tube and a Foley catheter are placed and the patient's skin is prepared and draped from the xiphoid process to the symphysis pubis and laterally to the iliac crests. A radiolucent operating table is mandatory when C-arm fluoroscopy is needed for pin and cage placement. (*Adapted from* Sachs and Schwaitzberg [4]; with permission.)

Anesthesiologist

First assistant (Laparoscopic surgeon)

Second assistant

Spine surgeon

Monitor

Scrub nurse

Mayo stand

Monitor

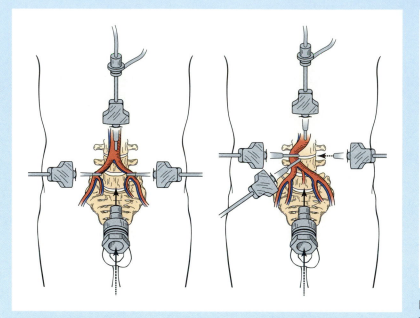

FIGURE 23-2.

A Hasson trocar is placed into the peritoneal cavity via a periumbilical incision. Insufflation of the abdominal cavity with CO_2 gas to a pressure of 15 cm H_2O is initiated, and the table is placed into a 30° Trendelenburg position to facilitate cephalad movement of the bowel. Two 5-mm trocars are positioned lateral to the inferior epigastric artery midway between the umbilicus and the pubis. Retractors are inserted through these ports to retract the bowel from the sacral promontory. Once the L4-5 and L5-S1 interspaces are identified and the vessels retracted, an 18-mm suprapubic port is placed parallel to the desired disc space. A percutaneous Steinmann pin is placed initially into the desired disc place before placement of the 18-mm port. (*Adapted from* Sachs and Schwaitzberg [4]; with permission.)

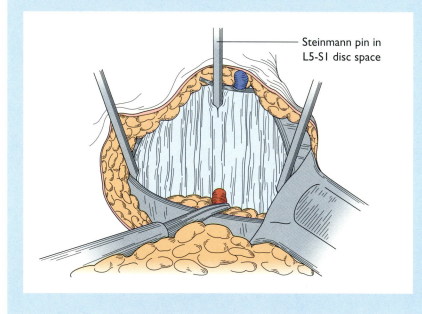

Steinmann pin in L5-S1 disc space

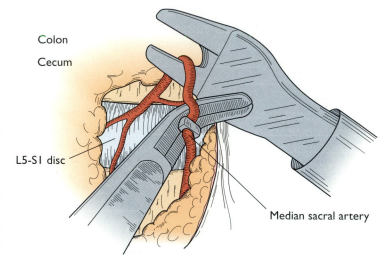

Colon

Cecum

L5-S1 disc

Median sacral artery

FIGURE 23-3.

The sigmoid colon and cecum are retracted laterally to expose the peritoneum overlying the L5-S1 interspace. The peritoneum overlying the L5-S1 interspace is carefully divided. By use of blunt dissection with a Kitner dissector and atraumatic graspers, the retroperitoneal tissue is spread in a longitudinal direction and the iliac and median sacral vessels are identified. Cautery is used sparingly to avoid injury to the parasympathetic chain and the iliac vasculature. The median sacual vessels are ligated with clips or are divided by using bipolar cautery. (*Adapted from* Sachs and Schwaitzberg [4]; with permission.)

FIGURE 23-4.

The dissection then proceeds transversely along the L5-S1 interspace. The annulus is cleaned laterally by using a Kitner dissector to mobilize the left iliac vein and right iliac artery. Steinmann pins are then carefully placed into the L5-S1 interspace, thereby fixing the lateral exposure of the disc to facilitate lateral retraction of these vascular structures. (*Adapted from* Sachs and Schwaitzberg [4]; with permission.)

Procedure

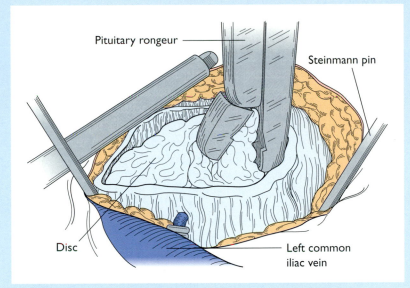

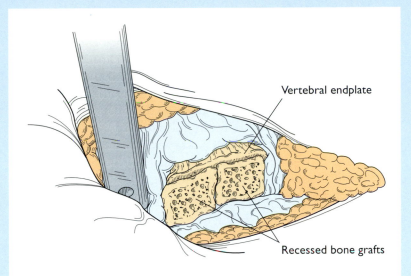

FIGURE 23-5.

The disc is excised by sharply excising the anterior longitudinal ligament and overlying annulus in a box-like fashion. A long modified Cobb is used to release the attachments within the disc space. The released disc is then removed by using a pituitary rongeur. After complete extraction of the disc contents and full distraction of the disk space, the disc space is examined and measured. (*Adapted from* Sachs and Schwaitzberg [4]; with permission.)

FIGURE 23-6.

An autograft of iliac crest bone is harvested and cut to the proper dimensions. The bone graft should be fashioned in a trapezoid shape with a central hole to allow the passage of a single suture within the fragment to facilitate manipulation of the bone graft within the abdomen. The tricortical bone is then placed in the abdomen and inserted into the disc space with the aid of a distractor that is placed in the interspace, followed by a bone tamp. After one bone graft is seated, the distractor is removed and a second bone graft is positioned to fill the remaining space. The suture material that was used to manipulate the bone graft is cut and removed from the abdomen. Along with allograft material, synthetic cages stuffed with autologous bone are being used for spinal fusion. These cages are placed laparoscopically and verified under fluoroscopy. Fusion occurs via the bone graft. (*Adapted from* Sachs and Schwaitzberg [4]; with permission.)

FIGURE 23-7.

The operating table is taken out of flexion, and the Steinmann pins are removed. Hemostasis is verified, and the overlying peritoneum is reapproximated for closure. The fascia of all laparoscopic ports greater than 5 mm is closed by using an exit device. The patient is taken out of Trendelenburg position, and the pneumoperitoneum is released. (*Adapted from* Sachs and Schwaitzberg [4]; with permission.)

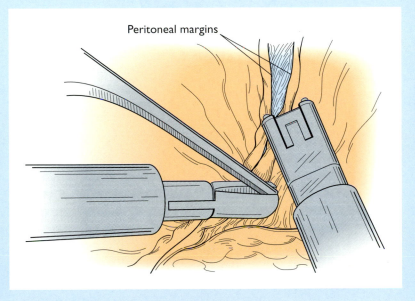

Postoperative Care

After surgery, the patient should wear a premolded plastic orthosis that prevents hyperflexion, extension, and dislodgement of the bone grafts. The nasogastric tube can be removed in the operating room or postanesthetic care unit, and the diet can be advanced as appropriate. The Foley catheter is removed in the operating room or when the patient is ambulating. Patients are discharged from the hospital when they can ambulate without difficulty, tolerate a regular diet, and void without difficulty. Many patients, and particularly those undergoing discectomy, can be released from hospital on the day of surgery. However, it would be appropriate for surgeons new to these techniques to observe their patients in hospital for a longer period.

Summary

Laparascopic exposure to the lumbar spine for discectomy and fusion has shown great promise for reducing postoperative pain and length of hospital stay for patients undergoing operations on the lumbosacral spine. The technique is technically demanding, but in experienced hands it appears safe and beneficial in terms of short-term clinical outcomes. These techniques continue to improve and evolve as expertise grows and technology advances. Ultimately, critical evaluation of long-term patient outcomes will determine whether laparoscopy is the standard approach to the lumbosacral spine.

References

1. Cummings RS, Prodoehl JA, Hermantin FU, *et al.*: Percutaneous laser discectomy using a flexible endoscope: technical considerations. In: *Proceedings of the Eighth Annual Meeting of the North American Spine Society.* San Diego: October 1993.
2. Bonati AO: Arthroscopic nuclectomy. *Am J Arthrosc* 1001, 1:16–22.
3. Obenchain TG: Laparoscopic discectomy: case report. *J Laparoendosc Surg* 1991, 1:145–149.
4. Sachs BL, Schwaitzberg SD: *Lumbosacral (L5-S1) Discectomy and Interbody Fusion Technique: Atlas of Endoscopic Spine Surgery.* St. Louis: Quality Medical Publishing; 1995:275–291.

*L*aparoscopic Staging Pelvic Lymphadenectomy for Prostate Cancer

Robert R. Byrne
Philipp Dahm
David T. Price

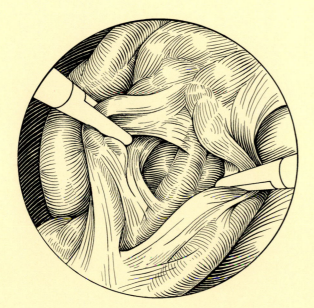

Since the first edition of this text was published, experience with the laparoscope in urology has broadened and matured. Laparoscopic techniques have been reported for many urologic procedures traditionally performed by using open approaches. Clinically established laparoscopic procedures in urology include pelvic lymphadenectomy, varicocelectomy, adrenalectomy, and simple nephrectomy [1]. Schuessler and coworkers [2] are credited with developing the technique of laparoscopic transperitoneal pelvic lymphadenectomy for staging of disease in patients with clinically localized prostate cancer. Subsequently, numerous articles described and reported on modifications of the procedure, in addition to analyzing its complication rate, learning curve, and cost-effectiveness [1]. These authors have concluded that laparoscopic pelvic lymph node dissection is a safe and minimally invasive alternative to open pelvic lymph node dissection.

Indications

Although pelvic lymph node dissection (PLND) remains by far the most commonly performed laparoscopic urologic procedure, indications for pelvic lymphadenectomy in prostate cancer have changed drastically over the past decade and remain controversial. Presumably because of earlier diagnosis, the incidence of positive lymph nodes identified by staging pelvic lymphadenectomy has decreased from approximately 20% to 4% in several retrospective studies [3,4]. Furthermore, refinements in the analysis of preoperative variables have subcategorized patients with clinically localized prostate cancer according to their calculated risk for positive lymph nodes. Such variables as prostate-specific antigen (PSA), clinical stage, and the Gleason score of prostate biopsy specimens have been used to generate nomograms that attempt to preoperatively predict pathologic stage, including the presence of lymphatic metastases (Table 24-1) [5,6]. Consequently, several authors have suggested that pelvic lymphadenectomy can safely be omitted in patients with low risk for extracapsular disease. This concept greatly affects patients undergoing radical perineal prostatectomy or radiation therapy for carcinoma of the prostate [7–11].

There is currently no consensus on the clinical criteria that necessitate pelvic lymphadenectomy. Some recommend performing staging PLND only in patients in whom the probability of identifying metastatic lymph nodes on the basis of probability nomograms is greater than 20% [12]. Rees and colleagues [11] generated a predictive model to identify a subset of patients at low risk for having lymphatic metastases; this model had a false-negative rate of less than 3%. Their model states that lymph-node dis-

Table 24-1. Nomogram for the prediction of pelvic lymph node involvement*

Gleason score	Clinical stage						
	TIA	TIb	TIc	T2a	T2b	T2c	T3a
PSA 0–4 ng/mL							
2–4	0	0	0	0	0	0	–
5	0	1	0	0	1	1	2
6	1	2	0	1	2	2	5
7	–	6	1	2	5	5	9
8–10	–	14	4	5	10	10	–
PSA 4.1–10 ng/mL							
2–4	0	1	0	0	1	1	1
5	1	2	0	1	2	2	3
6	3	5	1	2	4	4	9
7	8	12	3	4	9	9	15
8–10	18	23	8	9	16	17	24
PSA 10.1–20 ng/mL							
2–4	0	2	0	1	1	1	–
5	3	5	1	2	4	4	7
6	–	13	3	4	10	10	18
7	18	24	8	9	17	18	26
8–10	–	40	16	17	29	29	37
PSA >20 ng/mL							
2–4	–	4	1	1	3	–	–
5	–	10	3	3	7	7	11
6	–	23	7	8	16	17	26
7	–	–	14	14	25	25	32
8–10	–	51	24	24	36	35	42

PSA—prostate specific antigen.
*Numbers are percentage likelihood of nodal metastases [6].

section can be eliminated in patients with a PSA level not greater than 5 ng/mL or a Gleason score not more than 5 or a combination of PSA level not more than 25 ng/mL, Gleason score not more than 7, and a negative result on digital rectal examination. In *Campbell's Urology*, Carter and Partin state that laparoscopic PLND is indicated in patients with high suspicion of lymph node metastases on the basis of 1) enlarged pelvic lymph nodes seen on pelvic imaging (when percutaneous biopsy yields negative results or is not done), 2) serum PSA level greater than 20 ng/mL, 3) Gleason score of 8 to 10, or 4) a palpably advanced tumor [13]. Pelvic lymphadenectomy can easily be performed at the time of retropubic prostatectomy with little additional morbidity. However, patients at high risk for metastatic disease, in whom this is the only operation, may be served better by the low morbidity of laparoscopic PLND. Gill and coworkers define this group as patients with a PSA level greater than 40 ng/mL, a Gleason score of 8 or more, clinical stage T2b or higher (bilaterally palpable tumor), or failed or negative computed tomography (CT)–guided biopsy of CT-identified pelvic adenopathy [1].

At our institution, we discuss the probability tables with each patient and the controversies regarding lymphadenectomy. On the basis of these discussions and patient–physician comfort levels, we will perform laparoscopic PLND in patients with a greater than 5% to 10% chance of having positive nodes; in theory, by doing so we miss only about 10% of patients with lymph node metastases. We recommend laparoscopic lymphadenectomy in several scenarios. Before perineal prostatectomy or definitive radiation therapy, we recommend laparoscopic PLND to patients with normal findings on digital rectal examination but a PSA level greater than 20 ng/mL or a Gleason score of 8 to 10 and in patients with abnormal findings on digital rectal examination but a PSA level greater than 10 ng/mL or a Gleason score of 7 to 10. Before retropubic prostatectomy, we offer laparoscopic PLND to patients in whom the likelihood of lymphatic metastases is high and in whom the finding of lymphatic metastases would preclude prostatectomy (PSA level of 40 ng/mL or higher or Gleason score of 8 to 10). Finally, we offer laparoscopic PLND to patients with CT evidence of pelvic lymphadenopathy in whom percutaneous biopsy failed or yielded negative results.

Anatomy

The lymphatic drainage of the prostate usually occurs in a stepwise fashion to the ileopelvic nodes, although "skip" metastases that involve only the more proximal nodal regions have been seen in 14% to 29% of cases [1,14]. The primary landing site for metastases are the obturator nodes, followed by the hypogastric nodes (secondary site), external iliac nodes (tertiary site), and presacral nodes (quaternary site). The common iliac, presciatic, and periaortic nodes are usually involved with more advanced metastatic disease and, occasionally, with skip lesions. The obturator nodes are confined within the retroperitoneal obturator fossa, the borders of which are the external iliac vein laterally, the medial umbilical ligament (obliterated umbilical artery) medially, the pubic ramus caudally, the bifurcation of the common iliac vessels cranially, and the obturator nerve posteriorly. The bladder is medial to the medial umbilical ligament and the ureter courses over the common iliac vessels toward the bladder just cranially to the area of dissection (Figure 24-1).

Pathophysiology, Presentation, and Differential Diagnosis

Prostate cancer remains the principal cancer affecting men in the United States and is second only to lung cancer in causing cancer-related deaths, with 184,500 new cases and 39,200 deaths predicted for 1998 [15]. Adenocarcinoma accounts for most cases [16]. The cause of prostate cancer remains largely unknown: a variety of environmental factors, including heavy metals, dietary fats, and viral agents, have been proposed, and evidence exists for both hereditary and familial forms of prostate cancer. The only definitive factors associated with the development of prostate cancer are the presence of an intact hypothalamic-pituitary-gonadal axis and advancing age.

FIGURE 24-1.

Pelvic anatomy and the suggested incision.

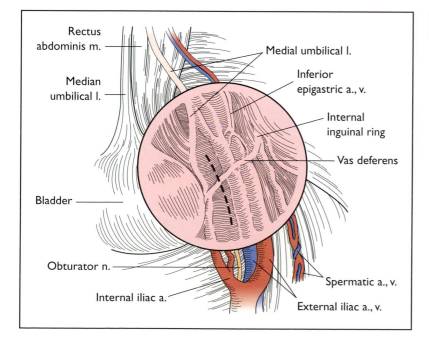

Rectus abdominis m.
Median umbilical l.
Bladder
Obturator n.
Internal iliac a.
Medial umbilical l.
Inferior epigastric a., v.
Internal inguinal ring
Vas deferens
Spermatic a., v.
External iliac a., v.

Prostate carcinoma, when clinically localized, is usually asymptomatic. Clinical symptoms, including low back pain, hip pain, abdominal pain, or hematuria, usually are not present in the absence of metastases. In most patients, prostate cancer is suspected on the basis of either abnormal findings on a digital rectal examination, an elevated PSA level, or both [13]. The differential diagnosis of a palpable prostatic mass and an elevated PSA level are listed in Tables 24-2 and 3. If prostate carcinoma is suspected and the patient is a candidate for definitive therapy, biopsy is indicated to obtain a histologic diagnosis. Biopsy of suspicious nodules should be performed with digital guidance, and random biopsies should be performed (usually sextant biopsies under ultrasonographic guidance) to detect nonpalpable tumors. Once the histologic diagnosis of prostate carcinoma has been established, the patient is evaluated for signs of metastatic disease and is clinically staged.

The extent of the work-up indicated to rule out metastatic disease in patients with prostate cancer is controversial. Because the proclivity of prostate cancer to spread to bones is well known, most urologists have evaluated for bony metastases using history and physical examination in addition to bone survey films or a radionucleotide bone scan before deciding on definitive local therapy. The bone scan is thought to be superior to radiographic survey in that at least 25% of patients with negative bone radiographs will have skeletal disease identified by bone scan [17]. Furthermore, the bone scan provides information on renal function or upper tract obstruction. Some studies suggest that clinical variables, including a negative history of bone pain and a PSA level less than 10 ng/mL, can identify a group of patients in whom bone scan is not cost-effective [18]. However, most believe that the added clinical information and the establishment of a baseline examination justify the bone scan as a preoperative clinical staging tool [13]. Pelvic CT or magnetic resonance imaging (MRI) has been shown to have low sensitivity for identifying lymphadenopathy associated with prostate carcinoma, and routine pelvic imaging is not recommended. The incidence of positive lymph nodes would have to be 32% for CT to be a cost-effective staging tool [19]. Although patients in this risk category could be inferred from probability tables (Table 24-1), Carter and coworkers suggest that pelvic imaging may be warranted in patients with markedly abnormal findings on digital rectal examination, PSA levels greater than 20 ng/mL, and Gleason scores of 8 to 10 [13]. If pelvic adenopathy is seen on CT or MRI, percutaneous biopsy is recommended. If the findings on either of these tests are positive, metastatic disease is confirmed; if findings are negative, pelvic lymphadenectomy is indicated.

Table 24-2. Differential diagnosis of a palpable prostate mass	
Prostate cancer	Granulomatous prostatitis
Benign prostatic hyperplasia	Prostatic tuberculosis
Prostatic infarction	Prostatic calculi

Table 24-3. Differential diagnosis of an elevated prostate-specific antigen level	
Prostate cancer	Prostatic infarction
Benign prostatic hyperplasia	Prostatitis

Surgical Technique

Figures 24-2 through 24-22 depict the surgical technique for laparoscopic pelvic lymphadenectomy.

Set-up

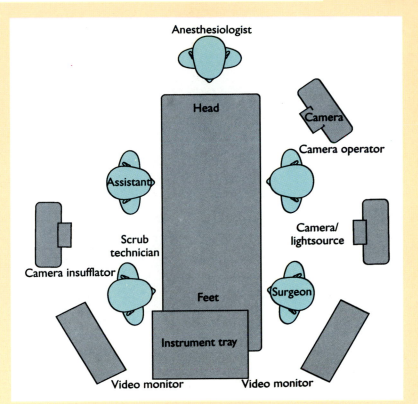

FIGURE 24-2.

Operative set-up for laparoscopic pelvic lymph node dissection (PLND). Two video monitors are positioned on the sides of the table, or a single monitor is positioned directly at the foot of the table in plain view for both the surgeon and the assistant.

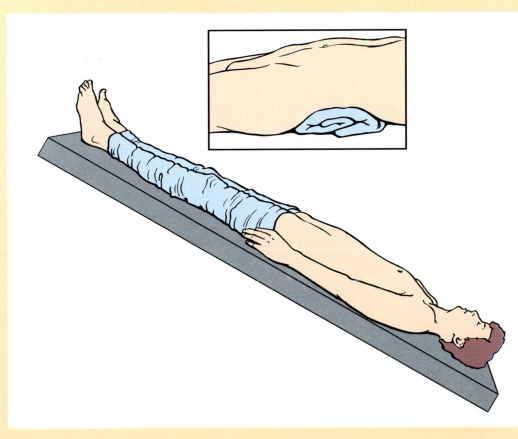

FIGURE 24-3.

A mechanical and antibiotic bowel preparation is administered the day before surgery on an outpatient basis. An antibiotic is administered before initiating the procedure, and both a nasogastric tube and Foley catheter are inserted after induction of general anesthesia. The patient is placed in a supine position. Intermittent pneumatic leg compression devices are used to decrease the risk for deep venous thrombosis. A towel is rolled and placed beneath the lower back (*inset*), and the patient is secured to the operating table with the arms placed along the side of the patient. The table is then placed in a 30° Trendelenburg position and rolled toward the surgeon to help gain better exposure to the area of dissection.

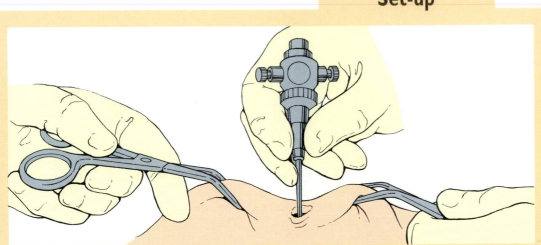

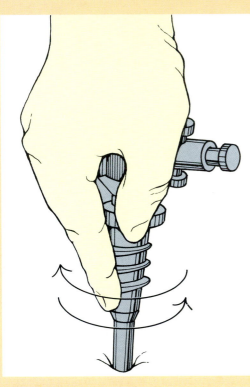

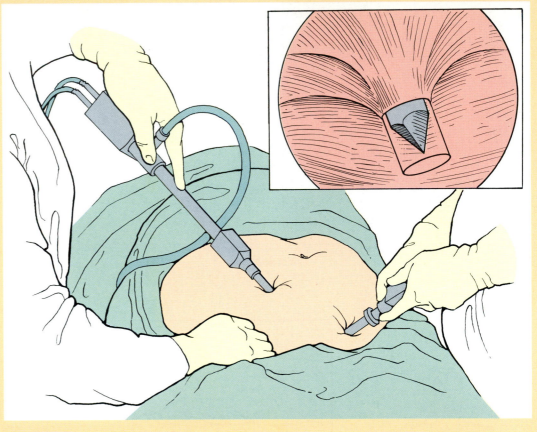

FIGURE 24-4.

Pneumoperitoneum is established by either the closed (Veress needle) or open (Hasson trocar) technique. The Veress needle is inserted through a small incision at the umbilicus at a 45° angle to the abdominal wall directed caudally. In the Hasson trocar technique, the initial trocar is placed into the peritoneal cavity under direct vision, thereby decreasing the chance of significant injury. This technique is useful in patients who have had previous abdominal surgery and are at increased risk for having bowel adhesions.

FIGURE 24-5

After pneumoperitoneum is established with carbon dioxide insufflation to 15 mm Hg, the initial trocar should be placed at the umbilicus as shown. The trocar is held securely in the surgeon's hand with one index finger extended, and with controlled downward pressure and a twisting motion the trocar is forced through the abdominal wall. It is important to have control of the trocar at all times to prevent injury to intraperitoneal structures.

FIGURE 24-6.

Additional trocars and ports are placed under direct laparoscopic vision to avoid injuring intra-abdominal organs. The laparoscope can also be used to transilluminate the abdominal wall to identify the inferior epigastric vessels before trocar placement.

Set-up

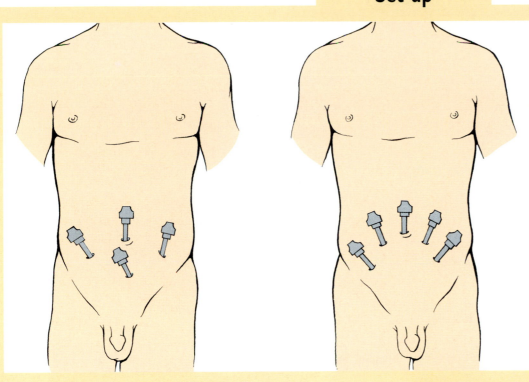

FIGURE 24-7.
The two most commonly used patterns of trocar or port placement for this procedure are the diamond (*left*) and fan (*right*) arrangement. In the diamond pattern, four ports are placed: one 11-mm port at the umbilicus, one 11-mm port in the midline half way between the umbilicus and the symphysis pubis, and two 5-mm ports, one on each side midway between the umbilicus and the anterior superior iliac spine. In the fan configuration, five ports are placed: an 11-mm port at the umbilicus, a 10-mm port on each side at the level of the anterior superior iliac spine, and a 10-mm port on each side midway between the umbilicus and the anterior superior iliac spine. At our institution, the fan arrangement is favored because it allows both the surgeon and the assistant to use both hands to operate and assist during the procedure.

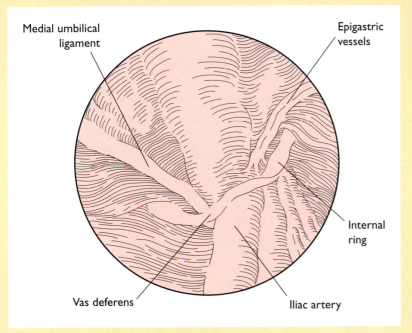

Medial umbilical ligament

Epigastric vessels

Internal ring

Vas deferens

Iliac artery

FIGURE 24-8.
Anatomic landmarks of importance that should be identified before the procedure begins include the bladder, medial umbilical ligament, and iliac vessels. The vas deferens may be visualized coursing medially beneath the peritoneum in some cases.

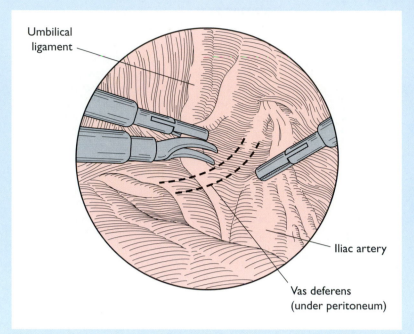

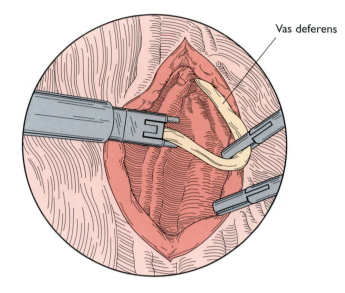

FIGURE 24-9.

The dissection begins over the obturator fossa on the surgeon's contralateral side. The right side should be investigated first unless there is a high suspicion of finding a positive node on the left. It is usually simpler to perform because of the redundancy of the sigmoid colon on the left. The peritoneum is grasped and lifted anteriorly by using an endoscopic dissector, creating a tent in the peritoneum just anterior to the vas deferens. An incision in the peritoneum is made lateral to the medial umbilical ligament extending from the point shown to the pubic ramus using endoscopic scissors.

FIGURE 24-10.

A combination of sharp and blunt dissection is used to identify the vas deferens medial to the iliac vessels and lateral to the umbilical ligament.

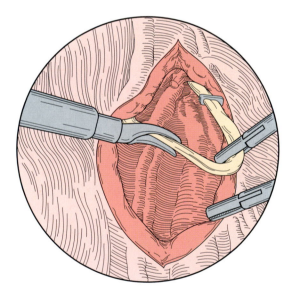

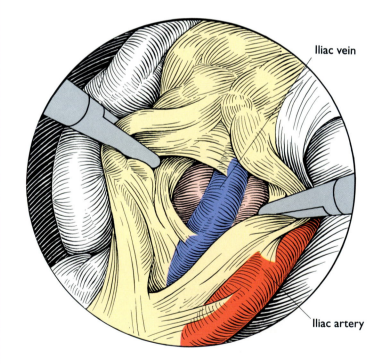

FIGURE 24-11.

The vas deferens is dissected from the surrounding tissues and clipped before it is divided with endoscopic scissors.

FIGURE 24-12.

The nodal fat and nodal tissue is carefully retracted in a medial direction while blunt dissection is used to identify the medial surface of the external iliac vein.

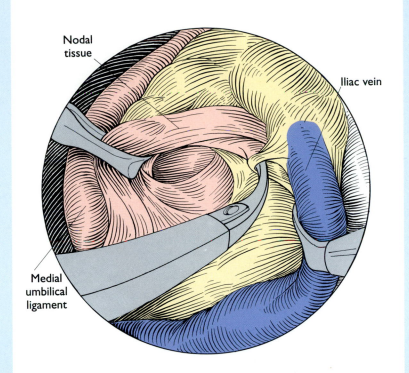

FIGURE 24-13.

After the external iliac vein is identified, a laparoscopic vein retractor can be used by the assistant to retract the vein laterally while the surgeon pulls the nodal package medially and dissects the nodal package off the medial surface of the vein and pelvic side wall. This dissection is continued caudally to the pubic ramus.

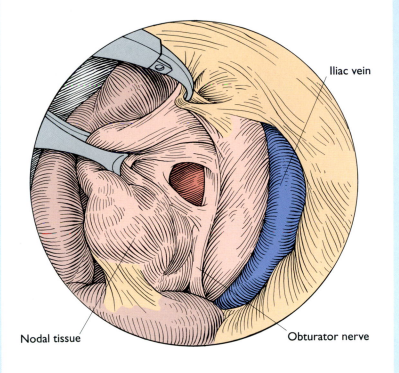

FIGURE 24-14.

The dissection continues caudally toward the pubic ramus and posteriorly down the pelvic side wall by using a combination of sharp and blunt dissection to identify the obturator nerve that is the limit of the posterior dissection. The use of cautery and sharp dissection in this region should be limited to avoid injury to the obturator nerve and vessels.

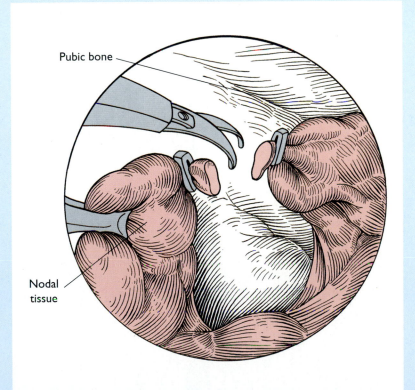

FIGURE 24-15.

The nodal tissue is then bluntly dissected from the pubic ramus and divided between clips. Care should be taken in this region to avoid injury of the aberrant obturator vein.

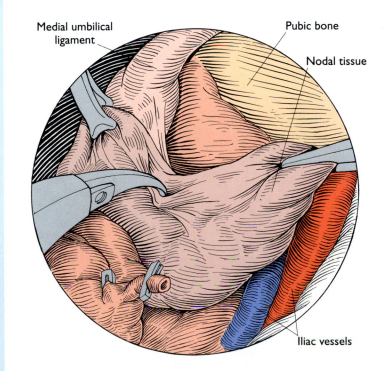

FIGURE 24-16.

The nodal package is then grasped by the assistant and pulled laterally while the surgeon develops the medial limits of the dissection that is just lateral to the medial umbilical ligament.

Procedure

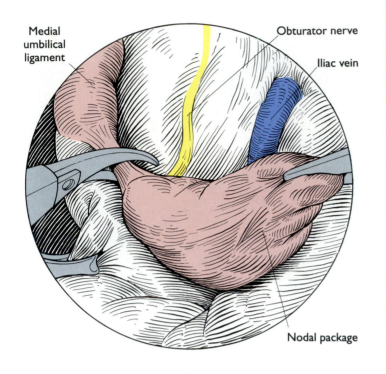

FIGURE 24-17.

The nodal package is bluntly dissected from the medial umbilical ligament and obturator nerve in a cephalad direction by using a gentle sweeping motion by the surgeon as the assistant holds traction in the lateral and cephalad direction. The cephalad limit of the dissection is the bifurcation of the common iliac vessels.

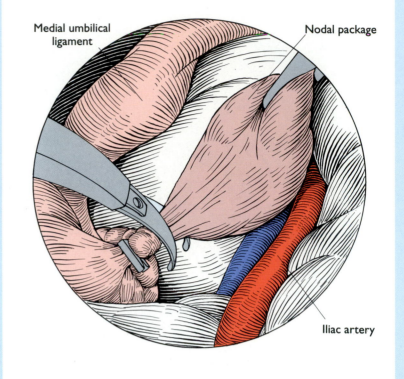

FIGURE 24-18.

Once the cephalad limit of the dissection is reached, the nodal package is divided above a clip. Care should be exercised in this region because of the proximity of the ureter.

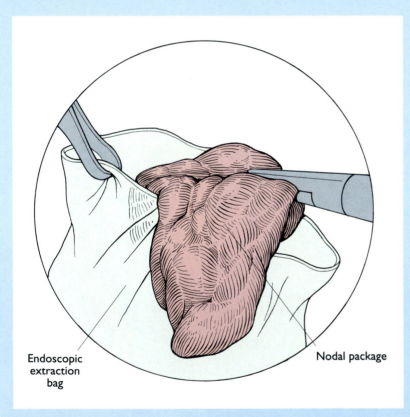

FIGURE 24-19.

The nodal package is placed in an endoscopic extraction bag, as shown before removing from the abdomen. An alternative method of removing the specimen is to use spring-loaded, self-locking, 10-mm spoon forceps to remove the specimen through an 11-mm port.

FIGURE 24-20.

The nodal package contained in an endoscopic extraction bag is removed under laparoscopic vision through a port site.

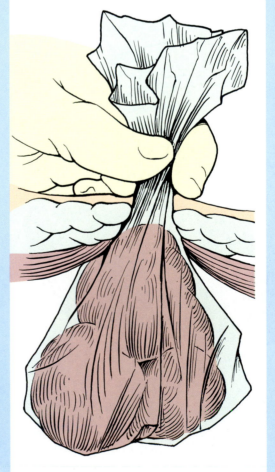

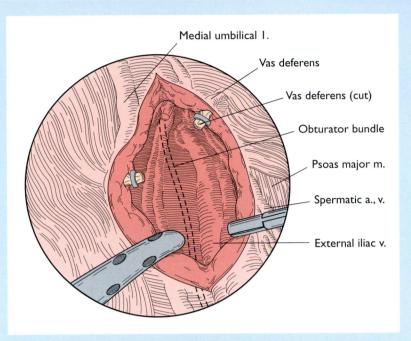

FIGURE 24-21.

The obturator fossa is irrigated with heparinized saline, and pneumoperitoneum is gradually decreased under laparoscopic visualization to identify small bleeding vessels. The procedure is terminated if cancer is detected on frozen section in the specimen from the initial side.

Labels: Medial umbilical l.; Vas deferens; Vas deferens (cut); Obturator bundle; Psoas major m.; Spermatic a., v.; External iliac v.

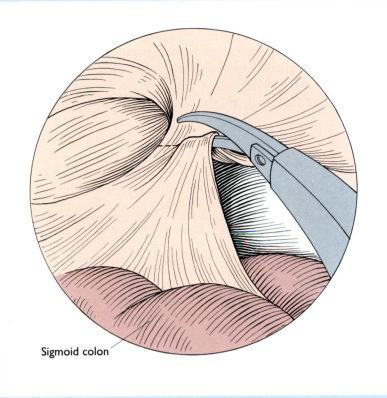

FIGURE 24-22.

Attention is then turned to the left obturator fossa and the procedure is conducted as described for the right. However, the peritoneal attachments of the sigmoid colon may need to be divided to gain access to the left obturator space. If this is the case, the assistant holds medial and cephalad traction on the sigmoid colon while the surgeon incises the peritoneal attachments. Otherwise, the dissection is identical as for the right side.

Label: Sigmoid colon

Several studies have indicated that the laparoscopic approach to pelvic lymphadenectomy was shown to be roughly equivalent to the open approach in the number of nodes retrieved and the node-positive rate [20,21]. Moreover, the laparoscopic approach resulted in decreased blood loss (100 mL compared with 212 mL), earlier resumption of diet (0.6 days compared with 2.2 days), decreased analgesic requirements (1.6 mg of morphine sulfate compared with 47 mg), and decreased hospital stay (1.7 days compared with 5.4 days) [1,21]. As with any laparoscopic procedure, a learning curve is recognized with regard to complication rates and operative times [22,23]. The overall complication rate is reported to be 15%, a rate similar to that seen with open lymphadenectomy, although most complications occurred in early cases [24]. The most common reported complications are listed in Table 24-4 [1,25]. Maneuvers such as inspecting the operative site under low-pressure pneumoperitoneum to identify small bleeding vessels, removal of trocars under direct vision, and the institution of pneumatic compression devices can help to reduce the incidence and morbidity of complications. An extraperitoneal laparoscopic approach has been described, with the theoretical advantages of a decrease in the risk for bowel injury and adhesions, but studies have not been able to demonstrate superiority over the transperitoneal approach [8,26].

Several studies have evaluated the medical economics of laparoscopic PLND and have concluded that the laparoscopic approach remains slightly more expensive than the traditional extraperitoneal operation, primarily because of longer operative times and disposable equipment. However, these studies could not completely include the financial benefits of a shorter convalescence [27–29].

In conclusion, laparoscopic PLND is an option whenever PLND is indicated and open exposure is not contemplated (ie, perineal prostatectomy or radiation therapy) and whenever an open retropubic procedure is contemplated but unlikely (ie, in patients at high risk for metastatic disease who opt for retropubic prostatectomy). Its diagnostic ability is similar to its open counterpart but has significantly lower postoperative morbidity. Its performance is associated with a well-documented learning curve, and the use of

Table 24-4. Complications of laparoscopic pelvic lymph node dissection
Intraoperative vascular injury
Postoperative urinary retention
Postoperative lymphocele or lymphedema
Postoperative ileus
Deep venous thrombosis
Intraoperative bowel or bladder injury

pelvic training devices and animal models is highly recommended until the surgeon has gained sufficient experience with laparoscopic techniques [30]. An experienced laparoscopic surgeon should then proctor the initial attempts at laparoscopic PLND. Several authors have suggested that the procedure can be performed safely and efficiently after approximately 20 to 30 cases [22,23]. Although the indications for pelvic lymph node dissection in prostate cancer management have decreased, patients still frequently fall into intermediate-risk categories. Until noninvasive preoperative methods become better at identifying those with metastatic disease, staging pelvic lymphadenectomy will remain an important procedure in the treatment of prostate cancer.

References

1. Gill IS, Clayman RV, McDougall EM: Advances in urological laparoscopy. *J Urol* 1995,154:1275–1294.
2. Schuessler WW, Vancaillie TG, Reich H, *et al.*: Transperitoneal endosurgical lymphadenectomy in patients with localized prostate cancer. *J Urol* 1991, 145:988–991.
3. Petros JA, Catalona WJ: Lower incidence of unsuspected lymph node metastases in 521 consecutive patients with clinically localized prostate cancer. *J Urol* 1992, 147:1574–1575.
4. Danella JF, deKernion JB, Smith RB, *et al.*: The contemporary incidence of lymph node metastases in prostate cancer: implications for laparoscopic lymph node dissection. *J Urol* 1993, 149:1488–1491.
5. Partin AW, Yoo J, Carter HB, *et al.*: The use of prostate specific antigen, clinical stage and Gleason score to predict pathological stage in men with localized prostate cancer. *J Urol* 1993, 150:110–114.
6. Partin AW, Kattan MW, Subong EN, *et al.*: Combination of prostate-specific antigen, clinical stage, and Gleason score to predict pathological stage of localized prostate cancer. A multi-institutional update. *JAMA* 1997, 277:1445–1451.
7. Bluestein DL, Bostwick DG, Bergstralh EJ, *et al.*: Eliminating the need for bilateral pelvic lymphadenectomy in select patients with prostate cancer. *J Urol* 1994, 151:1315–1320.
8. Kavoussi LR: Techniques for nodal staging in prostate cancer [Editorial]. *J Urol* 1994, 151:1324–1325.
9. Parra RO: Laparoscopic surgery in urology: refining indications and techniques [Editorial]. *J Urol* 1995, 153:1178.
10. Gingrich JR, Paulson DF: The impact of PSA on prostate cancer management. Can we abandon routine staging pelvic lymphadenectomy? *Surg Oncol Clin North Am* 1995, 4:335–344.
11. Rees MA, Resnick MI, Oesterling JE: Use of prostate-specific antigen, Gleason score, and digital rectal examination in staging patients with newly diagnosed prostate cancer. *Urol Clin North Am* 1997, 24:379–388.
12. Moore RG, Partin AW, Kavoussi LR: Role of laparoscopy in the diagnosis and treatment of prostate cancer. *Semin Surg Oncol* 1996, 12:139–144.
13. Carter HB, Partin, Alan W: Diagnosis and staging of prostate cancer. In: *Campbell's Urology*, v 3. Edited by Walsh PC. Philadelphia: Saunders; 1997:2519–2537.
14. McGlaughlin A, Saltzein SL, McCullough DL, *et al.*: Prostate carcinoma: incidence and localization of unsuspected lymphatic metastases. *J Urol* 1976, 115:89–94.
15. Cancer Facts and Figures—1998. Atlanta: American Cancer Society; 1998:1–36.
16. Wheeler TM: Anatomy of the prostate and the pathology of prostate cancer. In: *Comprehensive Textbook of Genitourinary Oncology*. Edited by Vogelzang NJ, Scardino PT, Shipley WU, Coffey DS. Baltimore: Williams & Wilkins; 1996:621–639.
17. Paulson DF, Uro-Oncology Research Group: The impact of current staging procedures in assessing disease extent of prostatic adenocarcinoma. *J Urol* 1979, 121:300–302.
18. Chybowski FM, Keller JJ, Bergstralh EJ, *et al.*: Predicting radionuclide bone scan findings in patients with newly diagnosed, untreated prostate cancer: prostate specific antigen is superior to all other clinical parameters. *J Urol* 1991, 145:313–318.
19. Wolf JSJ, Cher M, Dall'era M, *et al.*: The use and accuracy of cross-sectional imaging and fine needle aspiration cytology for detection of pelvic lymph node metastases before radical prostatectomy. *J Urol* 1995, 153:993–999.
20. Parra RO, Andrus C, Boullier J: Staging laparoscopic pelvic lymph node dissection: comparison of results with open pelvic lymphadenectomy. *J Urol* 1992, 147:875–878.
21. Kerbl K, Clayman RV, Petros JA, *et al.*: Staging pelvic lymphadenectomy for prostate cancer: a comparison of laparoscopic and open techniques. *J Urol* 1993, 150:396–398,discussion 399.
22. Guazzoni G, Montorsi F, Bergamaschi F, *et al.*: Open surgical revision of laparoscopic pelvic lymphadenectomy for staging of prostate cancer: the impact of laparoscopic learning curve. *J Urol* 1994, 151:930–933.
23. Lang GS, Ruckle HC, Hadley HR, *et al.*: One hundred consecutive laparoscopic pelvic lymph node dissections: comparing complications of the first 50 cases to the second 50 cases. *Urology* 1994, 44:221–225.
24. Gill IS, Clayman RV: Laparoscopic pelvic lymphadenectomy. *Surg Oncol Clin North Am* 1994, 3:323–337.
25. Kavoussi LR, Sosa E, Chandhoke P, *et al.*: Complications of laparoscopic pelvic lymph node dissection. *J Urol* 1993, 149:322–325.
26. Das S: Laparoscopic staging pelvic lymphadenectomy: extraperitoneal approach. *Semin Surg Oncol* 1996, 12:134–138.
27. Troxel S, Winfield HN: Comparative financial analysis of laparoscopic versus open pelvic lymph node dissection for men with cancer of the prostate. *J Urol* 1994, 151:675–680.
28. Troxel SA, Winfield HN: Comparative financial analysis of laparoscopic pelvic lymph node dissection performed in 1990-1992 v 1993-1994. *J Endourol* 1996, 10:353–359.
29. Winfield HN, Donovan JF Jr, Troxel SA, *et al.*: Laparoscopic urologic surgery. The financial realities. *Surg Oncol Clin North Am* 1995, 4:307–314.
30. Stewart SC: Pelvic trainer for laparoscopic pelvic lymph node dissection. *J Endourol* 1992, 6:121–122.

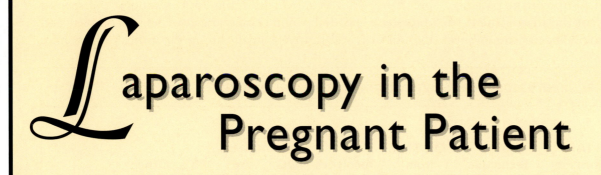

Laparoscopy in the Pregnant Patient

Cleveland W. Lewis
Steve Eubanks

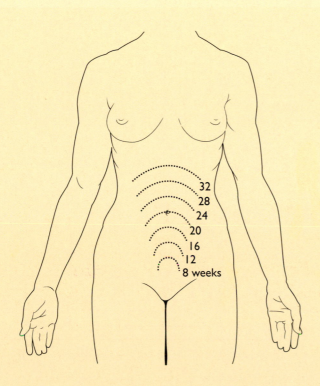

Since the mid 1980s, obstetricians have used laparoscopy in pregnant women as a diagnostic and therapeutic tool. For example, laparoscopy has been used to evaluate acute abdominal pain during pregnancy and has gained widespread acceptance for the diagnosis and treatment of ectopic pregnancy [1]. Nevertheless, general surgeons considered pregnancy a relative or even absolute contraindication to laparoscopic procedures, citing technical difficulty and an increased risk for fetal loss and maternal morbidity [2]. As surgeons became more skilled at performing laparoscopic cholecystectomy and appendectomy in nonpregnant patients, however, they began using laparoscopy in the management of pregnant patients with acute cholecystitis and appendicitis. Weber and coworkers [3] described the first laparoscopic cholecystectomy during pregnancy in 1991, and Schreiber [4] reported the laparoscopic appendectomy technique during pregnancy in 1990. Experienced surgeons have proven that with excellent perioperative planning and proficient technical skills, laparoscopic surgery can be performed safely in pregnant women without increased risks to fetus or mother [5,6].

Appendicitis, cholecystitis, and bowel obstruction are the leading nonobstetric indications for operative intervention during pregnancy [7]. As shown in Table 25-1, although the second trimester is the ideal period because organogenesis is complete and the uterus is still relatively small during this time, authors have

Table 25-1. Summary of reported laparoscopic cholecystectomies during pregnancy

First author	n	Trimester I	II	III	IAP (mm Hg)	Technique	OR Time (min)	Tocolytics	IOC	Spont Ab	PTL	Other
Abuabara	20	2	14	4		V				1*	0	2 CBDE
Adamsen	2	0	2	0				0	0	0	0	
Amos†	4	0	4	0	≤12	H	106	4		2		2 fetal death 2 incomplete Ab
Arvidsson	1	0	1	0	13	V	75	0	0	0	0	
Bennett	1	0	1	0		V		0	0	0	0	
Chandra	1	1	0	0	16	V		0	1	0	0	
Comitalo	4	0	4	0		H	90 (avg)	2	2	0	0	
Constantino	2	0	2	0	10	V	35 (avg)	0	0	0	0	
Csaba	1	0	1	0				1	0	0	0	
Curet‡	12				≤15		82			0	0	
Edelman	1	0	1	0	8	H			0	0	0	
Eichenberg	4	0	0	4	<10	V	70 (avg)	1	0	0	1	
Elerding	5	1	3	1	15	H		0	5	0	0	
Fabiani	1	0	1	0				0	0	0	0	
Hart	3	1	2	0	12	H		0	1	0	0	
Iafrati	1	0	1	0	0	H	<60		0		0	
Jackson	1	0	1	0		H		0	0	0	0	
Lanzfame	5	0	3	2	15	H(4), V(1)	69 (avg)	2	0	0	0	
Martin	3	0	3	0	10	H		0	1	0	0	
Morrell	5	0	3	2		H		0	5	0	0	
Pucci	1	0	0	1	14	H	40	0	0	0	0	
Rusher	1	0	1	0				0	0	0	0	
Schorr	2	0	2	0	15	H		0	0	0	0	
Shaked	1	1	0	0	15	V	50	0	0	0	0	
Soper	5	0	5	0		H(4), V(1)	51 (avg)	0	0	0	0	
Steinbrook	10	3	6	1	<15			1	0	0	0	
Weber	1	0	1	0		V		0	0	0	0	
Williams	1	0	1	0	12	H	65	0	0	0	0	
Wilson	2	0	2	0	12	H		0	0	0	0	
Wischner	6	0	5	1		V(3), H(3)		0	3	0	0	
Total	107	9	70	16		V(36), H(38)			18	3	1	6

Ab—abortion; avg—average; CBDE—common bile duct exploration; H—Hasson; IAP—intra-abdominal insufflation pressure; IOC—intraoperative cholangiogram; OR—operating room; PTL—preterm labor; Spont Ab—spontaneous abortion; V—Veress.
*Spont Ab 2 months post-laparoscopic cholecystectomy after laparotomy for small bowel obstruction related to Peutz-Jeghers syndrome.
†Study also includes patients undergoing laparoscopic appendectomy.
‡No breakdown by trimester for laparoscopic cholecystectomy group.
From Gouldman *et al.* [5]; with permission.

described laparoscopic procedures in all three trimesters of pregnancy [7,8]. Laparoscopy has become an efficient diagnostic and therapeutic tool for the surgeon evaluating patients with acute abdominal pain without obvious signs of peritonitis. Nausea, vomiting, and anorexia in a pregnant patient can present a challenging diagnostic question, and pregnancy can induce leukocytosis, similar to an infectious leukocytic response [9]. Insertion of the laparoscope allows confirmation of the preoperative diagnosis in a manner that is less invasive and does not harm the mother and fetus. The surgeon must carefully plan the operative strategy and work closely with the anesthesiologist and obstetrician to ensure a favorable outcome and to minimize the risk for preterm labor, spontaneous abortion, and maternal morbidity.

Successful outcome in laparoscopy in the pregnant woman begins during the induction period. General anesthesia is initiated via the rapid-sequence method because the gravid uterus creates increased risk for of aspiration (Table 25-2). Every precaution should be made to avoid periods of hypotension during induction. The pregnant patient is placed into a partially recumbent position at the time of induction to avoid venocaval obstruction. This maneuver is especially important in the third trimester, when the weight of the uterus may cause venocaval occlusion. Intensive maternal hemodynamic monitoring is instituted and continued throughout the perioperative period. Some earlier reports advocated mandatory intraoperative fetal monitoring during laparoscopic procedures in pregnant women [7]. At our institution, intraoperative fetal monitoring is used at the discretion of the obstetrician and during advanced laparoscopic procedures (*eg*, laparoscopic splenectomy).

Although some authors have described using the Veress needle puncture technique in the right upper quadrant, lateral to the midclavicular line [6], we uniformly use the supraumbilical open Hasson trocar method. Placement of the Hasson trocar is dictated by the size of the uterus, and the trocar is placed in the midline of the abdomen above the most superior aspect of the uterus. The abdominal cavity is insufflated to a pressure of 10 mm Hg. If mother and fetus remain hemodynamically stable, the pressure is gradually increased to 15 mm Hg. Maternal P_{CO_2} and end-tidal CO_2 levels are monitored during insufflation and throughout the operation. Acidosis during CO_2 insufflation has been implicated as a risk factor for spontaneous abortion and preterm labor after laparoscopic cholecystectomy [11]. Tocolytic agents (usually terbutaline) are given during induction at the discretion of the obstetrician, depending on the clinical status of mother and fetus and the complexity of the case.

Pregnancy is associated with an increased risk for cholelithiasis [12], and the incidence of biliary colic in pregnant women is about 0.05% to 0.1% [13]. Although most surgeons agree that the initial treatment for uncomplicated symptomatic cholelithiasis should be medical therapy [14], surgical intervention must be considered in the face of intractable biliary colic, severe acute cholecystitis, or complications of gallstones, such as pancreatitis [7]. Between 35% and 58% of pregnant patients with symptoms have refractory biliary colic [13,14,], and complications such as gallstone pancreatitis have historically been associated with a maternal death rate as high as 15% and a 60% fetal loss rate [15]. Three to eight of 10,000 pregnant women will require cholecystectomy during pregnancy [16]. The indications for intraoperative cholangiography are no different in the pregnant patient: elevated serum bilirubin level, common bile duct dilatation, or gallstone pancreatitis [7]. The standard laparoscopic cholecystectomy trocar placement is used except that the Hasson trocar is placed under direct vision above the dome of the gravid uterus. From this point, standard laparoscopic cholecystectomy is performed; the surgeon must ensure that the uterus is not touched or manipulated in any manner.

Advantages of successful laparoscopic cholecystectomy in the pregnant patient include less postoperative pain and shorter recovery time, leading to less fetal exposure to narcotics [17]. The patient can resume her regular diet on the first postoperative day, and the reduced immobility after laparoscopy reduces the risk for thromboembolic complications [3,18]. Risk for incisional hernia due to abdominal-wall strain during delivery is minimized with the laparoscopic procedure [18]. Finally, the laparoscopic approach minimizes manipulation of the uterus compared with the open procedure and reduces the risk for preterm labor [19].

Because the standard appendectomy incision is far less traumatic than the open cholecystectomy incision, the advantages of laparoscopic appendectomy are somewhat diminished. However, for the surgeon who is willing to use laparoscopy to evaluate acute abdominal pain in the pregnant patient, laparoscopic appendectomy for acute appendicitis is an excellent option for definitive operative management. Acute appendicitis is the most common nonobstetric indication requiring surgical intervention in the pregnant patient. Approximately 1 in 1500 pregnancies will be complicated by acute appendicitis, and 10% of these cases are further complicated by perforation. The incidence of fetal loss increases sharply from 1.5% in uncomplicated cases to 35% if the open perforation of the appendix has occurred [20]. Again, the open Hasson technique above the dome of the uterus is performed. During the first trimester of pregnancy, the working trocars are placed through stab incisions in the suprapubic region and the right upper and left lower quadrants. In women with more advanced pregnancies, the working trocars are placed higher in the epigastrium, more in the right upper quadrant (Fig. 25-1). Once the trocars are in place, standard laparoscopic appendectomy is performed.

The surgeon must consider several issues during the perioperative period. First, one must decide whether to use a Veress needle or to place the Hasson trocar under direct vision to begin insufflation of the abdominal cavity. The placement of either of these instruments must be tailored to each patient because the height of the fundus continues to increase with fetal growth, reaching the umbilicus by the 20th week (Fig. 25-2). Injury to the uterus, its

---

Table 25-2. Physiologic maternal changes in pregnancy relevant to the surgeon

1. Hyperventilation and earlier onset of hypoxia. This results in more rapid onset of anesthesia and greater necessity for oxygenation.
2. Reduction in cardiac output in the supine position (10% of women). The left partially recumbent position is advisable.
3. Delayed gastric emptying time, increasing the risk of aspiration.
4. Increase in fibrinogen and Factors VII, VIII, IX, and X, with decreased fibrinolysis, increasing the chance of thrombophlebitis.

From Newton [10]; with permission.

vasculature, or the fetus itself has been reported with use the Veress needle [21]. Uterine puncture could also result in uterine insufflation or CO_2 embolism. However, some authors have reported successful use of the Veress needle, especially in the first trimester, by inserting it through the umbilicus and aiming for the right upper quadrant [7]. We prefer placing the Hasson trocar under direct vision just above the dome of the uterus, regardless of the size of the uterus.

Second, manipulation of the uterus during the procedure is to be avoided, and the trocars should be placed such that the uterus does not have to be retracted away from the field of interest. The surgeon must also consider the potential for maternal and fetal acidosis caused by intraperitoneal CO_2 insufflation. Because the fetus absorbs CO_2 from the maternal circulation, maternal and fetal blood pH usually coincide. However, Hunter and coworkers [22] reported a significant delay in the development of maternal acidosis and elevated end-tidal CO_2 levels. Pucci and Seed [23] found no change in maternal arterial blood gas values during CO_2 insufflation for laparoscopy. We have discovered that monitoring maternal end-tidal CO_2 and PCO_2 by using serial arterial blood gas analyses gives the surgical team an accurate view of the pH status of the mother and fetus. If the mother becomes increasingly acidotic during the procedure or if signs of fetal hemodynamic instability appear, the pneumoperitoneum is immediately released. If both patients stabilize, the pneumoperitoneum is gradually increased to previous pressures. If the patient's condition continues to deteriorate or if reinsufflation is not tolerated, the procedure is converted to the open method.

Even though pregnancy was considered a contraindication to laparoscopy just 10 years ago, it has proven to be an excellent option for therapy in pregnant patients with acute cholecystitis and acute appendicitis. Surgeons have demonstrated that both procedures can be performed safely and effectively with little or no increased risk to mother or fetus. With laparoscopic cholecystectomy, laparoscopy has a distinct advantage over the open procedure. As experience with laparoscopy in pregnant patients grows, the indications will continue to expand and the techniques will become more advanced and challenging.

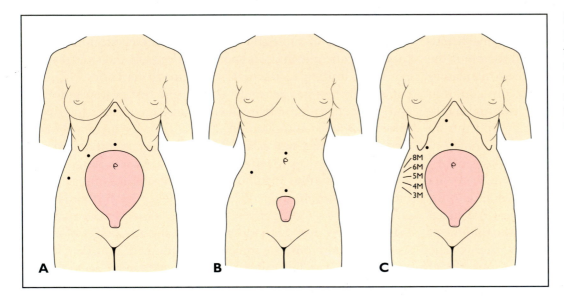

FIGURE 25-1.

Placement of ports for **A**, a laparoscopic cholecystectomy in a women 6 months pregnant. **B**, laparoscopic appendectomy in the early stages of gestation. **C**, Laparoscopic appendectomy at or after the sixth month of pregnancy. Position of appendix vermiformis in different stages of gestation is also shown. (*From* Gurbuz and Peetz [7]; with permission.)

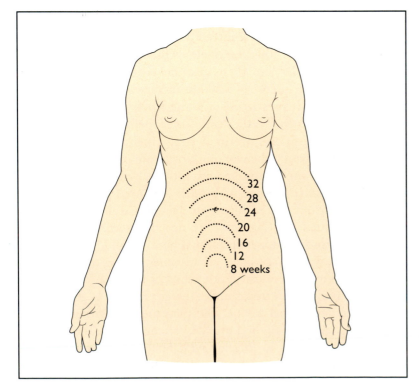

FIGURE 25-2.

Fundal height of the uterus based on gestational age in weeks. (*Adapted from* Lanzafame [6]; with permission.)

References

1. Tarraza HM, Moore RD: Gynecological causes of the acute abdomen and the acute abdomen in pregnancy. *Surg Clin North Am* 1997, 77:1371–1394.

2. Talamini MA, Gadacz TR: Laparoscopic approach to cholecystectomy. *Adv Surg* 1992, 25:1–20.

3. Weber AM, Bloom GP, Allan TR, *et al.*: Laparoscopic cholecystectomy during pregnancy. *Obstet Gynecol* 1991, 78:958–959.

4. Schreiber JH: Laparoscopic appendectomy in pregnancy. *Surg Endosc* 1990, 4:100–102.

5. Gouldman JW, Sticca RP, Rippon MB, *et al.*: Laparoscopic cholecystectomy in pregnancy. *Am Surg* 1998, 64:93–98.

6. Lanzafame RJ: Laparoscopic cholecystectomy during pregnancy. *Surgery* 1995, 118:627–633.

7. Gurbuz AT, Peetz ME: The acute abdomen in the pregnant patient. Is there a role for laparoscopy? *Surg Endosc* 1997, 11:98–102.

8. Schwartzberg BS, Conyers JA, Moore JA: First trimester of pregnancy laparoscopic procedures. *Surg Endosc* 1997, 11:1216–1217.

9. Smoleniec J, James D: General surgical problems in pregnancy. *Br J Surg* 1990, 77:1203–1204.

10. Newton ML, Jr:Gynecologic surgery. In *Hardey's Textbook of Surgery*. Editeds by Hardy JD, Kukora JS, Furs HI. Philadelphia: JB Lippincott; 1988:1306.

11. Bhavani-Shankar K, Steinbrook RA, Mushlin PS, *et al.*: Transcutaneous PCO$_2$ monitoring during laparoscopic cholecystectomy in pregnancy. *Can J Anaesth* 1998, 45:164–169.

12. Simon JA: Biliary tract disease and related surgical disorders during pregnancy. *Clin Obstet Gynecol* 1983, 26:810–821.

13. McKellar DP, Anderson CT, Boynton CJ, *et al.*: Cholecystectomy during pregnancy without fetal loss. *Surg Gynecol Obstet* 1992, 174:465–468.

14. Hiatt JR, Hiatt JG, Williams RA, *et al.*: Biliary disease in pregnancy: a strategy for surgical management. *Am J Surg* 1986, 151:263–265.

15. Printen KJ, Ott RA: Cholecystectomy during pregnancy. *Am Surg* 1978, 44:432.

16. Hill LM, Johnson CE, Lee RA: Cholecystectomy in pregnancy. *Obstet Gynecol* 1975, 46:291–293.

17. Bennett L, Estes E: Laparoscopic cholecystectomy in the second trimester of pregnancy: a case report. *J Reprod Med* 1993, 38:833-834. @Ref:18.   Hart RO, Tamadon A, Fitzgibbons RJ, *et al.*: Open laparoscopic cholecystectomy in pregnancy. *Surg Laparosc Endosc* 1993, 3:13–16.

19. Curet MJ, Allen D, Josloff RK, *et al.*: Laparoscopy during pregnancy. *Arch Surg* 1996, 10:511–515.

20. Kammerer WS: Non-obstetric surgery during pregnancy. *Med Clin North Am* 1979, 63:1157–1163.

21. Barnett MB, Lui DTY: Complications of laparoscopy during early pregnancy. *Br Med J* 1974, 23:328.

22. Hunter JG, Swanstrom L, Thornburg K: Carbon dioxide pneumoperitoneum induces fetal acidosis in a pregnant ewe model. *Surg Endosc* 1995, 9:272–279.

23. Pucci RO, Seed RW: Case report of laparoscopic cholecystectomy in the third trimester of pregnancy. *Am J Obstet Gynecol* 1991, 165:401–402.

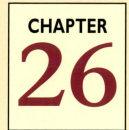

*L*aparoscopic-assisted Vaginal Hysterectomy With or Without Removal of the Adnexae

Mark W. Onaitis

John T. Soper

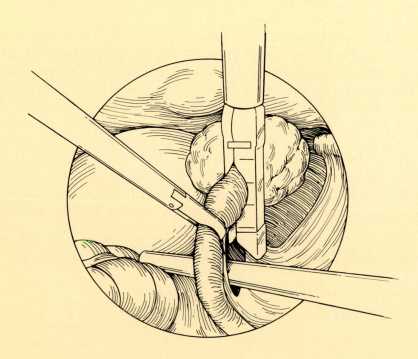

Although vaginal hysterectomies were described before the 18th century, it was not until the middle 19th century that the first successful abdominal hysterectomy was reported with survival of the patient [1]. Until the late 19th century, abdominal hysterectomy was rarely performed and remained an extremely morbid procedure until the principles of sterile technique, ligature of vascular pedicles for hemostasis, and basic anesthesia were widely applied in the 1890s and early 20th century. Initially, vaginal hysterectomy was more frequently performed than abdominal hysterectomy, but improvements in anesthetic techniques, antibiotics, and blood transfusion services in the mid-20th century, along with changing indications for hysterectomy, have resulted in a relative increase in the number of abdominal hysterectomies compared with vaginal hysterectomies.

Laparascopy has been widely used by obstetricians and gynecologists in the United States since the late 1960s for diagnostic purposes and for tubal sterilizations [2]. Until the development of videolaparoscopy, however, surgical procedures were generally limited to lysis of pelvic adhesions, fulguration of endometriosis, and simple procedures on adnexal structures.

Reich and coworkers [3] described the first laparoscopically assisted vaginal hysterectomy (LAVH) in 1989. Since this initial report, many anecdotal reports of LAVH using various techniques and instrumentation have appeared. It is only recently that series of patients have been reported rather than case reports; however, LAVH was widely embraced by gynecologists before the procedure was subjected to critical analysis in the literature. The use of laparoscopy along with a vaginal removal of the uterus would seem to yield many of the benefits of an abdominal approach without the morbidity of an abdominal incision and preserve the advantages of a vaginal approach. The purported benefits of LAVH are presented in Table 26-1.

Anatomy

The gynecologic anatomy pertinent to performance of the laparoscopic portion of LAVH will be considered; detailed gynecologic anatomy is presented elsewhere. Figure 26-1 depicts the gynecologic organs as viewed through the laparoscope. The uterus is situated between the bladder (anterior) and the rectosigmoid (posterior). The parietal peritoneum is applied directly to the uterus, fallopian tubes, and ovaries with little intervening adventitia. It reflects anteriorly over the bladder forming the anterior cul de sac, and posteriorly over the upper vagina onto the rectosigmoid forming the posterior cul de sac. Within loose areolar tissues along the endopelvic fascial planes are the potential vesicovaginal and rectovaginal spaces.

Lateral reflections of the visceral peritoneum applied to the adnexae and round ligaments bilaterally form the broad ligament. Condensations of perivascular fascia form the round ligaments. These pass anterolaterally from the anterior uterine cornu to exit the pelvis through the internal iliac rings. Sampson's artery, an anastomotic vessel arising from the uterine vasculature, accompanies the round ligament, and must be controlled when the round ligament is divided.

The anterior leaf of the broad ligament is the flat expanse of peritoneum extending from the round ligament to the bladder. The middle leaf of the broad ligament is the triangular portion of peritoneum bound by the round ligament anteriorly, the tube and infundibulopelvic ligament medially, and the pelvic sidewall laterally. When the anterior and middle leaves of the broad ligament are opened, the underlying loose areolar tissue can be easily dissected to expose the pelvic sidewall and retroperitoneal structures. The medial leaf of the broad ligament extends posterior to the fallopian tube, ovary, and infundibulopelvic ligament. In Figure 26-1, the peritoneum of the medial leaf of the left broad ligament has been removed to illustrate the relationships of the ureter, infundibulopelvic ligament, and uterine artery. The ureter is loosely adherent to the medial leaf of the broad ligament throughout its course through the pelvis and can be readily visualized through the peritoneum by the laparoscope. The posterior boundary of the medial leaf is formed by the uterosacral ligaments, which extend posterior from the lateral cervix, lateral to the rectum, to insert into the sacrum as the posterior rectal pillars.

The dominant uterine blood supply is from the uterine arteries that are anterior branches of the hypogastric (internal iliac) arteries. Each uterine artery rises and courses anteromedially, crossing anterior to the ureter approximately 2 cm lateral to the cervix. It divides into ascending branches, which supply the uterine fundus and anastomose with vessels from the mesosalpinx, and descending cervicovaginal branches. The uterine veins coalesce and descend as a plexus that drain into the hypogastric vein.

The vascular adventitia of the uterine vessels condense to form the cardinal ligament, which traverses laterally and pro-

Table 26-1. Purported advantages of laparoscopically assisted vaginal hysterectomy versus abdominal or vaginal hysterectomy

LAVH vs. vaginal hysterectomy	LAVH vs. abdominal hysterectomy
Superior visualization of abdominal contents	Abdominal incision avoided
Reliable removal of adnexae	Reduced ileus
Surgical approach to adhesions, endometriosis, and adnexal pathology	Reduced infectious morbidity
	Reduced postoperative adhesions
	Concomitant repair of vaginal relaxation
	Reduced hospital stay and convalescence

vides major lateral support to the uterine cervix. The ureter passes posterior to the uterine artery within the ureteric tunnel through the cardinal ligament (Figure 26-1).

The ovarian blood supply descends into the pelvis within the infundibulopelvic ligament. The ovarian arteries are direct branches from the aorta. The right ovarian vein drains into the inferior vena cava, while the left ovarian vein drains into the left renal vein. The ovarian artery continues medially forming the arcade of the mesosalpinx and terminates in anastomoses with ascending branches of the uterine artery adjacent to the uterine cornu. The ovaries are supported medially by the utero-ovarian ligaments.

The ureter enters the pelvis at approximately the level of the bifurcation of the common iliac artery in close proximity to the infundibulopelvic ligament. The pelvic ureter courses anterior and medial in a shallow arc. It is applied loosely to the medial leaf of the broad ligament and enters the ureteric tunnel under the uterine artery as previously described (Figure 26-1). The most common sites of injury to the ureter during hysterectomy are at the level of the uterine artery and at the level of the infundibulopelvic ligament. It is imperative that the ureter be isolated and visualized at all times during ligation of these structures.

Indications

A variety of disease processes are amenable to this hysterectomy [1]. It is beyond the scope of this chapter to discuss the pathophysiology of each of these. However, as in the use of any surgical technique, it is imperative that the surgeon be thoroughly familiar with the disease processes that might constitute indications for LAVH and have a thorough knowledge of the therapeutic options. It should be emphasized that it is inappropriate to use LAVH when a simple vaginal hysterectomy is indicated [4]. The major advantage to the use of LAVH lies in the potential to convert procedures that might otherwise be performed by laparotomy into vaginal procedures. A partial listing of both cervicouterine and adnexal diseases that might be approached with this technique appears in Table 26-2.

A normal uterus is often removed in conjunction with removal of adnexal pathology, particularly in women who do not desire to retain fertility or who are perimenopausal [1]. Conversely, elective removal of normal fallopian tubes and ovaries is often performed in conjunction with hysterectomy in perimenopausal women. In general, the lifetime risk of developing ovarian cancer in a retained ovary is approximately 1.5% at age 40 and increases threefold in women with a family history of ovarian cancer, but rare families may have a much higher risk for ovari-

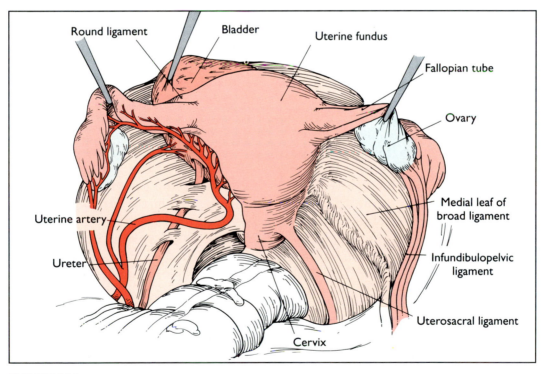

FIGURE 26-1.

Idealized laparoscopic view of the gynecologic pelvis. The medial leaf of the broad ligament has been removed to illustrate the relationships of the ureter, infundibulopelvic ligament, and uterine artery.

Table 26-2. Partial listing of indications for laparoscopically assisted vaginal hysterectomy	
Refractory dysfunctional uterine bleeding	Endometriosis
Adenomyosis	Refractory cervical dysplasia
Uterine leiomyomas	Endometrial adenomatous hyperplasia
Chronic pelvic inflammatory disease	Benign adnexal masses and ovarian neoplasms

an cancer among women. This risk and the risk of subsequent surgery for benign disease in a retained adnexum must be weighed against the risk of surgical castration of the patient and the need for estrogen replacement therapy in pre-menopausal women [1].

Relative contraindications for LAVH including the following: 1) Invasive cervical cancer: in these patients, radical surgery or radiation is appropriate, while simple hysterectomy of any type is generally inadequate therapy [1,5]. 2) Endometrial cancer: although usually treated with hysterectomy, this disease is surgically staged [5]. While the efficacy of laparoscopic staging of endometrial cancer is currently being evaluated [6], it often includes performance of pelvic and para-aortic lymphadenectomy, procedures that are beyond the capabilities of most laparoscopic surgeons. 3) Pelvic masses that are suspicious for ovarian cancer or are larger than approximately 6 to 8 cm in diameter: similar to patients with endometrial cancer, patients with early ovarian cancers usually require comprehensive staging laparatomies, including pelvic and para-aortic lymphadenectomies [5]. Furthermore, intra-abdominal rupture of an early ovarian malignancy increases the stage and may adversely affect survival [5]. Finally, management of advanced ovarian cancer is based on the principle of maximal tumor debulking at primary surgery [5]. Table 26-3 provides criteria that may aid in the identification of benign pelvic masses.

Surgical Technique

Several types of LAVH techniques have been reported, ranging in scope from simply using laparoscopy to confirm the feasibility of vaginal hysterectomy, to procedures that use laparoscopic ligation of all vascular pedicles and ligaments, development of the bladder flap, and entry into the vagina, leaving only removal of the uterus for the vaginal portion of the procedure [7]. We teach and use a modified LAVH technique: laparoscopic dissection is used to lyse adhesions, control the round ligaments, open the pelvic sidewall and control the infundibulopelvic ligament or utero-ovarian ligament and tube, and partially develop the bladder flap. The procedure is then converted to a standard vaginal hysterectomy with ligation of the uterosacral ligaments, cardinal ligaments, and uterine vessels

vaginally. We believe that this is the safest technique to learn and teach to physicians who do not have advanced laparoscopic skills. It avoids the potential for ureteral injury caused when endoscopic staplers or electrocautery are used for laparoscopic control of the uterine vessels [8].

Patients receive a mechanical bowel prep with clear liquids, magnesium citrate for 2 days before surgery, and perioperative prophylactic antibiotics. The patient is positioned in a modified lithotomy position using the candycane stirrups with the hips flexed 30° to 45°. The arms are tucked at the patient's sides. The vagina and perineum are sterilely prepped and draped but excluded from the abdominal field. A Foley catheter and uterine manipulator are placed. Figure 26-2 illustrates the operating room set-up that we use for LAVH. We usually use two lateral video monitors so that both the surgeon and assistant have an unobstructed view of the operation. An alternative placement of a single monitor at the foot of the operating table is also illustrated.

Peritoneal access is performed with a 10-mm sheath placed infraumbilically using closed (direct insertion and Veress needle) or open (Hasson trocar) techniques (Figure 26-3). CO_2 is insufflated with a high-flow (> 3 L/min) insufflator at pressures < 15 mm Hg. The laparoscope is inserted and upper abdominal contents are visualized. The patient is placed in 20° to 30° Trendelenburg position for visualization of the pelvic structures.

Additional sheaths are placed under laparoscopic guidance with transabdominal illumination and avoidance of the major vessels at the sites indicated in Figure 26-3. Two 5-mm sheaths are placed approximately 3 to 4 cm medial to and slightly above the level of the anterior superior iliac crests. The inferior epigastric vessels should be avoided when these sheaths are being placed. A 12-mm sheath is usually placed in the suprapubic location if endoscopic staplers or clips are to be used.

If additional exposure is required or a large uterus is encountered, the 12-mm trocar may be placed either above or below the umbilicus or an additional sheath may be placed at these sites (Figure 26-3). If these placements are used, the sheaths should be placed just off the midline to avoid interference between the instruments and the laparoscope.

The bowel is manipulated out of the pelvis with atraumatic forceps and the probe. Adhesions are taken down sharply

Table 26-3. Preoperative criteria suggesting benign pelvic mass	
Diameter < 7 cm	No evidence of ascites
Unilocular, simple cyst on ultrasound	Serum CA 125, < 35 μ/mL
Unilateral lesion	

(Figure 26-4) with endoscopic scissors. Electrocautery should not be used on adhesions involving the bowel. The course of each pelvic ureter should be visualized through the medial leaf of the broad ligament, and its relative position should be verified during each portion of the procedure.

The uterus is placed on lateral traction, and the round ligament on each side is elevated and divided with the endoscopic scissors using monopolar electrocautery (Figure 26-5) or divided after bipolar cautery with the Kleppinger forceps. The principles of traction-countertraction are used throughout the procedure. Although one operator can serve as the primary surgeon and the other as the camera operator/assistant, it is often easier for the two to alternate functions and serve as the primary surgeon for procedures on the opposite side of the pelvis.

The peritoneum of the broad ligament is opened lateral to the fallopian tube and infundibulopelvic ligament (Figure 26-6). Medial traction on the utero-ovarian ligament or ovary using atraumatic graspers and the use of endoscopic scissors with monopolar cautery expedite the dissection. The peritoneal incision parallels the tube and is lateral to the ovarian vessels. If salpingo-oophorectomy is to be performed, the peritoneal incision is extended cephalad, parallel to the infundibulopelvic ligament. The loose areolar tissue within the broad ligament and the pelvic sidewall are opened by blunt dissection. Occasional small perforators can be controlled with electrocautery. The ureter will remain adherent to the middle leaf of the broad ligament.

When salpingo-oophorectomy is performed, a window is created with endoscopic scissors above the level of the ureter in the middle leaf of the broad ligament (Figure 26-7). This extends from the infundibulopelvic ligament to approximately the uterine vessels. Electrocautery may be required to control bleeding from small vessels.

Ligation of the infundibulopelvic ligament can be performed with the endoscopic stapler by using the vascular staples. The instrument is placed through the 12-mm suprapubic port (Figure 26-8). The open stapler is advanced across the infundibulopelvic ligament though the window in the broad ligament. By closing the stapler and gently lifting the infundibulopelvic ligament before firing the stapler, the surgeon can ensure that the tips of the stapler are free, and the ureter is isolated from the pedicle (Figure 26-8).

An alternative technique using electrocautery with the bipolar Kleppinger forceps is illustrated in Figures 26-9A through 26-9C. The infundibulopelvic ligament is divided with endoscopic scissors after electrodesiccation (Figures 26-9A, 26-9B). Care must be taken to ensure that the ureter is at least 2 to 3 cm from the point of cautery. Additional assurance of hemostasis can be obtained by grasping the infundibulopelvic ligament through an open endoscopic loop suture (Figure 26-9B) as it is being divided. The endoscopic loop suture is then secured around the proximal pedicle (Figure 26-9C).

If the adnexae are to be preserved, the endoscopic stapler is passed through the suprapubic sheath and used to divide the utero-ovarian ligament and tube (Figure 26-10) using either the vascular or the tissue cartridge. The round ligament should be excluded from this pedicle and a tissue sizer used to determine the correct cartridge.

The fallopian tube/utero-ovarian ligament pedicle can also be divided after bipolar electrodesiccation with the Kleppinger forceps (Figure 26-11). The ureter is less likely to be damaged at this location than when the infundibulopelvic ligament is being divided.

The peritoneum and loose areolar tissues of the anterior leaf of the broad ligament and anterior peritoneal reflection of the uterus are opened with the endoscopic scissors using monopolar electrocautery for hemostasis (Figures 26-12 and 26-13). The bladder is reflected anteriorly with atraumatic forceps, and the bladder flap is developed with sharp dissection using monopolar electrocautery for hemostasis (Figure 26-13). Extensive mobilization of the bladder is not required because this will be completed during the vaginal phase of the procedure. The uterus should be elevated and directed toward the posterior pelvis during dissection of the bladder flap.

The instruments are removed from the sheaths and the patient repositioned in the lithotomy position with the hips flexed 45°. The uterine manipulator is removed. Hysterectomy is completed with a standard vaginal hysterectomy technique [1] and the vaginal cuff is closed. After completion of the hysterectomy, the peritoneal cavity is insufflated with CO_2 and the laparoscope reinserted to inspect all pedicles for hemostasis. The large fascial defects caused by 10- to 12-mm trocars should be closed to prevent hernia formation. The skin incisions are closed with subcuticular sutures of absorbable material.

Set-up

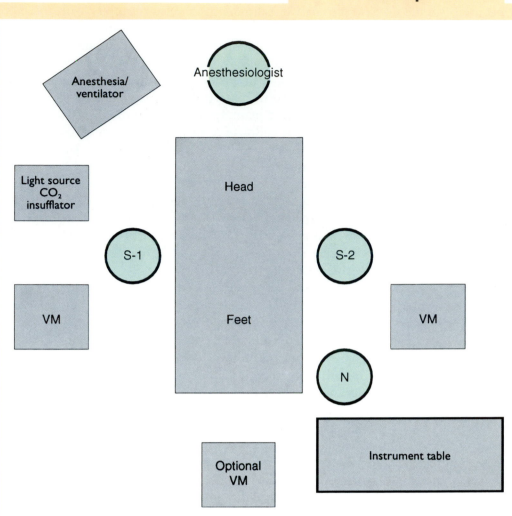

FIGURE 26-2.

Operating room set-up for laparoscopic-assisted vaginal hysterectomy. S-1—primary surgeon; S-2—surgical assistant; VM—video monitor; N—scrub nurse.

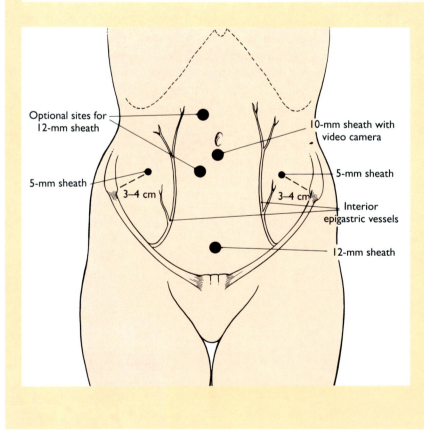

FIGURE 26-3.

Sites for placement of laparoscopic sheaths. If additional or superior placement of a 12-mm sheath is required, it should be positioned lateral to the midline to avoid interference with the laparoscope.

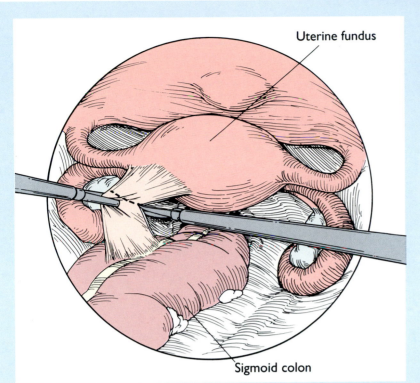

FIGURE 26-4.

Adhesions involving pelvic structures are frequently encountered. Adhesions involving the bowel should be taken down with sharp dissection, avoiding electrocautery.

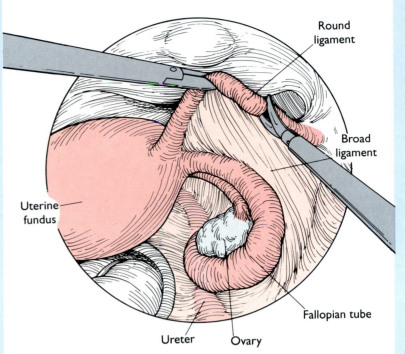

FIGURE 26-5.

Division of the round ligament using monopolar electrocautery and endoscopic scissors.

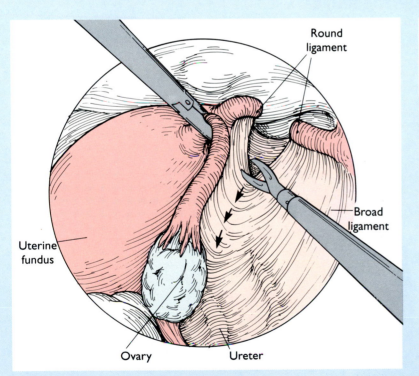

FIGURE 26-6.

Opening the peritoneum of the broad ligament lateral to fallopian tubes and infundibulopelvic ligament with endoscopic scissors.

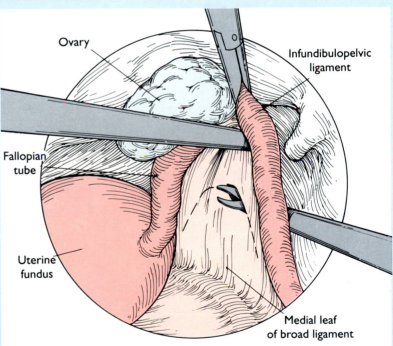

FIGURE 26-7.

Creating a window in the medial leaf of the broad ligament above the level of the ureter with endoscopic scissors. The peritoneal incision can be initiated with either a lateral approach, as shown, or with a medial approach and incising the peritoneum. In either case, the window is created only after the pelvic ureter is visualized. The peritoneal incision is extended from the infundibulopelvic ligament to the uterine arteries.

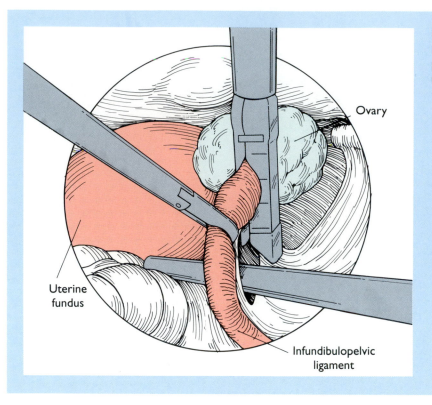

FIGURE 26-8.
Ligation and division of the infundibulopelvic ligament with an endoscopic stapler. A vascular cartridge is required in almost all cases when this technique is used. Illustration is of the right side.

Alternative Procedure

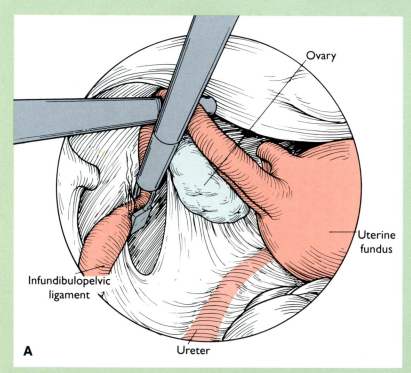

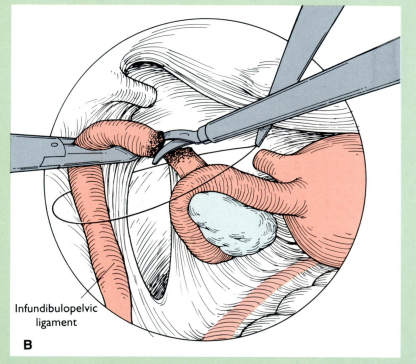

FIGURE 26-9.
Alternative technique using electrodesiccation with bipolar Kleppinger forceps (*panel A*) and division of the infundibulopelvic ligament with endoscopic scissors (*panel B*). Additional hemostasis may be obtained with an endoscopic loop suture applied to the proximal pedicle (*panels B and C*). (*Continued*)

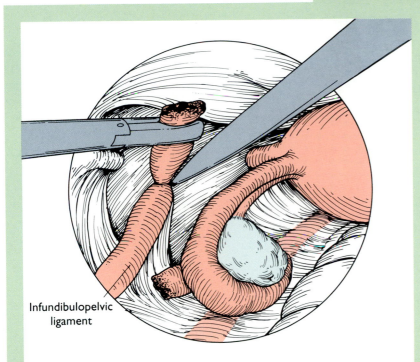

FIGURE 26-9. (*Continued*)
Illustration is of the left side.

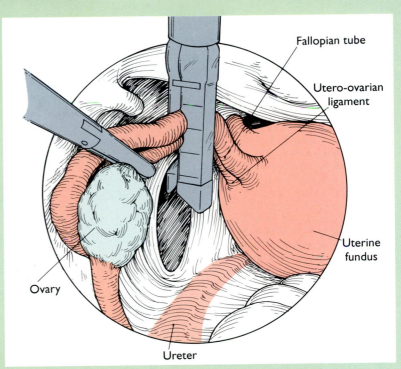

FIGURE 26-10.
Ligation and division of the tube and utero-ovarian ligament with an endoscopic stapler in patient desiring preservation of ovaries. The tissue sizer should be used to select the proper cartridge size.

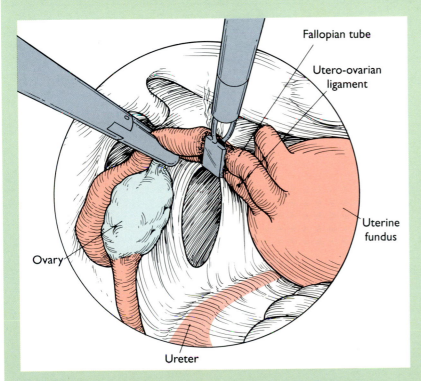

FIGURE 26-11.
Alternative use of bipolar electrocautery to control the fallopian tube and utero-ovarian ligament. These tissues are divided with endoscopic scissors after complete electrodesiccation.

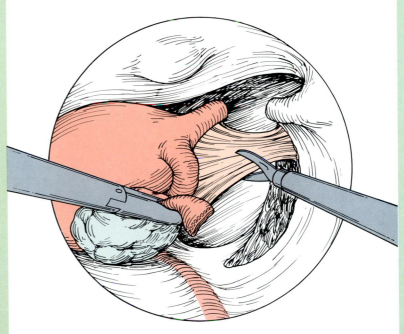

FIGURE 26-12.
Opening of the peritoneum and loose areolar tissue of the anterior leaf of the broad ligament using endoscopic scissors.

Alternative Procedure

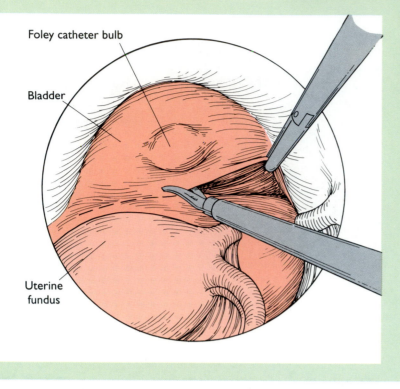

Foley catheter bulb

Bladder

Uterine fundus

FIGURE 26-13.
Opening the anterior peritoneal reflection of the uterus and beginning dissection of the bladder flap using endoscopic scissors. Extensive mobilization of the bladder is not performed because this will be completed during the vaginal phase of the procedure.

Table 26-4. Results of laparoscopically assisted vaginal hysterectomy from various studies.

Study	Total, *n*	Failed laparoscopy, *n*	Major complications, *n*
Summitt and coworkers [4]	29	2	1
Richardson and coworkers [9]	22	5	1
Raju and Auld [10]	40	1	0
Johns and coworkers [11]	839	0	1
Liu [12]	407	0	4
Deprest and coworkers [13]	385	12	60
Nezhat and coworkers [14]	361	1	3
Saye and coworkers [15]	167	4	1
Calandra [16]	153	6	7
Garcia-Padial and coworkers [17]	150	0	1
Johns and Diamond [18]	119	0	1
Harkki-Siren and Sjoberg [19]	100	0	5
Jones [20]	100	0	4
Mage and coworkers [21]	100	5	6
Hulka and Reich [22]	94	1	0
Puls and Henderson [23]	90	0	3
Lee and Soong [24]	82	3	2
Cristoforoni and coworkers [25]	78	8	0
Ou and coworkers [26]	75	0	0
Yuen and coworkers [27]	71	0	5
Daniell and coworkers [28]	68	6	0
Reich [29]	62	1	0
Arbogast and coworkers [30]	61	3	5
Lyons [31]	50	0	1
Boike and coworkers [32]	50	0	0
Bornstein and Shaber [33]	50	0	2
East [34]	50	3	0
	3853	61 (1.6%)	113 (2.9%)

Results

Three randomized studies have examined LAVH. Summitt and coworkers [4] compared LAVH with vaginal hysterectomy and concluded that patients undergoing LAVH had longer operative times and higher costs despite similar rates of blood loss and length of hospital stay. Thus, LAVH should not be used when vaginal hysterectomy is appropriate. Richardson and coworkers, in a slightly smaller study [9], found no significant differences between vaginal hysterectomy and LVAH in pain, complications, length of stay, and recovery and concluded that LAVH does not confer an advantage in most patients. Raju and Auld [10] compared LAVH with total abdominal hysterectomy and found that LAVH leads to a shorter hospital stay, a more rapid recovery, and an earlier return to usual activities. The results of these studies would seem to indicate that LAVH is an attractive alternative to total abdominal hysterectomy but should not be used in place of the vaginal hysterectomy when it is indicated.

Many studies have also included numbers of complications and numbers of conversions to total abdominal hysterectomy. Table 26-4 shows the results of several of the larger studies. These reveal that most of these cases can be completed laparoscopically. Definitions of complications vary, but most studies also have very low complication rates. In those with higher complication rates, postoperative fevers are usually one complication. These studies suggest that LAVH is safe if performed for appropriate indications.

References

1. Thompson JD: Hysterectomy. In *TeLinde's Operative Gynecology,* 7th ed. Edited by Thompson JD, Rock JA. Philadelphia: JB Lippincott Co; 1992:663–738.

2. Murphy AA: Diagnostic and operative laparoscopy. In *TeLinde's Operative Gynecology,* 7th ed. Edited by Thompson JD, Rock JA. Philadelphia: JB Lippincott Co; 1992:361–409.

3. Reich H, Decaprio J, McGlynn F: Laparoscopic hysterectomy. *J Gynecol Surg* 1989, 5:213–216.

4. Summitt RL Jr, Stovall TG, Lipscomb GH, Ling FW: Randomized comparison of laparoscopy-assisted vaginal hysterectomy with standard vaginal hysterectomy in an outpatient setting. *Obstet Gynecol* 1992, 80:895–901.

5. Disaia PJ, Creasman WT, eds.: *Clinical Gynecologic Oncology.* St. Louis: CB Mosby Co.; 1992.

6. Childers JM, Surwit EA: Combined laparoscopic and vaginal surgery for the management of stage I endometrial cancer. *Gynecol Oncol* 1992; 45:46–51.

7. Canis M, Mage G, Chapron C, *et al.*: Laparoscopic hysterectomy: a preliminary study. *Surg Endosc* 1993, 7:42–45.

8. Woodland MB: Ureter injury during laparoscopy-assisted vaginal hysterectomy with the endoscopic linear stapler. *Am J Obstet Gynecol* 1992, 167:756–757.

9. Richardson RE, Bournas N, Magos AL: Is laparoscopic hysterectomy a waste of time? *Lancet* 1995, 345:36–41.

10. Raju KS, Auld BJ: A randomized prospective study of laparoscopic vaginal hysterectomy versus abdominal hysterectomy each with bilateral salpingo-ophorectomy. *Br J Obstet Gynecol* 1994, 101:1068–1071.

11. Johns DA, Carrera B, Jones J, *et al.*: The medical and economic impact of laparoscopically assisted vaginal hysterectomy in a large, metropolitan, not-for-profit hospital. *Am J Obstet Gynecol* 1995, 172:1709–1715.

12. Liu CY: Complications of laparoscopic hysterectomy: prevention, recognition, and management. In: *Complications of Laparoscopy and Hysteroscopy. Edited by Corfman RS, Diamond MP, DeCherney AH. Boston: Blackwell Scientific Publications; 1993:160–166.*

13. Deprest JA, Cusumano PG, Donnez J, *et al.*: 1992 results of the Belcohyst register on laparoscopic hysterectomy. In: *Advanced Gynecologic Laparoscopy: A Practical Guide.* Edited by Cusumano PG, Deprest JA. New York: Parthenon Publishing Group; 1996:85–98.

14. Nezhat F, Nezhat CH, Admon D, *et al.*: Complications and results of 361 hysterectomies performed at laparoscopy. *J Am Coll Surg* 1995, 180:307–316.

15. Saye WB, Espy GB, Bishop MR, *et al.*: Laparoscopic doderlein hysterectomy: a rational alternative to traditional abdominal hysterectomy. *Surgical Laparoscopy and Endoscopy* 1993, 3:88–94.

16. Calandra C: Lararoscopically-assisted vaginal hysterectomy. *Austr N Z J Obstet Gynecol* 1995, 35:78–82.

17. Garcia-Padial J, Osborne N, Sotolongo J, *et al.*: Laparoscopically-assisted vaginal hysterectomy compared with abdominal hysterectomy. *J Natl Med Assoc* 1995, 87:288–290.

18. Johns DA, Diamond MP: Laparoscopically assisted vaginal hysterectomy. *J Reprod Med* 1994, 39:424–428.

19. Harkki-Siren P, Sjoberg J: Evaluation and the learning curve of the first hundred laparoscopic hysterectomies. *Acta Obstet Gynecol Scand* 1995, 74:638–641.

20. Jones RA: Laparoscopic hysterectomy: a series of 100 cases. *Med J Austr* 1993, 159:447–449.

21. Mage G, Wattiez A, Canis M, *et al.*: Hysteroscopie per coelioscopique. *Gynecologic Obstetrique* 1993, 1:126–135.

22. *Laparoscopic Hysterectomy: Textbook of Laparoscopy.* Edited by Hulka JF, Reich H. Philadelphia: WB Saunders; 1994:259–264.

23. Puls LE, Henderson RC: Small bowel herniation after laparoscopically assisted vaginal hysterectomy. *Acta Obstet Gynecol Scand* 1995, 74:307–309.

24. Lee CL, Soong YK: Laparoscopic hysterectomy with the Endo GIA 30 stapler. *J Reprod Med* 1993, 38:582–586.

25. Cristoforoni PM, Palmieri A, Gerbaldo D, *et al.*: Frequency and cause of aborted laparoscopic-assisted vaginal hysterectomy. *J Am Assoc Gynecol Laparosc* 1995, 3:33–37.1

26. Ou CS, Beadle E, Presthus J, *et al.*: A multicenter review of 839 laparoscopic-assisted vaginal hysterectomies. *J Am Assoc Gynecol Laparoscopists* 1994, 1:417–422.

27. Yuen *et al.*:2

28. Daniell JF, Kurtz BR, McTavish G, *et al.*: Laparoscopically assisted vaginal hysterectomy. *J Reprod Med* 1993, 38:537–542.

29. Reich H: Laparoscopic hysterectomy. In: *New Surgical Techniques in Gynaecology.* Edited by Sutton CJ. New York: Parthenon Publishing Group; 1992:91–99.

30. Arbogast JD, Welch RA, Riza ED, *et al.*: Laparoscopically assisted vaginal hysterectomy appears to be an alternative to total abdominal hysterectomy. *J Laparoendosc Surg* 1994, 4:85–90.

31. Lyons TL: Laparoscopic suracervical hysterectomy. *J Reprod Med* 1993, 38:763–767.

32. Boike GM, Elfstrand EP, DelPriore G, *et al.*: Laparoscopically assisted vaginal hysterectomy in university hospital: report of 82 cases and comparison with abdominal and vaginal hysterectomy. *Am J Obstet Gynecol* 1993, 1690–1701.3

33. Bornstein SJ, Shaber RE: Laparoscopically assisted vaginal hysterectomy at a health maintenance organization: cost-effectiveness and comparison with total abdominal hysterectomy. *J Reprod Med* 1995, 40:435–438.

34. East M: Comparative costs of laparoscopically assisted vaginal hysterectomy. *N Z Med J* 1994, 107:371–374.

Pediatric Endosurgery

Bryan C. Weidner
Samuel M. Mahaffey

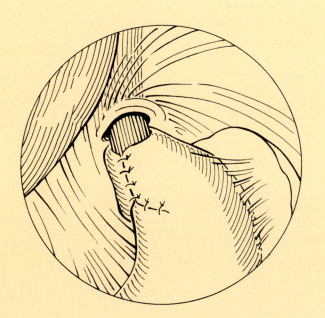

Minimally invasive surgical procedures have been enthusiastically received in adult patients. This enthusiasm has been driven by the appeal of shortened hospitalization, decreased perioperative pain, a more rapid convalescence, and an earlier return to work for the patients. Many of the same considerations make minimally invasive techniques appealing in pediatric patients (Table 27-1), especially the potential to decrease perioperative apprehension, discomfort, and respiratory complications, particularly in infants and children who have underlying respiratory conditions. Although pediatric peritoneoscopy and thoracoscopy were advocated in the 1970s [1–3], recent technical advances in imaging and downsizing of instrumentation in the past 5 years have made widespread use of these procedures feasible even in small patients. As a result, the use of these techniques has expanded dramatically, and imaginative new approaches to clinical problems are developing rapidly (Table 27-2).

A word of caution is in order, however. "Endoscopic" is not necessarily equivalent to "better." Many conventional procedures in pediatric surgery are already "minimally invasive," resulting in minimal morbidity and satisfactory cosmetic outcomes. The corresponding endoscopic procedures may be more lengthy and considerably more expensive. Under such circumstances, it may be difficult or impossible to demonstrate any advantage of endoscopic procedure over conventional techniques.

Special Considerations

Technical Considerations

Several modifications of the general technique for laparoscopy as performed in adults are listed in Table 27-3. The open technique of trocar sheath insertion is advocated for laparoscopy in children smaller than 15 kg. Because of their small size and the proximity of the very elastic anterior abdominal wall to the abdominal viscera and fixed retroperitoneal structures, and because the dome of the bladder is intraperitoneal, it is our impression that open trocar insertion is safer in infants and small children. In addition, the potential for an umbilical hernia that may contain bowel adherent to the peritoneal lining makes the open technique more appealing. These hernias are repaired by fascial closure upon removal of the trocar. Routine decompression of the urinary bladder and stomach is recommended to reduce the risk of trocar injury.

Trocar sheath placement is generally similar to that used for corresponding operations in adult patients. However, shorter

---

Table 27-1. Potential benefits of an endosurgical approach in pediatric patients

Improved cosmesis
Smaller incision
Decreased postoperative pain
Shorter hospital stay
Shorter convalescence
Decreased incidence of adhesive bowel obstruction*
Better intraoperative visualization
Fewer postoperative pulmonary complications*

*Not well-documented.

Table 27-2. Laparoscopic operations in pediatric surgery

Appendectomy	Pyloromyotomy
Meckel's diverticulectomy	Hirschsprung's disease
Adnexal detorsion	Biopsy
Nissen fundoplication	Colostomy
Inguinal exploration	Pullthrough
Cholecystectomy	Gonadectomy
Splenectomy	Orchiopexy
Diagnostic laparoscopy	Nephrectomy
Chronic pain	Varicocelectomy
Trauma	Ureterolysis
Hepatobiliary disease	Ureteral repair
Cancer diagnosis and staging	

Table 27-3. Modifications for pediatric patients

Smaller camera instruments and trocars
Wider spacing of trocar sites
Trocar placement at greater distances from operative site margin
Lower insufflation pressures
Smaller volumes for pneumoperitoneum
More frequent use of Hasson trocar
Foley and nasogastric catheter decompression

Table 27-4. Anesthetic considerations in pediatric endosurgery

Pneumoperitoneum/increased intra-abdominal pressure
  Decreased functional residual capacity
  Increased peak airway pressure
  Decreased systemic venous return
  Impaired return from lower-extremity intravenous lines
  Impaired splanchnic blood flow
Carbon dioxide insufflation
  Increased $PaCO_2$
  CO_2 gas embolus
Intraluminal gas
  Expands with N_2O
Single-lung ventilation

trocars are used, and if possible these sites are placed more widely apart and further from the operating field to prevent overlapping ("dueling") of instruments within the peritoneal cavity. The relatively large size of the liver, which may extend well below the right costal margin, demands great care when inserting trocars in the right upper quadrant in infants and small children.

The great elasticity of the abdominal wall in children generally means that a satisfactory pneumoperitoneum can be achieved with lower insufflation pressures than in adults. In general, only 5 to 10 mm Hg is required in infants weighing up to 15 kg. Whereas end tidal CO_2 tension may increase by 18% to 20% with insufflation pressures of 10 mm Hg, this change has been shown not to alter oxygen saturation or to cause hemodynamic instability [4]. The use of higher pressures can result in significant hemodynamic compromise or hypercarbia, and the operator is advised therefore to use the minimum insufflation pressure required to maintain adequate visualization of the peritoneal cavity.

Equipment

Perhaps the most significant technological advance leading to the widespread use of minimally invasive techniques is improved imaging. High-resolution monitors, true-color imaging, and high-sensitivity cameras (including the newer three-chip designs) allowed manufacturers to scale down telescopes to a size that is appropriate for infants and small children. Several companies are now introducing instruments designed specifically for pediatric patients. However, a prohibitive problem remains with stapling devices, which are often too large to fit within the limited space presented by the thoracic and abdominal cavities of infants and small children. Downsized stapling devices are not yet available.

Anesthesia

Major anesthetic considerations unique to endoscopic procedures are outlined in Table 27-4. These are related primarily to the mechanical effects of pneumoperitoneum and the requirement for single-lung ventilation during thoracoscopic procedures, which may be accentuated in infants and children compared with adults. Monitoring can be performed adequately by standard, noninvasive measurement of hemodynamics, airway pressure, ventilation, end-tidal carbon dioxide partial pressure, and intra-abdominal pressure.

Experimental models using piglets and neonatal lambs demonstrate decreased cardiac index and impaired perfusion of the kidneys, liver, and intestine when intra-abdominal pressures exceed 15 mm Hg [5,6]. Although children usually compensate well, they should be adequately volume resuscitated before laparoscopy, and intra-abdominal pressures should be maintained at the minimum level needed to safely visualize the operative field.

Elevation of the diaphragm by the pneumoperitoneum may decrease lung compliance, thereby adversely affecting minute ventilation. The resulting hypercapnia may be further accentuated by absorption of carbon dioxide across the peritoneum. These effects are usually manageable by modest increases in minute ventilation. During upper abdominal operations, accidental egress of carbon dioxide from the peritoneal cavity into the pleural space resulting in a pneumothorax may result in acute changes in ventilatory requirements. This complication mandates termination of the laparoscopic procedure and may require placement of a tube thoracostomy.

Thoracoscopic procedures may be performed under general or regional anesthesia with intravenous sedation. Regional techniques, such as a four-rib intercostal block, are potentially attractive for patients undergoing biopsy of mediastinal masses resulting in tracheal compression, where the risk of general anesthesia may be prohibitive. Single-lung ventilation is preferred for optimal thoracic exploration and may be achieved by use of the dual-lumen endotracheal tube in larger patients or selective bronchial intubation in smaller patients. This is usually well tolerated when the lung is intrinsically normal. During biopsies for interstitial lung disease (viral or fungal pneumonias, bleomycin toxicity, and so forth), gas exchange may not be adequate during single-lung ventilation, and the thoracoscopic approach may not be feasible.

Endosurgical Procedures

Cholecystectomy

Laparoscopic cholecystectomy is the most widely reported and universally accepted indication for minimally invasive surgery in children. Cholelithiasis associated with hematologic disease is the most common indication for cholecystectomy, followed by calculus and acalculus cholecystitis, parenteral nutrition–induced cholestasis, gallbladder dysfunction, and ileal resection.

The details of the operative procedure are nearly identical to those described for adults (see Chapter 14). As illustrated in Figure 27-1, trocar placement should emphasize wide separation to avoid overlap of instruments at the operative site. This is an issue of major technical importance. In smaller children this may necessitate placing the second right subcostal trocar in the right lower quadrant and the epigastric trocar in a left subcostal position. The 5-mm laparoscope can be used in infants. Intraoperative cholangiography should be used selectively but may be particularly useful when there is difficulty defining the anatomy, particularly the junction of the cystic duct with the common bile duct. Published results have uniformly been excellent, confirming shortened hospital stay and earlier return to school and normal activities [7–11].

Appendectomy

Appendectomy is the most common emergency intra-abdominal operation performed in children. The first laparoscopic appendectomy was performed by Semm in 1982 [12]. Subsequent reports describe successful application of the minimally invasive technique in children [13–15]. In both of these reports only two trocars, one in each of the lower quadrants, were used in addition to the camera port. An additional trocar may be placed in the left lower quadrant, through which a grasper may be placed for better retraction and exposure of the mesoappendix, particularly if acute periappendiceal inflammation is present (Figure 27-2). Placement of this trocar in the left lower quadrant in children will help avoid overlapping trocars and promote facile manipulation of the appendix. Dissection of the mesoappendix and appendiceal base (Figure 27-3) proceeds as in adults (see Chapter 11). The base of the appendix can be secured with either endoscopic loops or staples.

Recently a single trocar technique for laparoscopic appendectomy in children has been reported [16]. A 10 mm operative telescope is placed infraumbilically. The appendix is grasped with a 450 mm-operative atraumatic instrument introduced through the operative channel of the laparoscope, and then exteriorized through the umbilical cannula. The appendectomy is then performed using the traditional method outside the abdominal cavity. Whereas this approach appears safe in the referenced author's hands, it remains to be seen whether it will gain widespread acceptance.

Suspected perforation is not considered a contraindication to laparoscopic appendectomy. In fact, laparoscopy may permit better visualization of the right lower quadrant and pelvis with more thorough irrigation and aspiration of necrotic material. The laparoscopic approach also provides excellent visualization of abdominal and pelvic organs that must be investigated when the appendix is normal. This may be the primary advantage of the endosurgical approach compared with the open technique. Many of these other pathologic conditions can be managed laparoscopically (*eg*, adnexal torsion or Meckel's diverticulitis).

Early observations suggest that patients undergoing laparoscopic appendectomy may have shorter hospital stays and shorter convalescence than those undergoing a traditional open approach. This observation, and the hidden economic advantage of lost time for the parents of these children, might compensate for the increased cost of the laparoscopic procedure. However, the role of laparoscopic approaches in pediatric patients is not at all clear at present. Both open and laparoscopic appendectomies are effective, with limited morbidity that is roughly equivalent in current reports. As noted, an important argument for a laparoscopic approach is in the patient without a clear clinical diagnosis.

Antireflux Procedures

Gastroesophageal reflux is a common problem in infants and children, particularly those with impaired neurologic function. Antireflux procedures are unequivocally indicated for the management of complications of gastroesophageal reflux, which are

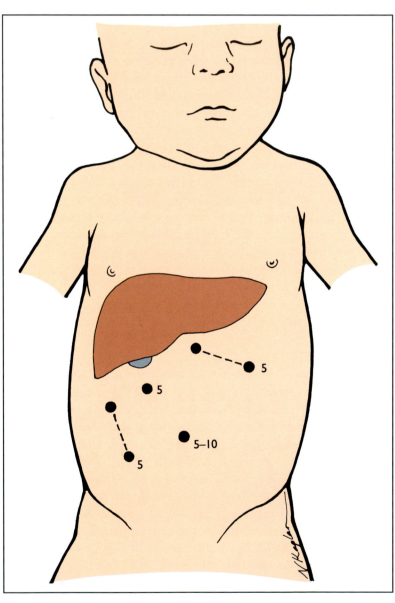

FIGURE 27-1.

Trocar placement for laparoscopic cholecystectomy. Note the inferior placement of the right upper quadrant trocars in order to avoid the liver and the wide spacing of the trocars for smaller children. The second 5-mm, right-sided trocar may even be in the right lower quadrant skin crease. A 5- or 10-mm umbilical port may be used depending on camera size availability.

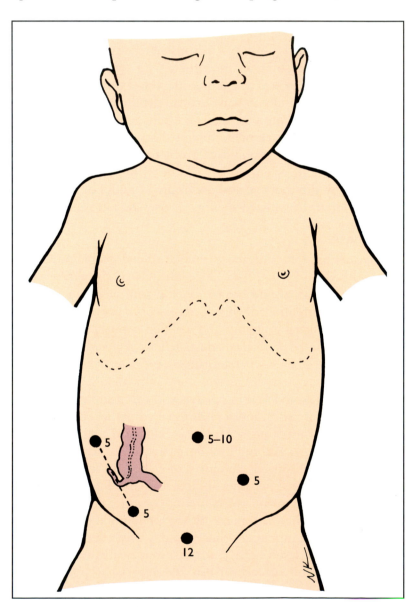

FIGURE 27-2.

Trocar placement for appendectomy. Adequate visualization can be achieved with either a right lower quadrant or suprapubic trocar through which a retractor is placed. However, use of both ports frequently provides superior retraction. The 10-mm trocar, through which the stapler is passed, can be placed in the suprapubic position, which is more easily hidden below the hairline, rather than in the left lower quadrant.

summarized in Table 27-5. A more difficult management decision is required in the neurologically impaired infant or child who requires placement of a gastrostomy for nutritional support. The authors generally advocate a selective approach to fundoplication in these patients, based on the outcome of upper gastrointestinal contrast studies and extended (24-hour) esophageal pH monitoring. It should be noted, however, that a significant number of these patients without demonstrable gastroesophageal reflux preoperatively develop symptoms attributable to reflux after fixation of the gastric wall to the anterior abdominal wall for gastrostomy placement [17].

The minimally invasive approach is particularly attractive in the neurologically impaired population, simplifying perioperative pain management and the management of other medications, particularly anticonvulsants. Neurologically impaired patients and other patient populations with compromised pulmonary function due to recurrent aspiration or frequent pneumonias potentially benefit by avoiding an upper abdominal incision. The theoretical possibility that the laparoscopic approach minimizes the development of adhesions and the potential for future intestinal obstruction is also very appealing, although unproven.

Many minor technical differences exist among surgeons on the particular details of fundoplication (Table 27-6). However, laparoscopic fundoplication can be performed in essentially the same manner as any conventional open approach, allowing for subtle differences in technique.

A nasogastric tube should be placed after endotracheal intubation to assure gastric decompression for safe trocar insertion and visualization of the left upper quadrant. It is particularly important to leave the nasogastric tube in place if a percutaneous endoscopic gastrostomy is to be placed after fundoplication. Distention of the fundic wrap during insufflation may preclude passage of the endoscope into the stomach if it is not decompressed via the nasogastric tube. Before dissection of the esophageal hiatus, an appropriate sized esophageal bougie is placed transorally into the stomach. This is used to calibrate the esophagus and the esophageal hiatus as well as to plan suture placement. It is withdrawn when

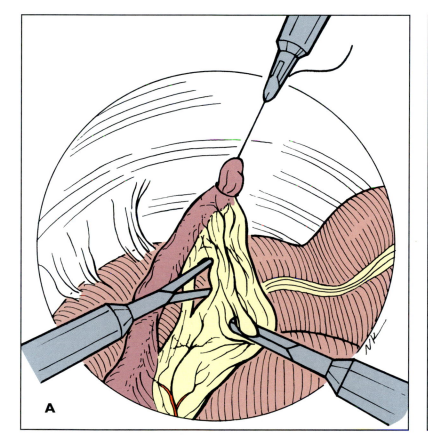
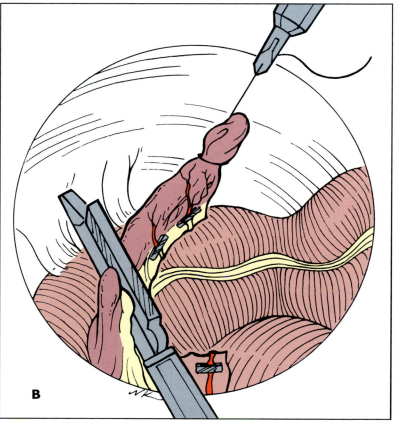

FIGURE 27-3.

A, The mesoappendix is dissected with blunt-tipped forceps. The mesoappendix can be secured with either endoscopic clips or an endoscopic stapler.

B, The base of the appendix can be divided with an endoscopic stapler or between endoscopic loop sutures.

Table 27-5. Indications for an antireflux procedure
Aspiration pneumonia
Refractory vomiting
Failure to thrive
Apnea or "near miss" sudden infant death syndrome
Reactive airway disease and temporally related reflux
Severe esophagitis or its complications (hemorrhage, stricture)
Failure of medical therapy

Table 27-6. Variations in Nissen fundoplication
Tightness of wrap (Bougie diameter)
Length of wrap (number of sutures)
Use of pledgets
Incorporating diaphragm with uppermost suture
Plication of crura
Division of short gastric vessels

the sutures are actually tied to facilitate tension-free tissue apposition. A loose, circumferential fundic wrap is the objective of the Nissen fundoplication; it is relatively easy to produce obstruction of the esophagus in an infant or small child, or a patient who has underlying esophageal dysmotility.

Trocar placement for Nissen fundoplication is illustrated in Figure 27-4. Again, we prefer an open technique for placement of the infraumbilical trocar, which is used for camera insertion and insufflation. The remaining ports are placed under direct vision. In general, an isosceles triangle is designed with the working ports inferior and the apex at the operative site (the esophageal hiatus). Again, in small children it is important to place the working ports far enough from the hiatus to allow facile manipulation. The remainder of the procedure is similar to that described for adults in Chapter 5. The completed Nissen fundoplication is seen in Figure 27-5.

Most infants and children require a gastrostomy. We prefer a conventional percutaneous endoscopic gastrostomy. Once again, it is important to avoid insufflation of the stomach without a nasogastric tube present to avoid esophageal compression by the wrap that may preclude passage of the endoscope.

Other antireflux procedures can be performed by using minimally invasive techniques, including the posterior gastropexy and anterior fundoplication. We have some experience with the anterior fundoplication described by Thal and used extensively by Ashcraft and coworkers [18]. This technique uses a partial fundic wrap, which appears to produce less symptomatic esophageal obstruction. This technique is useful in small infants in whom the size of the fundus may be inadequate to perform a circumferential wrap and in patients with significant esophageal dysmotility.

Long-term efficacy of the endoscopic technique has not yet been documented. Perioperative complications are reported in up to half of the patients undergoing conventional open fundoplication [19,20]. These include postoperative pulmonary compromise in approximately 15%, small bowel obstruction in 8% to 10%, and disruption of the fundic wrap in approximately 10%. Approximately one-fourth of the infants and children who require surgery for gastroesophageal reflux die of other causes within 5 years of their operation. Therefore, a minimally invasive technique that decreases this perioperative morbidity with equivalent safety and efficacy is particularly desirable.

Pyloromyotomy

Given that the traditional open technique for the treatment of infantile hypertrophic pyloric stenosis results in minimal morbidity, the use of the endosurgical approach for the management of this condition has been met with controversy. Increased expense, increased operative time, and a higher complication

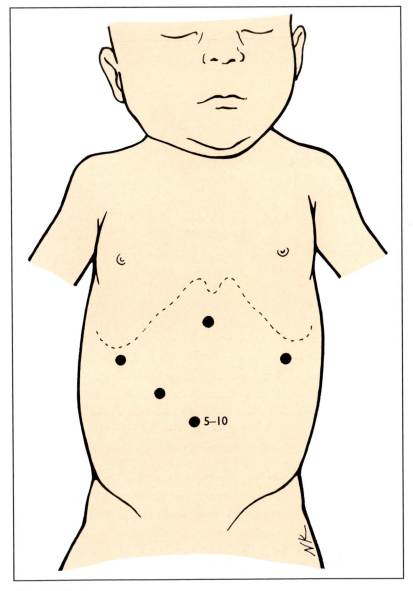

FIGURE 27-4.

Trocar placement for laparoscopic Nissen fundoplication. Emphasis is placed on wide separation of trocar sites to permit dexterous manipulation of the instruments and mobilization of the esophagus. In particular, the right flank trocar should be placed as far laterally as possible.

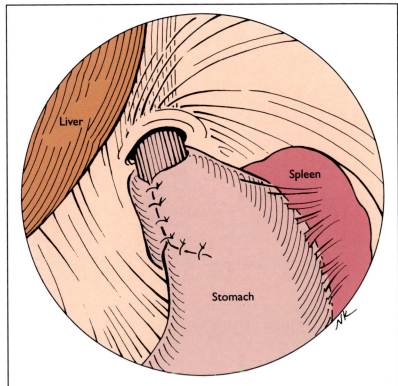

FIGURE 27-5.

Videoscopic appearance of a completed Nissen fundoplication.

rate have all been cited as reasons against laparoscopic pyloromyotomy [21,22]. Unrecognized duodenal perforation is a feared complication of the procedure significantly increasing morbidity and hospital stay.

Others, however, cite equal morbidity rates with improved cosmesis as well as improved postoperative course (average time to accept normal feeds and less time from feeding to discharge) as reasons to perform the procedure laparoscopically [23,24]. Bufo *et al.* [25] have recently described a technique for laparoscopic pyloromyotomy. A 5 mm periumbilical port is used for visualization along with the placement of two 2.7 mm instruments on either side for manipulation. The stomach is grasped from the left while a disposable arthroscopy knife is used from the right to incise the serosa and begin the myotomy. The myotomy is completed with a laparoscopic spreader. Using this technique, Bufo *et al.* report no statistically significant difference in results when the endosurgical technique is compared with the open Ramstedt pyloromyotomy. In summary, laparoscopic pyloromyotomy is a procedure that is gaining in popularity. In experienced hands, it may be performed with equal efficiency and safety as the open technique.

Inguinal Herniorrhaphy

Inguinal herniorrhaphy is the most common surgical procedure performed in children. The conventional open technique, which is essentially a high ligation of the hernia sac, is rapidly accomplished on an outpatient basis, with a small incision, minimal morbidity, and satisfactory cosmetic result. The potential risks to trocar placement and foreign body (mesh) placement probably outweigh any possible benefit. Not surprisingly, there are no reports of laparoscopic hernia repair in infants and young children.

An ongoing controversy exists over the necessity for contralateral groin exploration in infants with a unilateral hernia. The risk of a missed hernia in the asymptomatic groin that is normal on examination (approximately 10%) and the requirement for a second anesthetic must be weighed against the morbidity of a potentially unnecessary inguinal exploration, which may injure the testicular vessels or vas deferens. Several authors have reported their experience using laparoscopy to evaluate pediatric hernias [26–28]. Lobe and Schropp [29] have described their experience of laparoscopic contralateral inguinal exploration in pediatric patients undergoing conventional inguinal herniorrhaphy. In this technique, a 2-mm endoscope is passed through a 3-mm trocar after pneumoperitoneum has been established. Both internal rings are then examined (Figure 27-6). Standard open groin exploration is then performed in patients in whom a contralateral hernia is identified. Others have suggested passing the laparoscope into the peritoneum through the open hernia sac in the symptomatic groin [30]. Fuenfer *et al.* [31] have recently described a newer technique for the exploration of the contralateral groin in children. A pneumoperitoneum is produced by insufflation via a 14-gauge intravenous catheter placed into the hernia sac of the operated side. A 1.2 mm laparoscope is then passed through another 14-gauge intravenous catheter inserted through the abdominal wall of the contralateral side. This technique produces a direct view of the internal ring.

Abdominal Exploration

Diagnostic laparoscopy with or without biopsy can be easily performed in children and may spare the patient the need for open laparotomy. Examples include cases of trauma [32], hepatobiliary disease [33], or chronic pain of unclear cause [34]. Heloury and coworkers [35] have reported their experience with 27 children ranging in age from 8 to 16 years. Thirty diagnostic and therapeutic procedures were performed, including evaluation of adnexal abnormality, reduction of adnexal torsion, ovarian transposition before radiation therapy, gonadal ablation in cases of sexual ambiguity, drainage or biopsy of ovarian cysts, and evaluation of appendiceal abnormality.

Laparoscopic techniques have been used for cancer diagnosis and staging. Spinelli and coworkers [36] reported an extensive experience in pediatric patients aged 2 to 16 years. The primary indication for the laparoscopic procedure was staging of known neoplastic disease, particularly Hodgkin's disease. The laparoscopic examinations were accomplished with minimal morbidity (1.2%). There were some false-negative results on laparoscopic examinations, but in most cases the clinical and radiologic follow-up confirmed the reliability of the laparoscopic examination. The treatment of Hirschsprung's disease via a laparoscopic Duhamel pull through procedure has been reported [37,38]. Whereas the initial results appear promising, it remains to be seen whether broad acceptance of this technique will occur.

Splenectomy has also been described in children [39,40]. The technical aspects of this procedure are described in detail in Chapter 17.

Urologic Procedures

Evaluation of the child with cryptorchidism is a common problem in pediatric surgical practice, with impalpable testes making up about one-fifth of the cases. This condition is one in which evaluation and treatment using a laparoscopic approach is becoming increasingly popular. In 1976 Cortesi and coworkers [41] published the first description of the use of laparoscopy for localization of the undescended testis, and Scott [42] subsequently reported the use of this approach in a series of pediatric patients. Since these reports, many other groups have reported their experience using laparoscopy in the evaluation of the undescended testicle [43–46]. Figure 27-7 outlines an algorithm for managing patients with impalpable testes in which laparoscopy plays a prominent role as the initial diagnostic modality. This permits minimally invasive assessment of the presence, location, and size of an undescended testes, and the length and position of the vas deferens and gonadal vessels.

The testes are most reliably identified by locating their blood supply. After placing the laparoscope into the peritoneal cavity, the abdominal cavity should be systematically explored, as outlined in Figure 27-8. Patients found to have a normal vas and gonadal vessels entering the internal ring (*see* Figure 27-6) or blind ending or absent gonadal vessels (Figure 27-9) are spared a laparotomy (or retroperitoneal dissection).

The laparoscopic approach can also be used as an important therapeutic modality. A small, atrophic testis with a normal contralateral gonad can be excised as illustrated in Figure 27-10*A*, thereby precluding the need for laparotomy. Two additional trocars are required for orchiectomy. After the testis is located these should be placed appropriately to form the base of an isosceles triangle with its apex at the site of the gonad. The first stage of Ransley's modification of the Fowler-Stephens procedure, in which short testicular vessels supplying high intra-abdominal testes are divided, can also be performed laparoscopically (Figure 27-10B). This follows a similar approach as orchiectomy in identifying the testis and dividing the testicular artery, but the vas deferens and testis are left untouched. This avoids laparotomy or exten-

sive retroperitoneal dissection and accomplishes the goals of the first stage of the modified Fowler-Stephens procedure with minimal manipulation of the testis and better preservation of the important collateral blood supply. On the basis of the early observations of Clatworthy and coworkers [47], a more favorable outcome would be predicted for patients whose testes have been subjected to minimal manipulation. With the development of collat-

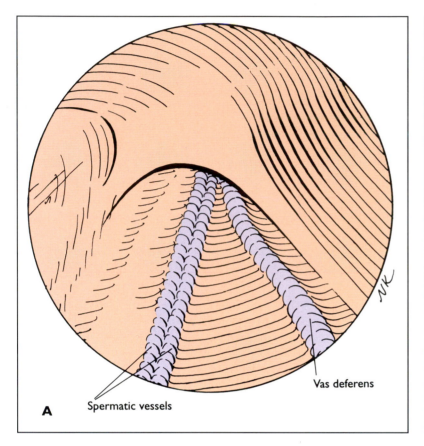

A Spermatic vessels Vas deferens

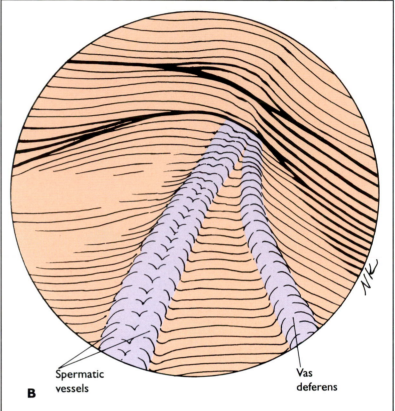

B Spermatic vessels Vas deferens

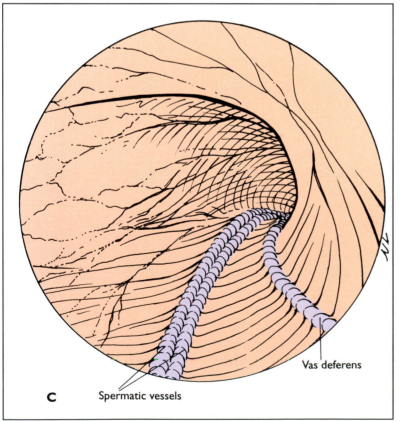

C Spermatic vessels Vas deferens

FIGURE 27-6.

Videoscopic appearance of the internal ring. **A**, A normal ring without a patent processus vaginalis. **B**, An internal ring with a patent processus vaginalis covered by a veil of peritoneum. **C**, A ring through which a large indirect hernia sac passes. Note the retroperitoneal vas deferens and spermatic vessels at the medial aspect of the ring.

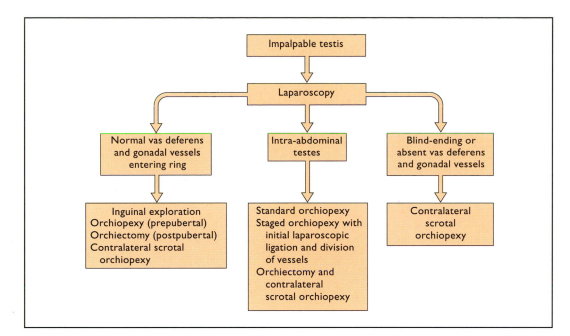

FIGURE 27-7.

Algorithm for initial laparoscopic evaluation and management of undescended testes.

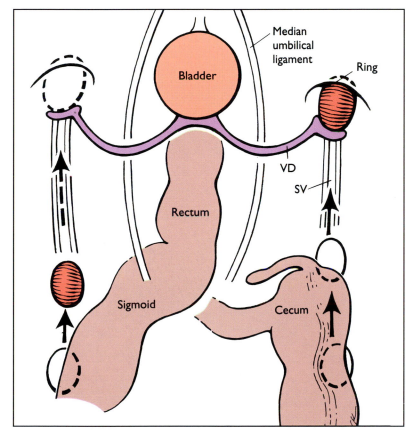

FIGURE 27-8.

Laparoscopic exploration for impalpable testes. After placing an infraumbilical trocar through which the laparoscope is passed, the normal, contralateral side and then the abnormal side is inspected. The median umbilical ligament and internal ring are identified and the vas deferens and spermatic vessels are sought. If they do not course into the internal ring, a systematic search is begun along the lateral paracolic gutter. This may require incising the lateral peritoneal attachments to the right or left colon by placing a suprapubic trocar for scissors and a contralateral lower quadrant trocar for a retractor, as in colectomy.

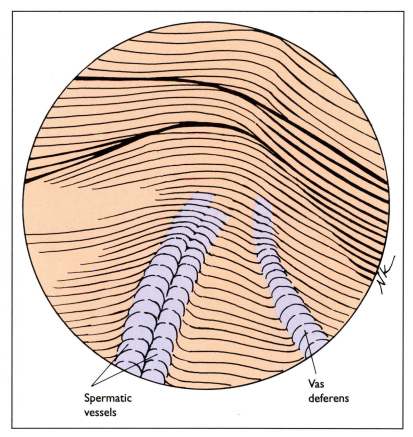

FIGURE 27-9.

Videoscopic appearance of internal ring with a blind-ending vas deferens and gonadal vessels.

eral blood flow to the testis through the vas deferens and gubernacular attachments, delayed orchiopexy can then be performed in the standard fashion.

Several case reports have detailed the use of the laparoscopic approach for other pediatric urologic procedures, including nephrectomy [48,49], varicocele management [50], ureterolysis [51], or extravesical ureteral repair for vesicoureteral reflux [52].

Thoracoscopic Procedures

Although thoracoscopy was first performed in 1910 by Jacobaeus, a significant series of thoracoscopic procedures in pediatric patients was not published until 1976 [53]. Since then, enthusiasm for the thoracoscopic approach to chest surgery in children has increased substantially as experience has been gained. A list of current indications for thoracoscopic surgery in children is given in Table 27-7. "Minimally invasive" surgery of the chest is especially appealing for the pediatric population because the pain and respiratory complications associated with a thoracotomy incision can be avoided, particularly when there is severe underlying lung disease.

Diagnostic thoracoscopy can be performed easily with a patient in a lateral decubitus position. Slight variations in patient positioning may be helpful during evaluations of particular regions of the thorax, such as the apices or mediastinum (Figure 27-11). The trocar for the thoracoscope is generally placed in the sixth intercostal space. A small skin incision is made at the selected site and the subcutaneous tissue and muscles are dissected bluntly until the parietal pleura is reached. Unlike the approach for standard tube thoracostomy, a tunnel through the subcutaneous tissue should not be created; a direct approach will help protect against injury to the visceral pleura that may be quite close in small patients and permits greater instrument mobility during the subsequent procedure. After pneumothorax has been created (in rare cases of noncompliant lungs, this may require minimal CO_2 insufflation), the trocars may be carefully placed. Additional trocars are placed in a similar fashion under direct vision as required. At the conclusion of a procedure, trocars are removed and sites are closed. A chest tube may be placed through one of the trocar sites to monitor drainage or if an air leak is anticipated. When these are not concerns, many surgeons simply evacuate the pneumothorax and cover thoracostomy sites with occlusive dressings without placing a chest tube.

Thoracoscopy has been shown to be effective in the diagnosis, evaluation, and management of intrathoracic lesions involving the lung parenchyma, pleura, and mediastinum in children [53–55]. Assistance in the evaluation of undiagnosed localized or diffuse pulmonary disease, especially in immunocompromised children, is frequently requested of pediatric surgeons, as is the diagnosis and staging of intrathoracic cancer. Thoracoscopic lung biopsy is sensitive, specific, and easily performed. A second trocar is placed over the area to be biopsied, through which a grasping instrument is passed, while a third trocar (12 mm) is placed as far away from the biopsy site as possible to allow complete entry of a linear stapler into the thoracic cavity (Figure 27-12). In very small patients, the stapler may not fit; biopsies are then taken directly through the trocar overlying the lesion with cup biopsy forceps. The lung parenchyma should be coagulated after deep biopsies. Thoracoscopic lobectomy has been reported in adults. The technique is described elsewhere in this text.

The differential diagnosis of a mediastinal mass is extensive and varied, as outlined in Table 27-8. Thoracoscopy can be used for both diagnosis and treatment. Patient and trocar positioning

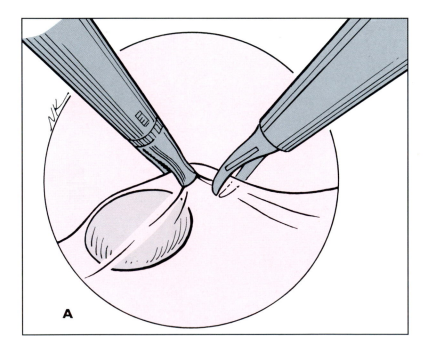

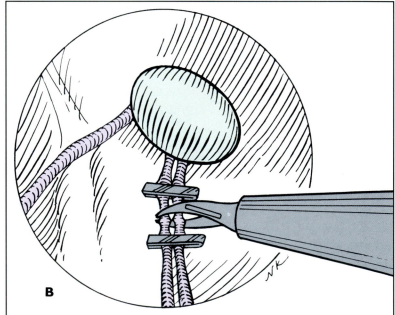

FIGURE 27-10.

Identification of intra-abdominal testes. **A**, Excision of atrophic intra-abdominal testis. The overlying peritoneum is incised and the testis is removed, usually by sharp dissection and electrocautery, because the blood supply is usually minimal. **B**, Ligation and division of testicular vessels. Placement of the two operating ports is based on localization of testes. The port for the instrument used to grasp the peritoneum is placed in the suprapubic region, and the second port for the dissecting instrument is placed as far away as possible in the contralateral lower quadrant. This trocar may need to be 10 mm to accommodate the clipping device.

for anterior and posterior mediastinal masses are shown in Figure 27-11. It is again important to place the operating trocar as far away from the lesion as possible in order to optimize mobility. The overlying pleura can be dissected with either scissor or hook cautery (Figure 27-13). As with mediastinoscopy, lesions should be aspirated before biopsy if there is a possibility that they are vascular structures.

Finally, there are reports of the successful use of thoracoscopy for the management of pleural disease in children, such as for effusions, empyema, and pneumothorax [50–58]. The techniques for pleural drainage, decortication, and pleurodesis (with or without bleb resection) are described elsewhere in this text.

Conclusions

The relatively small but rapidly expanding experience with pediatric laparoscopy and thoracoscopy is confirming the safety and efficacy of "minimally invasive" surgery in children. The potential benefits of improved visualization at the time of operation, decreased pain and ileus after surgery, shortened hospitalization, and improved cosmesis are especially attractive for the pediatric population. The specific indications and the operations best performed by an endosurgical approach are being evaluated. There should be a clearly demonstrated benefit of an endosurgical approach to an operation over the conventional, time-tested open technique. In addition, the risks of laparoscopy, such as trocar placement and pneumoperitoneum, as well as the loss of tactile sensation so important in the performance of many operations, should be carefully considered. There is no doubt that the role of these new approaches will undergo considerable evolution in the coming years.

Table 27-7. Common indications for thoracoscopic surgery in children
Diagnostic thoracoscopy
Lung biopsy
Evaluation and excision of mediastinal mass
Excision of bronchogenic cyst
Pleurodesis and bleb resection
Treatment of pleural effusion/empyema
Diagnosis and staging of cancer
Evaluation of chest wall and diaphragm

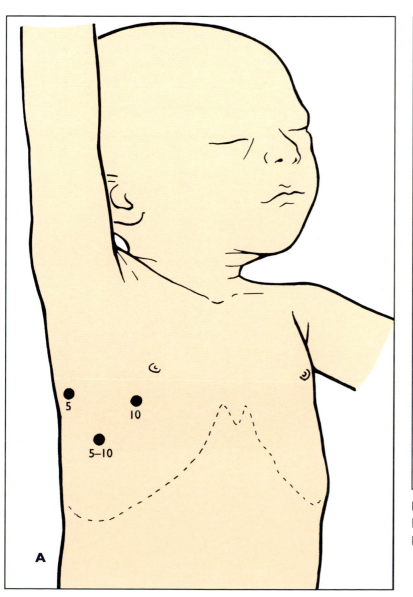

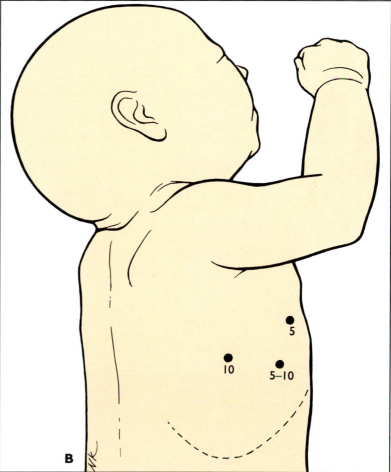

FIGURE 27-11.

Patient positioning for evaluation of lesions in the anterior mediastinum (A), and posterior mediastinum (B).

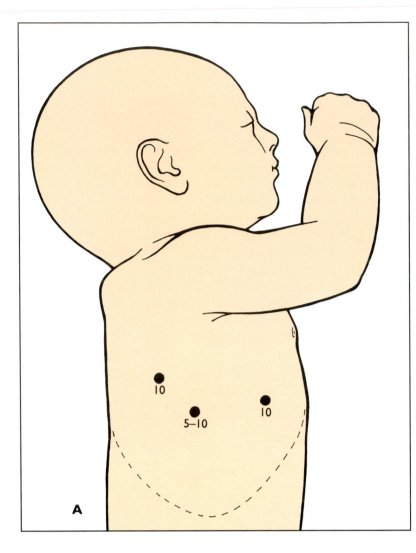

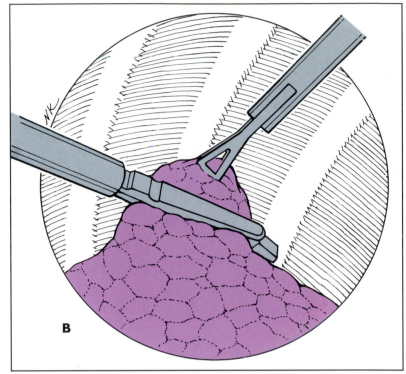

FIGURE 27-12.

A, Trocar positioning for the performance of lung biopsy. Specific trocar sites are dictated by the location of the lesion to be biopsied. **B,** Retraction of the lung and positioning of the stapling device for a thoracoscopic lung biopsy. It is essential that the trocar through which the stapler will pass be as far away from the anticipated biopsy site as possible to permit extended passage of the stapler into the chest so that the jaws may be opened fully. Inability to do this in a small infant may preclude a thoracoscopic approach. Several loads of staples may be required to remove an adequate biopsy specimen.

Table 27-8. Differential diagnosis of mediastinal mass		
Anterior	**Middle**	**Posterior**
Lymphoma	Enteric cysts	Neurogenic tumors
Teratoma	Bronchogenic cysts	
Thymic lesions	Lymphadenopathy	
	Lymphomas	
	Pericardial cysts	
	Lymphangioma	

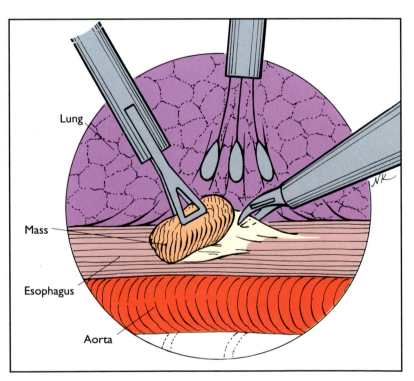

FIGURE 27-13.

Dissection of the pleura overlying a mediastinal mass before biopsy or excision of the mass.

References

1. Gans SL, Berci G: Advances in endoscopy of infants and children. *J Pediatr Surg* 1971, 6:199–234.

2. Gans SL, Berci G: Peritoneoscopy in infants and children. *J Pediatr Surg* 1973, 8:399–405.

3. Rodgers BM, Talbert JL: Thoracoscopy for diagnosis of intrathoracic lesions in children. *J Pediatr Surg* 1976, 11:703–708.

4. Hsing CH, Hseu SS, Tsai SK, *et al.*: The physiologic effect of CO_2 pneumoperitoneum in pediatric laparoscopy. *Acta Anaes Sinica* 1995, 33(1):1–6.

5. Lynch FP, Ochi T, Scully M, *et al.*: Cardiovascular effects of increased intra-abdominal pressure in newborn piglets. *J Pediatr Surg* 1974, 9:621–626.

6. Masey SA, Koehler RC, Buck JR, *et al.*: Effect of abdominal distention on central and regional hemodynamics in neonatal lambs. *Pediatr Res* 1985, 19:1244–1249.

7. Holcomb GW, Olsen DO, Sharp KW: Laparoscopic cholecystectomy in the pediatric patient. *J Pediatr Surg* 1991, 26:1186–1190.

8. Sigman HA, Laberge JM, Croitoru D, *et al.*: Laparoscopic cholecystectomy: a treatment option for gallbladder disease in children. *J Pediatr Surg* 1991, 26:1181–1183.

9. Newman KD, Marman LM, Attori R, *et al.*: Laparoscopic cholecystectomy in pediatric patients. *J Pediatr Surg* 1991, 26:1184–1185.

10. Moir CR, Donahoe JH, VanHeerden JA: Laparoscopic cholecystectomy in children: initial experience and recommendations. *J Pediatr Surg* 1992, 27:1066–1070.

11. Davidoff AM, Branum GD, Murray EA, *et al.*: The technique of laparoscopic cholecystectomy in children. *Ann Surg* 1992, 215:186–191.

12. Semm K: Endoscopic appendectomy. *Endoscopy* 1983, 15:59.

13. Valla JS, Limonne V, Valla V, Montupet P: Laparoscopic appendectomy in children: report of 465 cases. *Surg Laparosc Endosc* 1991, 166–172.

14. Ure BM, Spangenberg W, Hebebrand D, *et al.*: Laparoscopic surgery in children and adolescents with suspected appendicitis: results of medical technology assessment. *Eur J Pediatr Surg* 1992, 2:336–340.

15. Gilchrist BF, Lobe TE, Schropp KP, *et al.*: Is there a role for laparoscopic appendectomy in pediatric surgery? *J Pediatr Surg* 1992, 27:209–214.

16. Esposito C.: One-trocar appendectomy in pediatric surgery. *Surgical Endoscopy-Ultrasound & Interventional Techniques* 1998, 12:177–178.

17. Papaila JG, Vane DW, Colville C, *et al.*: The effect of various types of gastrostomy on the lower esophageal sphincter. *J Pediatr Surg* 1987, 22:1198–1202.

18. Ashcraft KW, Holder TM, *et al.*: The Thal fundoplication for gastroesophageal reflux. *J Pediatr Surg* 1984, 19:480–483.

19. Dedinsky GK, Vane DW, *et al.*: Complications and reoperation after Nissen fundoplication in childhood. *Am J Surg* 1987, 153:177–183.

20. Turnage RH, Oldham KT, Coran AG, Blane CE: Late results of fundoplication for gastroesophageal reflux in infants and children. *Surgery* 1989, 105:457–464.

21. Sitsen E, van der Zee DC, Bax NMA: Is laparoscopic pyloromyotomy superior to open surgery? *Surg Endosc* 1998, 12:813–815.

22. Ford WD, Holland AJ, Crameri JA: The learning curve for laparoscopic pyloromyotomy. *J Pediatr Surg* 1997, 32:552–554.

23. Scorpio RJ, Hutson JM, Tan HL: Pyloromyotomy: comparison between laparoscopic and open surgical techniques. *J Laparoendosc Surg* 1995, 5:81–84.

24. Alain JL, Terrier G, Grousseau D: Extramucosal pyloromyotomy by laparoscopy. *Surg Endosc* 1991, 5:174–175.

25. Bufo AJ, Lobe TE, Schropp KP, *et al.*: Laparoscopic pyloromyotomy: a safer technique. *Pediatr Surg Int* 1998, 13:240–242.

26. Rescorla FJ, West Kw, Engum SA, *et al.*: The other side of pediatric hernias-the role of laparoscopy. *American Surgeon* 1997, 63:690–693.

27. Miltenburg DW, Nuchtern JG, Jaksic T, *et al.*: Laparoscopic evaluation of the pediatric inguinal hernia—a meta-analysis. *J Pediatr Surg* 1998, 33:874–879.

27. Dubois JJ, Jenkins JR, Egan JC: Transinguinal Laparoscopic examination of the contralateral groin in pediatric herniorrhaphy. *Surgical Laparoscopy and Endoscopy* 1997, 7:384–387.

29. Lobe TE, Schropp KP: Inguinal hernias in pediatrics: initial experience with laparoscopic inguinal exploration of the asymptomatic contralateral side. *J Laparoendosc Surg* 1992, 2:135–140.

30. Yerkes EB, Brock JW, Holcomb GW, Morgan WM: Laparoscopic evaluation for contralateral patent processus vaginalis: part III. *Urology* 1998, 51:480–483.

31. Fuenfer MM, Pitts RM, Georgeson KE: Laparoscopic exploration of the contralateral groin in children: an improved technique. *J Laparoendoscopic Surg* 1996, 6 Suppl 1:S1–4.

32. Fabian TC, Croce MA, Stewart RM, *et al.*: A prospective analysis of diagnostic laparoscopy in trauma. *Ann Surg* 1993, 217:557–565.

33. Reich H, McGlynn F, De Caprio J, *et al.*: Laparoscopic excision of benign liver lesions. *Obstet Gynecol* 1991, 78:956–958.

34. Goldstein DP: Acute and chronic pelvic pain. *Pediatr Clin North Am* 1989, 36:573–580.

35. Heloury Y, Guiberteau V, Sagot P, *et al.*: Laparoscopy in adnexal pathology in the child: a study of 27 cases. *Eur J Pediatr Surg* 1993, 3:75–78.

36. Spinelli P, Pizzetti P, Lo Gullo C, *et al.*: Laparoscopy in oncological pediatrics. *Pediatr Med Chir* 1988, 10:99–101.

37. Smith BM, Steiner RB, Lobe TE: Laparoscopic Duhamel pullthrough procedure for Hirschsprung's disease in childhood. *J Laparoendoscopic Surg* 1994, 4:273–276.

38. Lagausie P, Bruneau B, Besnard M, *et al.*: Definitive treatment of Hirschprung's Disease with a laparoscopic Duhamel pull-through procedure in childhood. *Surg Lap & Endosc* 1998, 8:55–57.

39. Tulman S, Holcomb GW III, Karamanoukian HL, Reynhout J: Pediatric laparoscopic splenectomy. *J Pediatr Surg* 1993, 28:689–692.

40. Esposito C, Corcione F, Garipoli V, Ascione G: Pediatric laparoscopic splenectomy-are there real advantages in comparison with the traditional open approach? *Ped Surg Int* 1997, 12:509–510.

41. Cortesi N, Ferrari P, Zambarda E, *et al.*: Diagnosis of bilateral abdominal cryptorchidism by laparoscopy. *Endoscopy* 1976, 8:33–34.

42. Scott JES: Laparoscopy as an aid in the diagnosis and management of impalpable testis. *J Pediatr Surg* 1982, 17:14–16.

43. Mark SD, Davidson PJ: The role of laparoscopy in evaluation of the impalpable undescended testis. *Aust & New Zealand J Surg* 1997, 67:332–334.

44. Fahlenkamp D, Winfield HN, Schonberger B, *et al.*: Role of laparoscopic surgery in pediatric urology. *Euro Urology* 1997, 32:75–84.

45. Humke U, Siemer S, Bonnet L, Ziegler M: Pediatric laparosocopy for nonpalpable testes with new miniaturized instruments. *J Endourology* 1998, 12:445–450.

46. Hayashi Y, Mogami T, Sasaki S, *et al.*: Transinguinal Laparosocopy for nonpalpable testis. *Int J Urology* 1996, 3:274–277.

47. Clatworthy H Jr, Hollanbaugh R, Grosfeld J: The "long loop vas" orchiopexy for high undescended testis. *Am Surg* 1972, 38:69–73.

48. Clayman RV, Soper N, Kavoussi LR, *et al.*: Laparoscopic nephrectomy: laboratory and clinical experience. *J Urol* 1991, 145:421–425.

49. Koyle MA, Woo HH, Kavoussi LR: Laparoscopic nephrectomy in the first year of life. *J Pediatr Surg* 1993, 28:693–695.

50. Matsuda T, *et al.*: Laparoscopic varicocelectomy: a simple technique for clip ligation of the spermatic vessels. *J Urol* 1992, 147:636–638.

51. Kavoussi LR, Clayman RV, Brunt LM, Soper NJ: Laparoscopic ureterolysis. *J Urol* 1992, 147:426–429.

52. Peters CA: Laparoscopy in pediatric urology. *Urology* 1993, 41[suppl]:33–37.

53. Rodgers BM, Talbert JL: Thoracoscopy for the diagnosis of intrathoracic lesions in children. *J Pediatr Surg* 1976, 11:703–707.

54. Ryckman FC, Rodgers BM: Thoracoscopy for intrathoracic neoplasia in children. *J Pediatr Surg* 1982, 17:521–524.

55. Rogers DA, Lobe TE, Schropp KP: Video-assisted thoracoscopic surgery in the pediatric patient. *Chest Surg Clin North Am* 1993, 3:325–335.

56. Vanderschueren RG: The role of thoracoscopy in the evaluation and management of pneumothorax. *Lung* 1990, 168[suppl]:1122–1125.

57. Daniel TM, Tribble CG, Rodgers BM: Thoracoscopy and talc poudrage for pneumothoraces and effusions. *Ann Thorac Surg* 1990, 50:186–189.

58. Kern JA, Rodgers BM: Thoracoscopy in the management of empyema in children. *J Pediatr Surg* 1993, 28:1128–1132.

Index